Midwives, Research
and Childbirth

VOLUME 4

OTHER HEALTH SCIENCE TITLES AVAILABLE FROM CHAPMAN & HALL

Midwives, Research and Childbirth Volumes 1, 2 and 3
Edited by Sarah Robinson and Ann M. Thomson

Safer Childbirth?
A critical history of maternity care
Marjorie Tew

Delivered at Home
Julia Allison

Prenatal Diagnosis: The human side
Edited by Lenore Abramsky and Jean Chapple

Psychological Processes of Childbearing
Joan Raphael-Leff

Teaching Interactive Skills in Health Care
Ann Faulkner

Personal Computing for Health Professionals
Philip Burnard

Health Care Computing
Philip Burnard

Clinical Supervision and Mentorship in Nursing
Edited by Tony Butterworth and Jean Faugier

For more information and other titles please contact: The Promotion Department, Chapman & Hall, 2–6 Boundary Row, London SE1 8HN, Telephone 0171 865 0066

Midwives, Research and Childbirth

VOLUME 4

Edited by

Sarah Robinson

*Senior Research Fellow, Nursing Research Unit,
King's College, London*

and

Ann M. Thomson

*Senior Lecturer in Midwifery, School of Nursing Studies,
University of Manchester and Director, Health Care Research Unit,
Manchester College of Midwifery and Nursing*

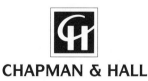

CHAPMAN & HALL

London · Glasgow · Weinheim · New York · Tokyo · Melbourne · Madras

Published by Chapman & Hall, 2-6 Boundary Row, London SE1 8HN, UK

Chapman & Hall, 2-6 Boundary Row, London SE1 8HN, UK

Blackie Academic & Professional, Wester Cleddens Road, Bishopbriggs, Glasgow G64 2NZ, UK

Chapman & Hall GmbH, Pappelallee 3, 69469 Weinheim, Germany

Chapman & Hall USA., 115 Fifth Avenue, New York, NY 10003, USA

Chapman & Hall Japan, ITP-Japan, Kyowa Building, 3F, 2-2-1 Hirakawacho, Chiyoda-ku, Tokyo 102, Japan

Chapman & Hall Australia, 102 Dodds Street, South Melbourne, Victoria 3205, Australia

Chapman & Hall India, R. Seshadri, 32 Second Main Road, CIT East, Madras 600 035, India

Distributed in the USA and Canada by Singular Publishing Group Inc., 4284 41st Street, San Diego, California 92105

First edition 1996

© 1996 Chapman & Hall

Chapters 3, 9 and 11 © Crown Copyright

Typeset in 9.5/11pt Times by Mews Photosetting, Beckenham, Kent
Printed in Great Britain by Page Bros (Norwich) Ltd

ISBN 0 412 45840 3   1 56593 289 7 (USA)

A Catalogue record for this book is available from the British Library

Library of Congress Cataloging Card Number: 95-74642

∞ Printed on permanent acid-free text paper, manufactured in accordance with ANSI/NISO Z39.48-1992 and ANSI/NISO Z39.48-1984 (Permanence of Paper)

Contents

Contributors

Jo Alexander — Principal Lecturer in Midwifery, University of Portsmouth

Janet Askham — Deputy Director, Age Concern Institute of Gerontology, King's College, London University

Rosaline Barbour — Senior Lecturer in Health Service Research, Department of Public Health Medicine, University of Hull

Marie Chamberlain — Assistant Professor, School of Nursing, Faculty of Health Sciences, University of Ottawa

Ruth M. Davies — Professional Officer (Midwifery), Welsh National Board for Nursing, Midwifery and Health Visiting

Diana Elbourne — Deputy Director, Perinatal Trials Service, National Perinatal Epidemiology Unit, Oxford

June Hannam — Head of History, Faculty of Humanities, University of the West of England, Bristol

Hazel E. McHaffie — Research Fellow, Institute of Medical Ethics, Edinburgh University, Department of Medicine

Robyn Phillips — Lecturer, School of Education, University of Wales, Cardiff

Sarah Robinson — Senior Research Fellow, Nursing Research Unit, King's College, London University

Ann M. Thomson Senior Lecturer in Midwifery, School of Nursing Studies, University of Manchester and Director, Health Care Research Unit, Manchester College of Midwifery and Nursing

Preface

This volume is the fourth in a series which brings together studies of particular relevance to the care provided by midwives for childbearing women and their families. The series is intended primarily for midwives but we hope that other health professionals involved in the maternity services, as well as those who use the services, will also find the series interesting and useful.

In undertaking this venture we have been fortunate in the support received from colleagues, friends and family. In particular we would like to thank the following: Rosemary Morris, Senior Editor, Health Sciences at Chapman & Hall; all the authors who have contributed to the series; colleagues at both the Nursing Research Unit, London University and the School of Nursing Studies, Manchester University; and Paul and Rachel Robinson. Special thanks are due to Sue Ankers, Julie Greenwood, Elaine Pacey and Geraldine Reast for secretarial support.

Sarah Robinson, *London*
Ann M.Thomson, *Manchester*
March 1995

CHAPTER ONE

Introduction

Sarah Robinson and Ann M. Thomson

MIDWIFERY RESEARCH AND THE 'MIDWIVES, RESEARCH AND CHILDBIRTH' SERIES

From the early 1970s onwards, the view has steadily gained ground in the UK that all aspects of midwifery – care during pregnancy, labour and the puerperium, together with the education, professional development and management of members of the profession – must have a knowledge base grounded in research. By the mid-1990s the profession can look back on considerable achievements in this respect: a substantial body of research on a diversity of subjects now exists; a literature on designs and methods appropriate to researching midwifery is being established; opportunities to learn about research methods and findings are firmly embedded in midwifery curricula and a diverse range of fora for dissemination of research has been established. The main events in the history of midwifery research, and the factors that have facilitated its development, have been summarized in earlier volumes in this series, as have those factors that constrain further progress (Robinson and Thomson 1989, 1991).

The aim of the Midwives, Research and Childbirth series is to bring together a proportion of this research base in a way that will be maximally useful to those who wish to use research findings in practice, teaching and management and to those who wish to undertake research themselves. Our policy is thus to provide authors with sufficient space to review relevant literature, discuss research strategies in detail, present a substantial proportion of findings, and consider their implications for the profession and for further research. The series aims to provide, therefore, a depth of detail and discussion, particularly about methods, that is usually available only in formats such as unpublished dissertations and reports to funding bodies.

The criterion for inclusion in the series is research that is of particular relevance to the care provided by midwives. This is a wide remit and includes studies concerned with midwifery practice, education and management and with the organization of the maternity services. In this introductory chapter we summarize the extent to which these subjects have been included in the series to date.

Turning first to practice, then, midwives in Britain are qualified to provide care on their own responsibility throughout pregnancy, labour and the puerperium, to recognize those signs of abnormality that require referral to medical staff, and to provide information, advice and support from early pregnancy to the end of the postnatal period. These three elements of maternity care – the clinical, the advisory and the supportive – have all been the subject of research. Some of the studies are descriptive, whereas others have sought to evaluate alternative policies or treatments; many have included users' views of the service.

Descriptive studies in the series include the following: the antenatal booking interview (Methven in Volume 1); providing care at a midwives' clinic (Thomson in Volume 2); experiences of women admitted antenatally (Kirk in Volume 3); the psychological effectiveness of antenatal and postnatal care (Porter and Macintyre in Volume 1); information-giving during labour (Kirkham in Volume 1); pain relief in labour (Niven in Volume 3); aspects of postnatal care (Ball, Laryea and Thomson in Volume 1, Murphy-Black and Levy in Volume 3) and women's views of childbirth (MacIntosh in Volume 1). Topics that have been the subject of evaluation include placental grading (Proud in Volume 1), the giving of enemas (Drayton and Rees in Volume 1), and aspects of perineal care and management (Sleep and Logue in Volume 2).

As evidenced by reports from MIRIAD (the midwifery research database produced by the National Perinatal Epidemiology Unit) the volume of research into midwifery practice, and users' views of care, is considerably greater than that on either midwifery education or management (National Perinatal Epidemiology Unit, 1990, 1991; Sims *et al.*, 1994). This is reflected in the Midwives, Research and Childbirth series in that more than half the studies included to date are concerned with the nature of, and views about, aspects of care.

One of the major themes in the history of the maternity services has been the extent to which the role that midwives are qualified to fulfil has been constrained by the involvement of medical staff in normal maternity care. The division of responsibility between these two groups of professionals has been the subject of three large-scale studies in England and Wales, all of which are included in this series (Robinson in Volume 1, Garcia and Garforth in Volume 2, and Green, Kitzinger and Coupland in Volume 3).

Recognition of the extent to which their role had been eroded led many midwives not only to attempt to regain lost ground but also to develop and expand their role to meet more effectively the needs of childbearing women and their families. Many of the innovative schemes devised have been the subject of evaluation, and have been reported in this series: providing individualized care (Bryar in Volume 2); continuity of care (Flint in Volume 2) and providing support for women with particular needs (Davies and Evans in Volume 2 and Oakley in Volume 3).

The quality of care that midwives are able to provide for childbearing women and their families depends not only on the extent to which the service facilitates the deployment of their skills but also on the education that they receive. Analysis and evaluation of educational processes, in the various contexts in which they occur, are therefore essential components of a programme of midwifery research. While it is the case that much less research has focused on midwifery education than on midwifery practice, a number of major studies have been completed. To date this series includes the following: evaluation of a post-basic course for antenatal education teachers (Murphy-Black in Volume 2); the educational experiences of student midwives (Lewis and Robinson in Volume 2 and Mander in Volume 3) and the implementation of pre-registration midwifery education (Radford and Thompson in Volume 3). Recent years have seen an increase in the number of educational studies, and this is reflected in the current volume.

The third strand of research focuses on midwives themselves. If the service is to be adequately and appropriately staffed, then midwives have to perceive that it offers them opportunities for career progress and professional development. The research base upon which strategies in these respects might be developed is, as yet, relatively small. In this series such studies are represented by Lewis's study of male midwives (Volume 2), Robinson and Mander's studies of student midwives' career intentions (Volume 2) and Robinson and Owen's work on career pathways and development in the profession (Volume 3). Taken together these studies have made a start on identifying factors that facilitate and constrain careers in midwifery.

A fourth area of research, as yet little developed, is that of historical studies. Although the history of midwifery has been the subject of quite extensive research, for example Donnison's (1977) study of events that led to the passing of the 1902 Midwives Act, the volume of historical research overall is small in comparison with that on present-day practices and events. Recognition is increasing, however, of the extent to which many of the issues that faced midwives in the past are relevant to events today, and that understanding the former is an important precursor to confronting the latter. A number of accounts of the main events in the history of the profession have been produced (e.g. Bent, 1982; Towler and Brammall, 1986; Cowell and Wainwright, 1981; Robinson, 1990). Recently, however, a more detailed and analytical approach to history has been evident. This includes attempts to understand experiences of midwives at a local level, by accessing personal and institutional records and by interviewing retired midwives (Walmsley, 1991; Leap and Hunter, 1993); secondly, by seeking to understand policy-making at a national level in the context of the social and political environment of the time (Heagerty 1990).

A number of contributors to the Midwives, Research and Childbirth series have written brief historical accounts as a background to their research (e.g. Robinson in Volume 2, Radford and Thompson in Volume 3, Murphy-Back in Volume 3) but no specifically historical studies have been included to date. However, the number of such studies is now increasing. We plan to include a proportion in the series; this volume marks a beginning with Hannam's study of the history of the Royal College of Midwives.

Much of the research undertaken falls broadly into one of four categories: practice, education, management or history. At the same time, however, many studies are relevant to more than one of these categories. Consequently, we rejected an approach that brought together studies pertaining, for example, to antenatal care in one volume, education in another and midwives' careers in a third. Moreover, such an approach is in opposition to the holistic way in which midwifery is now developing. Our approach is for each volume to contain studies that together reflect not only a diversity of subject, but also a diversity of method. As mentioned, authors are provided with sufficient space to write in detail about relevant literature, methods and findings. Consequently, the first two volumes contained just 10 studies. In the third and subsequent volumes we decided to include one or two review chapters. This is because a number of studies that have not been widely disseminated hitherto contain important findings, but are not of sufficient size to warrant a separate chapter. (Thomson on care in labour in Volume 3).

CONTENT OF VOLUME 4

This fourth volume in the series is similar to the preceding three in that it also contains 10 chapters on a diversity of subjects that together have entailed the use of a wide range of methods. In Chapter 2 Hannam presents two aspects of a historical study of the Royal College of Midwives (Hannam and Maggs, 1992); namely, the aims and motivation of the leadership of what was then the Midwives Institute and the relationships between these leaders and rank and file midwives. The research drew on documents from national and local archives and Hannam discusses the problems of obtaining and evaluating source materials for a historical account of this kind.

In the previous section, attention was drawn to the three large-scale studies that have analysed the level of responsibility exercised by midwives in England and Wales, and the constraints imposed on this by the degree of involvement of medical staff in normal maternity care. In Chapter 3, Askham and Barbour report on a similar study undertaken in Scotland, thus completing the picture for Britain as a whole. By means of questionnaires and observation they documented the extent to which the English and Welsh findings were reflected in the Scottish context. Using interviews they also identified the ways in which midwives maintained professional integrity and satisfaction, often in circumstances of considerable constraints on professional freedom.

This volume reflects the steady growth in the number of studies on midwifery education that have now been completed. Phillips (Chapter 4) focused on a little-researched topic, yet one of potentially great importance to the profession – the criteria upon which student midwives are selected. By means of a questionnaire sent to all senior midwife teachers she demonstrated the wide range of criteria and diversity of view that are brought to bear on this first stage in determining the composition of the profession. Although questionnaires are often the method of choice in midwifery research, reports do not always include an account of the potential complexity of designing the questionnaire and the means of ensuring instrument validity and reliability. Phillips, however, provides a detailed account of these processes.

Davies (Chapter 5) and Chamberlain (Chapter 6) both focus on the experience of student midwives and both adopted an ethnographic approach which entailed periods of observation and semi-structured interviews. Davies' concern was to understand the way in which students made sense of the disparity between the role of the midwife as independent practitioner, as promulgated by the education staff, and the reality of practice in a medically dominated obstetric unit. Davies provides a detailed account of the process of gaining admission to the research setting and the means whereby she gained sufficient acceptance by the students to be able to undertake the research.

Chamberlain's research focused on the education of student midwives in the clinical environment. It is here that students develop and gain confidence in their clinical skills and, as many have maintained, it is the extent to which students feel confident in this respect that may determine whether or not they decide to practise after qualification (Stewart, 1981). By means of some 360 hours of observation of students in clinical settings, Chamberlain disentangled the diversity of teaching and learning styles in operation and identified those that students found most helpful. As well as contributing to the research base on midwifery education, the work by Davies and Chamberlain also adds to the small, albeit growing, volume of midwifery studies that adopt the general logic of 'grounded theory' as advocated by Glaser and Strauss (1967) and of 'analytic induction' (Denzin, 1978). The need for this approach, as the most appropriate way of exploring the nature of little-understood processes and encounters, has gained increasing recognition amongst midwives in recent years. In Chapter 7 Robinson provides a broad perspective on research into midwifery education. In a review of published work she identifies directions pursued and methods adopted, the main findings to emerge and views as to which aspects of the education of midwives should take priority for future research.

Two chapters in this volume represent one of the major components of research into midwifery, namely, the evaluation of procedures by means of a randomized controlled trial. In Chapter 8, Alexander reports on her evaluation of alternative treatments for inverted and non-protractile nipples, and in Chapter 9 Elbourne focuses on research into management of the third stage of labour. Alexander and Elbourne both demonstrate how the success of research of this kind depends on the support of midwives in the clinical setting, and on their willingness to adhere to the trial protocol. Both chapters demonstrate the importance of continuing programmes of research in midwifery, with one study building on another. Alexander's work led to a subsequent study which sought to replicate her design on a larger scale (Main Trial Collaborative Group, 1994). Elbourne shows how the Bristol trial on active versus physiological management arose from a systematic review of existing research evidence on the subject and has in turn resulted in a number of other studies on aspects of the third stage of labour.

Chapter 10 by Thomson continues our policy of including one or two review chapters. The studies that Thomson reviews are all concerned with aspects of postnatal care: the six-week postnatal examination, the mother–child relationship, and early postnatal transfer.

The volume concludes with an account by McHaffie (Chapter 11) of a study of support for families of very low birthweight babies. The needs of parents of these babies for support from health professionals in hospital and in the community is well documented. McHaffie's study, however, broke new ground in this respect in that she focused on the needs of grandparents as well as parents, and on the kind of support that the two generations provided for, and wanted from, each other. Shared and differing perspectives on the subject were elucidated by means of questionnaires sent to midwives and doctors on the one hand and to parents and grandparents of very low birthweight babies on the other.

As with the three previous volumes, this fourth one demonstrates the depth and breadth of research relevant to midwifery. Findings from the studies presented are relevant to all members of the profession: midwives in practice can draw on clinical findings and on those that relate to learning experiences of students in clinical settings; midwife educators can use clinical findings in their teaching and educational findings as a basis for teaching and learning strategies; those responsible for management can draw on findings about those factors that facilitate and constrain the work of midwives; and student midwives will find much of relevance to the theoretical and practical components of their course.

FUTURE CHALLENGES FOR MIDWIFERY RESEARCH

Despite the growing volume of midwifery research, much of everyday practice, education and management is not documented or evaluated. Midwives' views as to priorities in this respect have been canvassed by a number of means (Robinson, Thomson and Tickner, 1989; Sleep and Clark, 1993).

Moreover, the next few years will see the impact of current changes on many aspects of midwifery, all of which will generate a new agenda for research. Midwifery practice is at a particularly exciting juncture. The publication of *Changing Childbirth* (Department of Health, 1993) saw government endorsement of a position advocated in the 1992 House of Commons Health Committee Report and one that many midwives have long argued for; namely, maternity care organized in a way that places women at the centre of the service, and enables midwives to make full use of their knowledge and skills. In particular the report's authors maintain that resources should not be duplicated and that the care of women with an uncomplicated pregnancy should increasingly be led by midwives.

At the time of writing midwives up and down the country have been instituting schemes to facilitate care in the manner outlined in these reports (see, for example, Page, 1995). As described earlier, research demonstrated the way in which the organization of maternity care in previous decades had eroded the midwife's role. Similarly it is essential that research is undertaken in due course to examine the way in which the recommendations of *Changing Childbirth* are implemented and the extent to which individual midwives feel adequately prepared and supported to practise in the way envisaged. The earlier studies of the organization of maternity care and the role of the midwife provide not only a benchmark against which subsequent findings can be compared, but also a detailed account of appropriate designs and methods for research of this kind.

The education and management of midwives similarly have been characterized by considerable change in recent years. Pre-registration midwifery courses have been introduced, there has been a growing emphasis on assessment of competence and on opportunities for continuing education, and many midwifery colleges have merged with nursing colleges and then been incorporated into higher education institutions. What impacts will these developments have on the nature and quality of curricula and on the careers of midwifery practitioners and educators? Again, research is required to provide at least some of the answers, and several projects are already underway (e.g. Worth-Butler, Murphy and Fraser, 1994).

The management structures and lines of professional accountability for midwives have changed as a result of health service changes that have separated the purchasers of the service from the providers. The impact of these changes on the representation of midwifery issues at various policy-making levels requires research, as does the impact of the growing independence of health care trusts on the career structures and conditions of service for midwives.

All in all, midwives in Britain currently face a period of considerable challenge and change, and the need for a vigorous programme of analysis and evaluation has, perhaps, never been greater.

REFERENCES

Bent, E.A. (1982) The growth and development of midwifery. In Allan, P. and Jolley, M. (eds), *Nursing, Midwifery and Health Visiting Since 1990*. Faber & Faber, London.

Cowell, B. and Wainwright, D. (1981) *Behind the Blue Door: The History of the Royal College of Midwives 1881–1981*. Baillière Tindall, London

Denzin, N. (1978) *The Research Act* (2nd edn). McGraw-Hill, New York.

Department of Health (1993) *Changing Childbirth: Report of the Expert Maternity Group Parts 1 and 2,* (Cumberledge Report). HMSO, London.

Donnison, J. (1977) *Midwives and Medical Men: A History of Interprofessional Rivalries and Women's Rights*. Heinemann, London.

Glaser, B. and Strauss, A. (1967) *The Discovery of Grounded Theory: Strategies for Qualitative Research*. Aldine, Chicago.

Hannam, J. and Maggs, C. (1992) *A history of the Royal College of Midwives*. Unpublished report to the Royal College of Midwives, London.

Heagerty, B. (1990) *Class, gender and professionalization: the struggle for British midwifery 1900–1936*. Unpublished PhD thesis, Michigan State University.

House of Commons Health Committee (1992) *Second Report, Session 1991–1992 Maternity Services* (Winterton Report). HMSO, London.

Leap, N. and Hunter, B. (1993) *The Midwife's Tale: An Oral History from Handy Woman to Professional Midwife*. Scarlet Press, London.

Main Trial Collaborative Group (1994) Preparing for breast-feeding: treatment of inverted and non-protractile nipples in pregnancy. *Midwifery*, **10**(4), 200–2.

National Perinatal Epidemiology Unit (1990, 1991) MIRIAD– *The Midwifery Research Database*. National Perinatal Epidemiology Unit, Oxford.

Page, L. (ed.) (1995) *Effective Group Practice in Midwifery: Working with Women*. Blackwell Science, Oxford.

Robinson, S. (1990) Maintaining the independence of the midwifery profession: a continuing struggle. In Garcia, J., Kilpatrick, R. and Richards, M. (eds), *The Politics of Maternity Care*. Clarenden Press, Oxford.

Robinson, S. and Thomson, A.M. (1989) Research and midwifery. In Robinson, S. and Thomson, A.M. (eds), *Midwives, Research and Childbirth*, Vol. 1. Chapman & Hall, London.

Robinson, S. and Thomson, A.M. (1991) Research and midwifery: moving into the 1990s. In Robinson, S. and Thomson, A.M. (eds), *Midwives, Research and Childbirth*, Vol. 2. Chapman & Hall, London.

Robinson, S. and Thomson, A.M. and Tickner, V. (1989) Midwives' views on directions and developments in midwifery research. In Robinson, S. and Thomson, A.M. (eds), *Research and the Midwife Conference Proceedings for 1988.* Nursing Research Unit, King's College, London.

Sims, C., McHaffie, H., Renfew, M. and Ashurst, H. (1994) *The Midwifery Research Database MIRIAD*. Books for Midwives Press, Hale.

Sleep, J. and Clark, E. (1993) Major new survey to identify and prioritise research issues for midwifery practice. *Midwives Chronicle*, **106**(1265), 217–18.

Stewart, A. (1981) The present state of midwifery training. *Midwife, Health Visitor and Community Nurse*, **17**(7), 270–2.

Towler, J. and Bramall, J. (1986) The Midwife in History and Society. Croom Helm, London.

Walmsley, W. (1991). The change in workload of Manchester domiciliary midwives 1960–1972. In Robinson, S., Thomson, A.M. and Tickner, V. (eds), *Research and the Midwife Conference Proceedings for 1990*. Department of Nursing Studies, University of Manchester.

Worth-Butler, M., Murphy, R.J.L. and Fraser, D.M. (1994) Towards an integrated model of competence in midwifery. *Midwifery*, **10**(4), 25–31.

CHAPTER TWO

Some aspects of the history of the Royal College of Midwives

June Hannam

INTRODUCTION

The Royal College of Midwives (RCM) is the leading professional body for midwives in the UK and has helped to shape the nature of midwifery practice and the type of midwife with which we are familiar today. In order to understand the nature of the profession, and to be able to consider whether alternatives to that nature are either possible or desirable, it is necessary to explore the history of the RCM, in particular its aims, policies and leadership.

The research on which this chapter is based was originally commissioned by the RCM; it was undertaken on a part-time basis by two full-time academics and addressed a wide range of themes (Hannam and Maggs, 1992). The starting point for the work was to review existing literature which covered, either directly or indirectly, aspects of the history of the RCM and then to decide on the themes and questions which needed to be explored. This chapter focuses on two themes: the aims and motivation of the leadership of the Midwives' Institute (the organization that became the Royal College of Midwives) and on the relationships between these leaders and rank and file midwives. The period in question is up to and including the First World War; brief reference is also made to the inter-war years. The chapter concludes with consideration of how some of the issues of these periods have been echoed in more recent times.

PREVIOUS STUDIES OF THE ROYAL COLLEGE OF MIDWIVES

The RCM originated from a small organization, the Matron's Aid Society and Midwives' Institute, which was formed in 1881. It quickly became known as the Midwives' Institute (MI) and retained this name until receiving a Royal Charter in 1947. As early as 1923 members of the Institute expressed an interest in learning more about the history of their organization. This prompted Emma Brierly, editor of *Midwives Chronicle and Nursing Notes*, to write a series of short articles about the early years of the Institute (Brierly, 1923a, 1923b, 1923c, 1923d). These articles must form the starting point for anyone interested in the history of the RCM. Not only do they provide unique insights from those who participated in the development of the organization, but they created a particular view of the aims and achievements of the MI which have influenced the approach of subsequent studies. The emphasis is on the hard work of the founding members in pressing for legislation to improve the status of the midwife and in seeking to foster professional unity, and on their achievements as a pressure group. Brierly concludes that 'the Institute watches over the interests of the certified midwife politically, municipally, socially and educationally. It is managed by midwives, for midwives, and is a self governing body of professional women' (Brierly, 1923d).

This approach is followed to a large degree in the main study of the RCM, *Behind the Blue Door*, by Betty Cowell and David Wainwright, which gives a narrative account and provides much useful information (Cowell and Wainwright, 1981). Even as a descriptive piece, however, there are a number of problems. The study emphasizes periods around key pieces of legislation – themselves somewhat arbitrarily selected – which results in an uneven coverage of the College's history. For example, there are only 12 pages on the inter-war years, a period when there was widespread interest in questions of health status and health care provision (Lewis, 1980). There is a tendency to emphasize the importance of selected leaders of the organization and to state rather than to analyse their influence on events. The impression given throughout is one of linear progress towards greater professional strength and status. Many of these historiographical problems stem from a failure to consider systematically which questions need to be considered when looking at the history of an organization and then to analyse the material within that framework.

Other studies take a more complex view of the role of pressure groups such as the RCM, their overall aims and the extent to which they had an influence in the shaping of social policy. For example, Jean Donnison examines the demand of the MI during the 1890s for midwife registration and professional status in the context of the women's movement of the period (Donnison, 1977). She explores the way in which arguments around the registration and status of midwives were inextricably linked to the fears of male doctors about their own professional status and exclusivity. Donnison argues that in order to ensure that midwifery remained a female occupation based on training, the leaders of the MI needed the co-operation of key members of the medical profession. Thus they accepted measures which limited the midwife's sphere of competence and agreed to a system of strict supervision by a body, the Central Midwives' Board, which was not required to contain a single midwife member (Donnison, 1977).

Donnison also suggests that such compromises were made because the leaders of the Institute were keen to get registration in order to ensure that poor women had the services of a trained midwife. It was for these reasons, namely the limitation of the autonomy of midwives entailed by the provisions of the 1902 Act, that the women's rights movement of the period was very reluctant to support the Institute. Nonetheless, Donnison argues that the Act was 'a triumph for women' since an all-male parliament was at last willing to take an interest in midwifery. Moreover, the Act ensured that the midwife would survive and would increase her status.

In her account Donnison emphasizes the importance of pressure group politics in the achievement of changes in the status and definition of midwives. She argues that through using political skill, economic power or moral force the leaders of the MI were able to persuade policy-makers to accede to their demands. This interpretation has been questioned by Dingwall, Rafferty and Webster (1988), who suggest that more attention should be given to the attitude of government and policy-makers who were often reluctant to increase the monopoly of power of professional groups. When legislation was introduced the intentions behind it could be quite different from those of the pressure groups involved and it could have unforeseen results. External factors could also influence the status of midwives and the nature of their work practices. In the inter-war years, for example, the declining birth rate, the provision of antenatal care in clinics and the increase of hospital deliveries put pressure on the survival of independent midwives despite the attempts by the Institute to ensure their continued existence.

This more searching analysis of the role of a pressure group of professionals in influencing policy-makers is also paralleled by more recent studies which question the aims and motivation of the leadership of such organizations. Until recently a growing literature on professionalization has tended to view professionalism as representing progress for both the employee and the client (Melosh, 1982). In a recent, stimulating thesis on the Midwives' Institute, Brooke Heagerty criticizes this interpretation. Instead she uses Melosh's work on American nursing as a basis for her argument that social élites dominate professional groups and often conflict with the rank and file (Heagerty, 1990). She suggests that the leaders of the MI, who were trained in prestigious hospitals and held positions of power, for example as matrons, were mainly interested in reforming working-class family life. They were drawn from the same middle-class backgrounds as the leaders of the women's movement and shared their values and aims. In their view the midwife would play a key role in transforming working-class child-rearing practices and therefore it was imperative that she should be drawn from the middle class and properly trained. Thus, Heagerty argues, they were keen to keep control of the Institute so that they could pursue their aim of eliminating the working-class midwife and consequently could not be seen as working for the interest of most midwives (Heagerty, 1990).

It is suggested, therefore, that in seeking to raise the status of midwives and to attract well-educated women to the profession the leaders of the MI developed a particular view about the practice of midwifery and its relationship to other health workers, in particular nurses and health visitors. Midwives were the first group to establish a legal definition of their membership and activities and to create a monopoly of practice. The aims of the leaders of the MI were to create an independent practitioner who would be distinct from the nursing profession and who would work autonomously in her own sphere of competence. In practice, however, external factors which made it difficult for the independent practitioner to make a living, the increasing number of nurses who were also midwives, in particular after the establishment of a salaried service in 1936 and the trend towards hospital births after the 1930s, all militated against the aims of the MI. Dingwall, Rafferty and Webster (1988) argue that the RCM in the 1990s might maintain the fiction of the midwife as a 'practitioner in her own right', but that this is not comparable to the pre-war independent practitioner, since there are now so many limits to her area of discretion.

QUESTIONS CONSIDERED IN RESEARCHING THE HISTORY OF THE ROYAL COLLEGE OF MIDWIVES

Each of these more recent studies suggests that issues around the development of the RCM politics should not be seen as unproblematic. In approaching the writing of our own history of the RCM therefore, we set out with a number of questions which we thought should be asked about any organization. These included how the organization works, what its policies are, how policy is arrived at and who has the most power within it. The influence that the organization has had in helping to shape the external environment, in particular government policies, also needs to be examined and assessment made of the influence of that external environment on the success or otherwise of the organization and the nature of midwifery practice. Such questions can then help to give shape and balance to any narrative.

In order to move beyond the descriptive, however, the history of the RCM must be explored in relation to broader historical debates about professionalism, the nature of the women's movement, the development of social policy and the labour process. The MI was not alone, for example, in seeking to realize professional status in the period before the First World War. Nurses and teachers also sought professional recognition and debated similar concerns about state regulation, registration and what to do about the unqualified worker (Abel-Smith, 1960; Holcombe, 1973).

Locating the history of midwifery and of midwife organizations in the literature on professionalization has yielded valuable insights, in particular of a comparative nature. On the other hand, the history of the midwifery organizations has only rarely been placed in the context of labour history or women's history (e.g. Donnison, 1977) and yet these fields of enquiry can suggest new themes for study. Labour history, for instance, draws attention to the relationship between trade unionism and professionalism, to definitions of skill and the tactics used by skilled workers to maintain and enhance their position. This approach to labour history can enhance our understanding of women's work (Rose, 1993). These issues are as relevant to the history of the RCM as to the history of a trade union. The working practices of midwives were subject to considerable pressure and change during the period prior to the First World War and these encouraged them to protest and at times to take more vigorous action than the leadership of the Institute would have advised.

Both labour history and women's history have focused on 'history from below', drawing attention to the need to examine the experiences and attitudes of the rank and file. In studying the development of an institution, where most records are of an official character, it is a useful corrective to question whether the aims and objectives of the leadership necessarily matched those of the rank and file, or indeed whether they matched those of only one section of the workforce. A recent example of such an approach is Carpenter's study of the role of the Asylum Workers' Union in the history of psychiatric nursing (Carpenter, 1980).

Recent studies in women's history have also provided insights into the motivations and attitudes of middle-class women who were active in a range of organizations and political movements which can enhance our understanding of the outlook of leading figures in midwifery. They have also shown the importance of friendship networks between women in helping to sustain their political activity, enthusiasm and the organization of which they were a part (Levine, 1987; Rendall, 1987; Caine, 1992). Of particular relevance for the history of the RCM are studies of women's philanthropic and social reform activities in the late nineteenth and early twentieth centuries. These suggest that the ideas of such women and their contribution to redefining women's role in the public sphere were complex.

For instance, social reformers did not always directly challenge women's social role, but their work in the public sphere was an implicit challenge to contemporary definitions of femininity and could have led some of them to join the women's movement. Their ideas were often rooted in notions of sexual difference which coexisted, if somewhat uneasily, with a belief in equal rights. Concepts of duty, citizenship and the desire to bring about social regeneration, which developed from contemporary views of a woman's sphere and of her special qualities, gave an impetus to many women to take social action so that they could lead purposeful lives and help to bring about social change. They usually acted on a voluntary basis, but took the work as seriously as if they had received payment and gave it a single-minded commitment (Parker, 1988; Lewis, 1991).

The leaders of the Institute, in particular in the early years, were drawn from the same social class as members of the women's movement and had both friendship and family links with them. There was strong support from the MI for the campaign for women's suffrage and a commitment to raise the status and scope of women's work (Hannam, 1993). In their belief that they had a mission to improve the lives of poorer women the leaders of the Institute also shared the concerns of other women engaged in social work. There could be a tension, however, between this emphasis on social reform and the Institute's parallel aim to enhance the status and working conditions of the midwife which continued well into the twentieth century.

In approaching the history of the RCM, therefore, we identified a number of themes which would inform the study throughout: firstly, an examination of midwifery as an area of women's work which would be described and analysed in relation to more general debates concerning women's employment, skill and professionalism, including the relationship with other health practitioners. A second major theme is the consideration of the aims of the leadership and the tensions within their policies. Allied to this are issues arising from the potential conflict between leadership and rank and file and between the outlook of a professional group and trade unionism. Finally, a key theme must be the extent to which the MI/RCM was able to contribute to and influence not only government policy on the midwife herself but also more general social questions related to improved health care and the position of women.

SOURCE MATERIAL FOR THE RESEARCH

A variety of sources are available for such a study. The RCM has, to a large extent, been able to maintain its own archives and to make these available to scholars. They contain minutes of the main committees of the organization, with supporting papers, and reports from the annual general meetings. Of particular interest are the supporting papers for the Committee of Representatives (a body composed of midwives from various parts of the country) which contain invaluable material on the work of the regions. For anyone interested in the day-to-day practice of midwifery there are some case-books in the archives as well as miscellaneous ephemera, including letters and photographs, which can add a different perspective to the more standardized organizational material.

In addition, the *Midwives Chronicle and Nursing Notes*, while formally independent of the MI/RCM, provides a major source for the history of the organization and of midwifery. It contains full reports of all the committee meetings, letters from members and articles on issues of the day that were seen as of vital importance for midwives. It provided a platform for the leadership to express their views on key questions as well as detailing a range of other related activities in which they were involved. The close relationship between the journal, midwives, midwifery and the MI/RCM make it an important record of change. In addition, official government reports and enquiries can be used to show the way in which the MI, and now the RCM, have sought to influence policy in midwifery, maternity care and professional development.

Historians are well aware of the problems of sources for studies such as this (Bedoe, 1983; Davin, 1992). Much of the documentary evidence has been created by and for the organization and its leadership. The vagaries of archival collections limit the opportunities for broader or contrary views to survive. Local branches have, in some instances, kept their own records and these can be useful in providing an insight into the relationship between the centre and the practising midwife, although the leadership in local areas often mirrored the leadership nationally in terms of social background, status within the profession and outlook. It is difficult, therefore, to find material of the experiences of the rank and file midwife, although oral history raises the possibility of finding out more about her life and work (Roberts, 1984; Leap and Hunt, 1993).

In the more recent past, the issues which can be seen with some clarity in the early years are still being worked through and may not yet be resolved. While it is relatively easy to comment on the role of now-dead leaders and individuals, the fact that those involved in the development of the organization today are themselves actors in the unfolding historical events necessitates some reticence in using contemporary material.

The MI/RCM has been in existence for over a hundred years and therefore any account of its development, policies and characteristics must, given the short space available in this chapter, necessarily be selective. As stated at the outset the intention, therefore, is to concentrate on an examination of two related themes: the aims and motivation of the leadership, and the relationship between the leaders and the rank and file. The discussion will focus on the period up to and including the First World War and concludes with a brief survey of changes in the inter-war years. It will be suggested that many of the developments in this early period helped to shape the concerns of the RCM in more recent times and it is hoped that the discussion will illustrate some of the key questions raised in the review of secondary literature as outlined above.

LEADERSHIP

Key figures in the early years

From its inception until the First World War the MI was led by a number of well-educated women who fell roughly into two groups: those who lent their support to the Institute, but had to devote most of their time to their own occupation, and the officers, who were largely unpaid but who gave a full-time commitment to the MI. For example, in 1910 Paulina Ffynes-Clinton had an honorarium of £55 as organizing secretary and the assistant secretary received £60 (Midwives' Institute, 1910a). The Council of the Institute drew its membership from the most prestigious leaders and managers in the field. For example, in 1893 they were nearly all matrons, superintendents or inspectors of the Queen Victoria Jubilee Institute for Nurses (QVJIN), while there were two doctors among the vice-presidents. The Council addressed broad policy issues, but day-to-day affairs were run by an executive group who in turn helped to formulate policy.

The president, treasurer and secretary exercised considerable influence over the shape of the Institute's development since they gave most of their time to its affairs and there was a great deal of continuity in leadership up to the 1920s. For example, between 1890 and 1919 there were only three presidents. Zepherina Smith, the first treasurer of the Institute, acted as president from 1890 until her death in 1894. The daughter of a clergyman, she trained as a nurse in 1867 and gained the London Obstetrical Society (LOS) certificate in 1873. Although she withdrew from nursing when she married the surgeon Henry Smith in 1876 she was active in establishing the Institute and in seeking to improve the status of midwives (*Nursing Notes*, 1894), Jane Wilson took over as president in 1894 and held the position until 1911, when she was succeeded by Amy Hughes for the period 1911–1919. Jane Wilson was a founder member of the MI and was honorary secretary of the Workhouse Infirmary Nursing Association, which took an interest in the training of Poor Law midwives. Amy Hughes trained as a nurse at St Thomas' under Mrs. Wardroper and became a superintendent of the QVJIN.

A key figure from the 1880s through the inter-war years was Rosalind Paget, treasurer of the Institute and a driving force behind its development. Born in 1855, Rosalind Paget was the daughter of a barrister and police magistrate. Her uncle, William Rathbone, the Quaker shipowner and MP for Liverpool, who had played an important part in developing nursing services in the city, appears to have been instrumental in awakening his niece's interest in the nursing profession. Like so many young women who grew up in families who were active in social reform questions, Rosalind Paget wanted to do something useful with her life and trained as a nurse at the Westminster Hospital in 1875. After working in the Children's Hospital and the London Hospital she was appointed Inspector General of the QVJIN in 1889. While working at the London Hospital she took time off in 1885 to qualify as a midwife at Endell Street Lying In Hospital and subsequently became involved in the affairs of the MI. In 1897 the officers were strengthened when a close friend of Rosalind Paget, Paulina Ffynes Clinton, took over the role of secretary of the Institute. The two women had nursed together at the London Hospital and shared a flat until Paulina died in 1918 (Rivers, 1981).

The aims of the Institute's leaders

From the beginning the Institute made two major claims: firstly that midwifery was essential to the health of mothers and babies, and therefore to the health of the nation; and secondly, that midwives were distinct from other professionals even where the latter had some role to play in providing maternity services. While it laid claim to represent the interests of midwives and, at times, to voice the views and concerns of the majority of midwives whether they were members of the Institute or not, such claims were not made to effect a monopoly of representation but in support of its defence of these two core aims.

These varied aims were not always necessarily compatible. At the end of her speech to the AGM in 1899 the president, Jane Wilson, claimed that the MI aimed to 'forward the interests of trained midwives, and to help raise the status of midwives generally' (Midwives' Institute, 1899). The thrust of the Institute's policies, therefore, was towards the recruitment of well-educated young women to train as midwives to replace a more working-class, untrained labour force. To this extent the leadership was, in common with many members of the women's movement, attempting to extend and develop employment opportunities for middle-class women which would receive social status and respect. As part of this they defended the continued existence of the independent midwife practitioner who could make a free contract with her client.

A second set of objectives, which intertwined with the demand for professional status, was the aim of the leadership to provide an improved midwifery service for the poor. They were convinced that ignorant, untrained midwives were a danger to the health of mothers and babies. Beyond this, however, they felt that midwives should set a good example in their own behaviour and seek to be an 'influence for good' on the family lives of the poor (e.g. *Nursing Notes*, 1903a, 1904, 1906). This was a constant theme in issues of *Nursing Notes* at the time. In taking such a view they shared many of the assumptions of other women engaged in social reform work, who according to Jane Lewis linked 'the solution of social problems firmly to the family and to social work performed voluntarily by middle-class women' (Lewis, 1991).

This was particularly important at a time when the government was taking an increasing interest in the health of mothers and babies. After 1900 attention was drawn to problems of infant mortality and child health and welfare, while in the inter-war years maternal mortality and general health of mothers received most attention. These concerns were evidenced in Ministry of Health reports at the time (Campbell, 1923, 1924, 1927; Ministry of Health, 1929, 1930, 1937). In both contexts the MI argued that midwives had a crucial role to play:

> When we think of the enormous importance to the nation of the health of its mothers and of the infants who will be its future workers and fighters, it is borne upon us what an important and honourable

calling should be that of a midwife. In conclusion we cannot do better than remind our readers of the beautiful motto of the Midwives' Institute: Vita Donum Dei'.

(Nursing Notes, 1903a)

The leaders of the Institute believed that a role for midwives as health missioners, an improved service for poor mothers and an enhanced professional status could all go together. Commenting on a proposed Midwives' Bill in the late 1890s the officers claimed:

> though we are a body of women vitally concerned with this legislation, we can also see beyond the narrow outlook of a mere trades unionism, and we are able to consider what is the most effectual Bill for the protection of the lying-in woman as well as what is an advantage to ourselves, and we can feel assured that what is the best for her will in the end be best for us.

(Nursing Notes, 1899)

RELATIONSHIPS BETWEEN THE LEADERS OF THE MIDWIVES' INSTITUTE AND PRACTISING MIDWIVES

In practice there were difficulties in reconciling the various objectives held by the Institute leaders. Heagerty (1990), in particular, argues that the class differences between the leaders and the rank and file meant that their aims, objectives and needs were very different. The middle-class leadership, motivated by a particular set of political and social ideas and values, sought to push for an 'ideal' midwife who would transform the lives of the poor. She concludes that the MI

> had manipulated evidence to construct a self-serving analysis of the profession's problems in order to replace rank and file midwives with a new breed. The Institute did not represent the rank and file of midwifery. To the extent that it did so, it represented an ideal: women who were educated, who were nurses, and who were young and unmarried. For the Institute, the majority of the rank and file were millstones who dragged down the profession and drove the ideal away.

(Heagerty, 1990)

Many elements of this analysis ring true, but it will be argued in the rest of this chapter that the outlook of the leadership and their relationship to the rank and file were far more complex than this would suggest. The leaders of the Institute did not all speak with one voice; officers such as Rosalind Paget often had very different views on a range of issues from many matrons and inspectors on the Council, while some of the newer provincial representatives who joined Institute committees before the First World War occasionally challenged the actions of the officers. Moreover, Institute leaders were flexible enough to modify their political strategies in response to external and internal pressures, while attempting to keep the balance between their two main concerns; that midwifery was essential to maternal and child welfare, and that the contribution of the midwife was distinct from that of other professions.

Recruiting members for the Midwives' Institute

A major problem which had to be faced from the beginning, and which threatened to undermine the effectiveness of the organization, was the difficulty in attracting members. The leadership was aware that their lack of members could hamper them in attempting to pressurize for legislation or on claiming to speak on behalf of midwife interests, but, given their emphasis on the importance of trained midwives, membership rules were strict. Members had to be over the age of 25, of good character and the holders of an LOS diploma. By 1892 only 1000 women held this diploma and therefore it is hardly surprising that membership figures were low (25 in 1885). From 1886 membership was widened to include associate members, who were trained nurses, and lay members. By 1894 membership totalled 240 but increases were slow throughout the 1890s. After the passing of the Midwives' Act in 1902 greater interest was shown in the organization and membership finally topped 1000 in January 1908, rising to 1235 on the eve of the First World War. Of these 1235 members 782 were midwives, but they only represented a small proportion of the 5500 trained midwives whose names appeared on the roll in 1914 (Midwives' Institute, 1914a). Under the provisions of the 1902 Midwives' Act, midwives could only practise if their names were entered on the roll of Midwives maintained by the Central Midwives' Board.

These figures raise questions about why the Institute failed to attract more members and the consequences of this for its effectiveness as a pressure group. The Institute had clear aims: to raise the efficiency and improve the status of midwives and to facilitate discussion about the profession. It set out to offer a range of services to members; there was a lending library and the Institute operated as a centre of information. Members could, for example, have their names placed on an employment register to facilitate their search for work. In keeping with an organization which put such weight on training, the Institute helped its members prepare for the LOS examination by providing classes of instruction, and by the turn of the century had begun to develop schemes for other benefits, including insurance.

Although membership growth was slow the Institute did manage to expand its premises, and hence the services offered, during the 1890s as well as employing a part-time secretary. The finance for this appears to have come from friends and patrons since the income from members was so low.

Rosalind Paget complained throughout the period about the financial problems of the MI, which were exacerbated by members who paid their subscriptions late or who allowed them to lapse altogether (Midwives' Institute, 1906, 1910b).

The difficulty in recruiting members must have had a number of causes; practising midwives were extremely busy and for practical reasons were largely drawn from London, while only a small proportion fulfilled the entry requirements. Even after the turn of the century, when more became qualified, it was difficult to build up a sense of professional identity among them, although this was a key aim of the Institute from its inception. At the end of every annual prospectus there was a paragraph which noted that 'the knowledge that they belong to a large organization to which they have the right to apply for advice and help in practical difficulties will do so much to further the feeling of *esprit de corps* so advantageous to isolated workers' (Midwives' Institute, 1892).

Differing concerns of the Midwives' Institute leaders and practising midwives

Despite these calls for solidarity and sense of professional identity the concerns of the leadership could seem far removed from the interests of practising midwives, whether qualified or not. The preoccupation with seeking recognition was not necessarily shared even by those midwives who were already trained. In 1902 the editors of *Nursing Notes* complained that practising midwives had taken little interest in the Midwives' Bill and that this had undermined the case for a midwife representative on the Central Midwives' Board (*Nursing Notes*, 1902). Three midwives were members of the Board, but not by virtue of the fact that they were midwives; Rosalind Paget represented the QVJIN, Dorothea Oldham represented the Royal British Nurses' Association, and Jane Wilson was appointed by the Privy Council to represent the public interest. The representative of the MI had to be a doctor (*Nursing Notes*, 1902).

The social reform aims of the Institute could also conflict with the needs of practising midwives. The emphasis on the midwife's 'influence for good' meant that her character was seen as all important. Recognizing that it would be difficult to attract sufficient numbers of well-educated middle-class women to midwifery, the leaders of the MI sought to 'ensure that the midwife of the future is, in the first place, a clean and sober woman possessed of sufficient elementary education to enable her to pass an examination in midwifery and to be trained for attendance on normal labour' (*Nursing Notes*, 1903b).

In a context in which infant health was seen as vital for the nation's wellbeing the Institute welcomed the more efficient supervision and inspection of midwifery practice which came with the Midwives' Act of 1902. Midwives themselves, however, often resented the strict, detailed regulations and discipline under which they had to work, which seemed to undermine their claim that they were competent to act independently and responsibly. The Institute recognized that midwives might find the new rules onerous, but argued that they should welcome supervision. If the midwife put 'her patients' welfare before her own dignity' she would raise her own professional standing and her work would be treated with respect (*Nursing Notes*, 1903a).

The three midwives on the Central Midwives' Board (CMB) in the early 1900s – Rosalind Paget, Jane Wilson and Dorothea Oldham – who were all active in the affairs of the MI, always supported initiatives to enforce disciplinary actions which involved a woman's moral character. For example, in July 1914 Mary Stock, a qualified midwife, was struck off the roll for misconduct. There was no suggestion that she had been incompetent, but she had had a child and lived with a man who was not her husband. On appeal to the High Court against the decision she won her case, but the leaders of the MI sent a memorial to the CMB supporting the original decision and requesting it to continue to 'support the moral as well as the professional status of the practising midwife' (Midwives' Institute, 1915).

Defending the interests of midwives and women

On the other hand, the midwife members of the CMB fought hard to protect the interests of midwives when they appeared to be under threat, and were not afraid to contest the views of medical members of the board, including the doctor who represented the MI. There were frequent disagreements about the relationship between doctors and midwives. For example, on one occasion the Medical Officer of Health from Bolton wrote to the CMB for advice about whether a doctor could dismiss a midwife from a case after he had been summoned by her. The Board gave a very unclear answer from which Rosalind Paget dissented. She claimed that only the patient or the supervisory authority could cancel the services of a midwife, but failed to obtain a seconder for this view. The newly appointed representative of the Institute, Dr Atkinson, moved the next question which the other Institute members found to be particularly unhelpful since it meant that the issue would be postponed indefinitely (*Nursing Notes*, 1909a).

Other questions which affected midwives, such as who should pay the doctor's fee, or the inclusion of Poor Law midwives under the supervisory clauses of the Act, were pursued by the leaders of the Institute outside the auspices of the CMB. Rosalind Paget, in particular, worked hard in lobbying local authorities, giving evidence to official enquiries and acting with other interested groups to put pressure on the government when new pieces of legislation were suggested. In 1910 and 1911, for example, the officers of the Institute spent most of their time in seeking amendments to the proposed

National Insurance Bill. One clause proposed that insured persons should receive maternity benefit to cover the doctor's fee, but there was no mention of the midwife. The Institute sought support, therefore, for an amendment which would give the woman the right to decide who should attend the birth and thus who would receive the fee. The Institute joined with groups such as the QVJIN, the Association for Promoting the Training and Supply of Midwives and the National Union of Women Workers to pressurize the government, and the amendment was accepted (Midwives' Institute, 1911a).

Discussions over proposed legislation in the pre-war years suggested that the ideas of the Institute's leaders about the relationship between the midwife and working-class women and between state responsibility, professional social workers and voluntary action were complex. Although the Institute was largely staffed by voluntary workers its aim to provide a trained, paid professional midwifery service for working-class women ensured that the views of the MI leadership did not necessarily mirror those of the majority of philanthropists.

Although the Institute could be critical of some of the habits of the poor, its general tone was one of sympathy for the difficulties faced by poorer women. In reacting to proposals for legislation which aimed to reduce infant mortality the attitudes of the leadership show a mixture of dislike for state intervention and concern that the working-class woman was being penalized. In 1908 an editorial in *Nursing Notes* proclaimed 'Who would be a mother!':

> She is not allowed to earn her bread before her baby is born – nor afterwards – in fact, a married woman is never, apparently, to earn at all. Within thirty-six hours of lying-in the mother is to be visited by a Health Visitor (competent or not as the case may be). She is to breast-feed as those theorizers judge fit ... above all, she is to breast-feed her child whether she can fitly do so or not.
>
> (*Nursing Notes*, 1908a)

In the paper it was argued that if women could not earn income they would turn to crime, 'and who shall dare to be hard upon women driven by starvation? For we do not hear of State Support for these mothers' (*Nursing Notes*, 1908b).

Rosalind Paget, in particular, welcomed the Insurance Act as a step away from notions of philanthropy towards self-reliance and independence for both midwife and mother. She thought that too often the midwife had been inadequately paid and expected to do other people's charitable work, but this would now be 'totally out of place with insured persons' (Midwives' Institute, 1912a). She also argued that the marital status of women was irrelevant to their entitlement to have a competent practitioner at childbirth. Aware that her views were not shared by all members of the Institute she made a special effort to persuade midwife members of advisory committees not to adopt the 'specious arguments of some rescue society ... it is not a question of morals, but of common honesty' (Midwives' Institute, 1912b).

The leaders of the Institute were also concerned to exert political influence and to seek legislation to achieve their aims. They were conscious that, as an all-female group concerned with the health of women and children, they were taken less seriously by legislators than if they had been men. They therefore gave wholehearted support to the women's suffrage campaign and any attempts to increase women's representation on public bodies. They argued that the Midwives' Act had been postponed time and again in a way 'that would have been impossible had women had voting power behind them, instead of being able to wield that "indirect influence" so revolting to the straightforwardly minded, but which some misguided persons consider to be more feminine' (*Nursing Notes*, 1908c).

Representing the views of practising midwives

The Institute's complex views about its role as representative of a professional group of workers and its social reform aspirations also affected the organization's outlook towards its own membership. As already noted, membership grew only slowly up to 1914 and the leadership was aware from early on that this could reduce their effectiveness as a pressure group. The close-knit group who led the Institute no longer practised midwifery and Rosalind Paget, in particular, was concerned to be more in touch with the views and needs of midwives on the ground. Therefore, in 1900 she argued that the best way to do this was through their direct representative on the Midwives' Council. Until then the election to the post had not been taken seriously and the representative had played only a minor role in the affairs of the Institute.

Rosalind Paget now called for at least four nominations, to be accompanied by electoral addresses, and persuaded the Sectional Committee of Midwives to accept that there should be two direct representatives. Diplomatically she assured her audience that the help they gave her as trainers and supervisors was invaluable since they were able 'to look at the matter from a wider point of view than the practising midwife' (*Nursing Notes*, 1901a). Nonetheless she would find it personally very useful, as a member of the Midwives' Bill Committee, if she had a couple of midwives who could advise her about particular clauses in the Bill. Two midwives were selected and one of their first actions was to organize a system of centres in different districts in London 'for interesting and helping local midwives and bringing them in touch with the Institute' (*Nursing Notes*, 1901b).

Relations at the Midwives' Institute between officers and committee members

However, as the organization began to grow and the Midwives' Act in many respects enhanced the status and importance of the Institute in speaking for midwives, there were increasing tensions both about the way in which the affairs of the Institute were run and also about the extent to which it had been successful enough in attracting members. In theory the Midwives in Council Sectional Committee became more important after the Act. This committee consisted of all the midwife members of the Council and the midwife vice-presidents and was usually summoned when important matters affecting midwives needed consideration. In 1908 Rosalind Paget claimed that the Midwives in Council meetings had become a 'real power', able to suggest amendments to any possible legislation and to develop policy. In reality the executive subcommittee took the initiative about policy between meetings, while the officers frequently took action on their own.

On most occasions Council members endorsed actions which had been taken, but there were times when members expressed discontent at the failure to call full committee meetings. For example, during the First World War, Elsie Hall, a midwife teacher and direct representative of midwives on the Council, objected to the actions taken by the president, treasurer and secretary in sending a letter to the *Daily Telegraph* in reply to three articles on the midwife question. Miss Hall considered that the Council should have been called to draw up the letter: 'as direct representative she had known nothing about it and she thought she ought to have been informed' (Midwives' Institute, 1916).

Rosalind Paget objected to the fact that the officers appeared to be under censure while acting within the rules and argued that there had simply not been enough time to call a meeting. Nonetheless the incident led to a resolution being passed which clarified the powers that officers had to take action during emergencies and indicated that the relationship between the officers and the committees needed some re-examination. Before the First World War, however, the financial problems of the Institute and the reliance on a small group of largely unpaid officers to run the organization meant that decisions tended to rest with the latter. For example, when Paulina Ffynes Clinton resigned as secretary in 1912 because of ill health, she and Rosalind Paget decided on her successor themselves. They thought that Miss Goodlass, a midwife and trained nurse who had been known to them for a number of years, was so suitable that they only needed to send her name to the Council for approval (Midwives' Institute, 1914b). However, in some situations the officers did not have time to consult widely. For example, when the Institute was asked to nominate people to sit on provincial insurance committees in counties and county boroughs, nominations had to be provided within a week (Midwives' Institute, 1912c). Any disagreements about the actions of the officers were rare, and tended to arise when a strong-minded individual on the Council was discontented about one of the decisions made.

Development of local organizations

The main challenge to the authority of the officers before the war, therefore, came not from within the Institute but rather from outside groups which claimed to represent the interests of midwives. The labour unrest of 1909–1914, when men and women from a variety of occupations took action to improve pay and conditions, provided the context in which a number of local associations of midwives were formed, some of which had very different policies from those pursued by the MI. Plans were also put forward to establish an organization for midwives along trade union lines.

The first stirrings of local action came in January 1907 when a Manchester Association of Midwives was formed to watch over new legislation and to provide legal aid for midwives. A conference of the Association was held in Liverpool in 1909 when a Mrs Aldridge from Manchester claimed that legislation aiming to reduce infant mortality had laid greater emphasis on the midwife 'and all that was for the benefit of child or mother they wished to support, but the midwives required protection as well as parents' (*Nursing Notes*, 1909b).

Rosalind Paget attended this conference and directly afterwards the Institute announced that it was conscious of the greater need for organization among practising midwives. It was recognized that the MI was overwhelmingly London based in its membership and concerns and that there was little communication with midwives in the provinces. It was suggested, therefore, that a Committee of Representatives should be formed to keep in touch with local midwives.

This development seemed even more urgent when it was announced in the *Midwives Record* that there would be a meeting in December 1909 to form a Union of British Midwives. This finally took place in March 1910 with Mary Macarthur of the National Federation of Women Workers in the chair (*Nursing Notes*, 1910a).

Other local groups began to form; claiming to be organized on trade union lines they called for fixed and higher fees, direct representation for midwives on the CMB and raised criticisms of members of the medical profession.

The leaders of the MI began to feel that the position of their own organization as the leading representative of midwives was under threat and reiterated that the MI was 'not just the private concern of a few Club members' but that it spoke for all midwives (*Nursing Notes*, 1909c). They were careful not to give the impression that they were against the new societies, but reminded them of their own efforts to gain representatives on the CMB. They were also firm in their opposition to trade unionism. Mrs Glanville, chairman of the Committee of Representatives, claimed that

we are in no sense a trades union. For we do not believe that any society ever won greatness by self seeking ... as a professional body we prefer to try and raise the whole tone and status of midwives. And while in full sympathy with such methods (trades unionism) applied to bodies of workers engaged in manufacture or supply, I, personally, and

I believe the Institute generally, feel that work which lies wholly in the realms of birth, sickness and death, should be exempt from the restrictions and limitations of a trade union.

(Midwives' Institute, 1911b)

To forestall this interest in trades unionism in the provinces the leaders of the Institute aimed to use the Committees of Representatives to increase their own membership. In October 1909 a scheme was launched to form local Midwives' Associations (MA) which would affiliate to the MI and send representatives to the Committee of Representatives. Local secretaries and delegates to the Committee had to become members of the MI but the rest did not.

Large associations which were already in existence, such as Liverpool with 120 members, were asked to affiliate, but it was more usual for organizers from the Institute to take the initiative in contacting potential local sympathizers and in setting up and speaking at inaugural meetings.

In September 1910, for example, Mrs Glanville held a successful meeting in Nottingham with 150 in the audience, and 60 midwives agreed to form an association. She then travelled to Stafford where the Medical Officer of Health, George Reid, offered to help set up a local group (*Nursing Notes*, 1914). By 1914 there were 53 associations, although many had suffered a decline in members. The emphasis throughout was on finding prestigious local midwives to take the lead and gain the co-operation of medical men. In Bristol, for example, a preliminary meeting to discuss the formation of an association was held in the Bristol Royal Infirmary with the permission of Miss Baillie, the matron. A committee was formed a few months later and the group was addressed by Miss Du Sandoy, County Superintendent and Inspector of Midwives, who spoke on the amendments to the Midwives' Act (Bristol Midwives' Association, 1913).

Although in most local areas matrons were selected as delegates to the Committee of Representatives, in Plymouth a practising midwife was chosen. Local groups also varied in the composition of their membership and in the nature of midwives' problems and concerns. In Plymouth local midwives found it difficult to make a living because the QVJIN and another charity took cases for low fees, whereas in Norwich the main concern was that the health visitor attended midwifery cases before the end of the 10-day period.

Strategies adopted locally mirrored those at a national level, including delegations and petitions to local authorities and voluntary groups. When the Bristol MA found that a local charity was paying very low fees to midwives the officers sent a letter to the charity and were invited to a meeting with the secretary. The charity agreed that the fee was inadequate and it was raised to 7 shillings and 6 pence (Bristol Midwives' Association, 1913).

The more vigorous groups came up with new initiatives; the Liverpool MA co-operated with the local medical officer of health to establish a guarantee fund to cover doctors' fees when called by a midwife. The Liverpool group also devised a scheme to involve their members more directly in the work of the Association (*Nursing Notes,* 1915, 1916). Apart from minor differences of opinion local groups tended to support policies from the centre and to seek friendly relations with the medical profession. This is hardly surprising given that the local leadership was drawn from similar social and professional groups, such as matrons and inspectors, as the leaders of the MI. For many provincial midwives the local groups provided the same kind of support that the Institute had long provided for those based in London. It gave them a place to meet others, provided a redress for some of their grievances and helped to develop an *esprit de corps.*

Other midwives, however, were dissatisfied with the Institute's approach and continued to look for organization on trade union lines. In one letter to *Nursing Notes* a practising midwife argued: 'Why should a midwife be expected to uphold the dignity of her calling on the miserable pittance she is too often obliged to take in payment for her services?' Recognizing that poor women could not afford high fees she ventured to suggest that someone else should pay, and not necessarily the Poor Law authorities. In conclusion she argued that midwives should combine and insist on good pay. In 1914 two members of the Committee of Representatives thought that 'Union' should be added to the title of the Institute, but this was rejected (*Nursing Notes,* 1910b; Midwives' Institute, 1914c).

THE MOVE TO A SALARIED SERVICE

After the First World War these tensions still remained but were negotiated within a different context, which affected both the structure of the organization and its policies. In the inter-war years, for example, outside pressures, including an increase in the number of local authority clinics with their own midwives and the low pay and long hours of midwives working on their own account, posed a threat to the role of the independent midwife. By the end of the 1920s, therefore, the Institute leaders were flexible enough to realize that they would have to abandon their commitment to the independent practitioner. They argued instead that a salaried service was the only way to ensure an improvement in the professional status of midwives and the maintenance of a domiciliary service which now became their main concern (Midwives' Institute, 1928).

In her presidential address of 1935 Edith Pye was aware that some members 'may think your Council has gone back on its old principles' but her arguments were very reminiscent of those put forward before the 1902 Act, combining concern for the interests of midwives with social reform objectives. She warned her audience that the economic problems faced by midwives could lead to their demise and 'the sufferers will be the mothers and babies they serve' (Midwives' Institute, 1935).

The 1936 Act which created a salaried service for midwives, also had an impact on the organization of the Institute and on its role in relation to members. Membership grew and with this came demands for greater representation on central committees and more say in decision-making. The number of paid officers also increased and they had a key role in negotiating salaries and conditions of service for members who were now employed by organizations rather than by individual clients.

CONCLUSIONS

It has been argued throughout this chapter that, from the beginning, the MI made two highly charged claims: firstly, that midwifery was essential to the health of women and babies and therefore to the health of the nation; and secondly, that midwives were distinct from other professions. The MI set out not only to raise the status of the midwife, but also to improve health conditions for women and babies. In attempting to carry out these two aims, which at times could be in conflict with each other, the leaders of the Institute expressed complex views. Influenced by their own class position they nonetheless did not fit easily into categories such as social reform or philanthropist. Although they were anxious to improve health and conditions they also wished to develop a branch of women's work which affected their outlook on the needs of working-class women and the role of the state. They could also be flexible in approach, for example over the need for a salaried service, if they thought that this would protect the overall position of the midwife.

Although the context has changed it can be argued that the aims of the founders of the MI continue to influence the RCM today. Two recent examples of this are cited here. Firstly, prior to the passing of the Nurses, Midwives and Health Visitors Act in 1980 the RCM worked with government and other relevant bodies to ensure that the profession of midwifery remained separate to that of nursing, and that the control of midwifery remained with the midwifery profession (Mee, 1978; *Midwives' Chronicle and Nursing Notes*, 1978; RCM Headquarters, 1978). Secondly, the RCM was very prominent in giving evidence to the House of Commons Health Committee (1992) on the Maternity Services in England and the Policy Review Group of the Health Policy and Public Health Directorate of the Scottish Office Home and Health Department (1993). The reports produced by both these groups (House of Commons Health Committee, 1992; Scottish Office, 1993), and which in England culminated in a report of the Expert Maternity Group (DoH, 1993), confirmed that the midwife had a major role to play in the provision of maternity services. However, the tensions between the aims of the founders also still remain. This has meant that at times the RCM has been criticized by its own membership for its ability (or lack of ability) to protect their professional and material interests. On the other hand, the College continues to speak with authority on any issue relating to maternity and midwifery and continues to ensure that the midwifery perspective is heard throughout the professional world.

REFERENCES

Abel-Smith, B. (1960) *A History of the Nursing Profession*. Heinemann, London.
Bedoe, D. (1983) *Discovering Women's History*. Pandora, London.
Brierly, E. (1923a) In the beginning: a retrospect. *Nursing Notes*, **XXXVI**(421), 10.
Brierly, E. (1923b) In the beginning: a retrospect. *Nursing Notes*, **XXXVI**(422), 21.
Brierly, E. (1923c) In the beginning: a retrospect. *Nursing Notes*, **XXXVI**(423), 34.
Brierly, E. (1923d) In the beginning: a retrospect. *Nursing Notes*, **XXXVI**(431), 40–1.
Bristol Midwives' Association (1913) *Minutes of Meeting 8/12/1913*.
Caine, B. (1992) *Victorian Feminists*. Oxford University Press, Oxford.
Campbell, J.M. (1923) *The Training of Midwives*. Ministry of Health Reports on Public Health and Medical Subjects 21. HMSO, London.
Campbell, J.M. (1924) *Maternal Mortality*. Ministry of Health Reports on Public Health and Medical Subjects 25. HMSO, London.
Campbell, J.M. (1927) *The Protection of Motherhood*. Ministry of Health Reports on Public Health and Medical Subjects 48. HMSO, London.
Carpenter, M. (1980) Asylum nursing before 1914: a chapter in the history of labour. In Davies, C. (ed.), *Rewriting Nursing History*. Croom Helm, London.
Cowell, B. and Wainwright, D. (1981) *Behind the Blue Door: The History of the Royal College of Midwives, 1881–1981*. Ballière Tindall, London.
Davin, A. (1992) Redressing the balance or transforming the art? The British experience. In Kleinberg, S.J. (ed.), *Retrieving Women's History*. Berg, Oxford.
Department of Health (1993) *Report of the Expert Maternity Group* (Chairperson Julia Cummberledge). HMSO, London.
Dingwall, R., Rafferty, A.M. and Webster, C. (eds) (1988) *An Introduction to the Social History of Nursing*. Routledge, London.
Donnison, J. (1977) *Midwives and Medical Men: A History of Interprofessional Rivalries and Women's Rights*. Heinemann, London.
Hannam, J. (1993) Rosalind Paget: class, gender and the Midwives' Institute, c. 1886–1914. *History of Nursing Society Journal*. **5**(3), pp. 133–49.
Hannam, J. and Maggs. C. (1992) *A History of the Royal College of Midwives*. Unpublished Report to the Royal College of Midwives.
Heagerty, B.V. (1990) *Class, Gender and Professionalisation. The Struggle for British Midwifery, 1990–1936*. Unpublished PhD thesis, Michigan State University.
Holcombe, L. (1973) *Victorian Ladies at Work: Middle-Class Working Women in England and Wales,1850–1914*. Hamden, Connecticut.
House of Commons Health Committee (1992) *Report on the Maternity Services (Chairperson Nicholas Winterton)*. HMSO, London.
Leap, N. and Hunt, B. (1993) *The Midwives' Tale: An Oral History from Handywoman to Professional Midwife*. Scarlet Press, London.
Levine, P. (1987) *Victorian Feminism, 1850–1914*. Hutchinson, Oxford.
Lewis, J. (1980) *The Politics of Motherhood*. Croom Helm, London.

Lewis, J. (1991) *Women and Social Action in Victorian and Edwardian England*. Edward Elgar, Aldershot.

Mee, B. (1978) A letter on the Briggs legislation. *Midwives' Chronicle and Nursing Notes*, **91**(1083), 79–80.

Melosh, B. (1982) The Physician's Hand: Work, Culture and Conflict in American Nursing. Temple University Press, Philadelphia.

Midwives' Chronicle and Nursing Notes (1978) The Briggs Controversy, letters and comment. 91(1091), 368–9.

Midwives' Institute (1892) *Report of the Annual General Meeting*. Royal College of Midwives, London.

Midwives' Institute (1899) *Report of the Annual General Meeting*. Royal College of Midwives, London.

Midwives' Institute (1906) *Report of the Annual General Meeting*. Royal College of Midwives, London.

Midwives' Institute (1910a) *Council Minutes 7/1/1910*. Royal College of Midwives, London.

Midwives' Institute (1910b) *Report of the Annual General Meeting*. Royal College of Midwives, London.

Midwives' Institute (1911a) *Minutes of the Advisory Committee 1/6/1911*. Royal College of Midwives, London.

Midwives' Institute (1911b) *Report of the Annual General Meeting*. Royal College of Midwives, London.

Midwives' Institute (1912a) *Emergency Council Minutes 2/12/1912*. Royal College of Midwives, London.

Midwives' Institute (1912b) *Council Minutes 22/4/1912*. Royal College of Midwives, London.

Midwives' Institute (1912c) *Council Minutes 21/6/1912*. Royal College of Midwives, London.

Midwives' Institute (1914a) *Report of the Annual General Meeting*. Royal College of Midwives, London.

Midwives' Institute (1914b) *Council Minutes 16/2/1914*. Royal College of Midwives, London.

Midwives' Institute (1914c) *Minutes of the Committee of Representatives*. Royal College of Midwives, London.

Midwives' Institute (1915) *Council Minutes 11/6/1915*. Royal College of Midwives, London.

Midwives' Institute (1916) *Council Minutes 1/2/1916*. Royal College of Midwives, London.

Midwives' Institute (1928) *Minutes of Advisory Board 15/5/28 and Minutes of Parliamentary Subcommittee 1/6/28*. Royal College of Midwives, London.

Midwives' Institute (1935) *Report of the Annual General Meeting*. Royal College of Midwives, London.

Ministry of Health (1929) *Report of the Departmental Committee on Training and Employment of Midwives*. HMSO, London.

Ministry of Health (1930) *Interim Report of the Departmental Committee on Maternal Mortality and Morbidity*. HMSO, London.

Ministry of Health (1937) *Report of an Investigation into Maternal Mortality*. HMSO, London.

Nursing Notes (1894) Mrs Henry Smith. **VII**(76), 41–2.

Nursing Notes (1899) Midwives in Council. **XII**(143), 147.

Nursing Notes (1901a) Report of the meeting of the Midwives' Sectional Committee. **XIV**(157), 12–13.

Nursing Notes (1901b) Midwives conference. **XIV**(158), 29.

Nursing Notes (1902) Notes on the midwife question. **XV**(172), 144.

Nursing Notes (1903a) The rules of the Central Midwives' Board. **XVI**(190), 135.

Nursing Notes (1903b) The midwife of the future. **XVI**(185), 64.

Nursing Notes (1904) The workings of the Midwives' Act. **XVII**(203), 169–70.

Nursing Notes (1906) The nurse and midwife as citizen. **XIX**(228), 173.

Nursing Notes (1908a) The penalising of motherhood. **XXI**(244), 73.

Nursing Notes (1908b) Mothers and the State. (Editorial.) **XXI**(245).

Nursing Notes (1908c) Votes for women: why we ask for them. **XXI**(247), 138.

Nursing Notes (1909a) Northern midwives' meeting. **XXII**(259).

Nursing Notes (1909b) Midwife Notes: Central Midwives Board. **XXII**(264), 242–3.

Nursing Notes (1909c) Linking up. **XXII**(264), 235.

Nursing Notes (1910a) Union of Midwives. **XXIII**(267), 56.

Nursing Notes (1910b) Letters. **XXIII**(267).

Nursing Notes (1914) Liverpool and District Trained Midwives' Association. **XXVII**(319), 202.

Nursing Notes (1915) Midwives notes: Liverpool's scheme to supply medical assistance for midwives' cases. **XXVIII**(326), 38–9.

Nursing Notes (1916) Reports from Associations. **XXIX**(342), 140.

Parker, J. (1988) *Women and Welfare: Ten Victorian Women in Public Social Service.* Macmillan, London.

Rendall, J. (ed.) (1987) *Equal or Different: Women's Politics, 1800–1914.* Blackwell, Oxford.

Rivers, J. (1981) *Dame Rosalind Paget: A Short Account of Her Life and Work.* Midwives Chronicle, London.

Roberts, E. (1984) *A Woman's Place: An Oral History of Working-Class Women 1890–1940.* Blackwell, Oxford.

Rose, S.O. (1993) Gender and labour history: the nineteenth-century legacy. *International Review of Social History*, **38**, 145–62.

RCM Headquarters (1978) A view on Briggs. *Midwives' Chronicle and Nursing Notes*, **91**(1091), 351.

Scottish Office (1993) *Provision of Maternity Services in Scotland: A Policy Review.* Report to the Health Policy and Public Health Directorate. HMSO, Edinburgh.

CHAPTER THREE

The negotiated role of the midwife in Scotland*

Janet Askham and Rosaline Barbour

This chapter represents findings from a study funded by the Scottish Home and Health Department, which looked at the role and responsibilities of the midwife in Scotland. Although it is now some time since the data were collected (1983–1985), the findings are still relevant for understanding the position of the midwife within the maternity care system of the 1990s.

BACKGROUND TO THE STUDY

The late 1970s and early 1980s were characterized by concerns about the erosion of midwives' responsibilities and alleged lack of opportunities for the midwife to work 'as a practitioner in her own right' – developments seen as resulting from the increased dependence on technology, the continuing encroachment of medical staff and the growing reliance on proscriptive unit policies. These concerns were expressed by prominent members of the midwifery profession and reflected in the professional literature (Bent, 1978; Barnett, 1979; Brain, 1979; Maclean, 1980; Thomson, 1980). Meanwhile the under-utilization of midwives' clinical skills – particularly with respect to antenatal care – were recognized in several influential reports (Social Services Committee, 1980; Royal College of Obstetricians and Gynaecologists, 1982; Maternity Services Advisory Committee, 1982). A report produced by the Central Midwives' Boards for the UK and Eire and published in February 1983 (as pilot work for our study began) highlighted the more general under-utilization of midwives' skills within the maternity care team (Central Midwives Board for Scotland *et al.*, 1983).

Incomplete use of the midwife's skills, combined with low rates of retention, were issues of concern to the midwifery profession in Scotland and to the Scottish Home and Health Department.These concerns, together with the recognition that lack of responsibility may perhaps be a cause of poor retention, led to the commissioning of the study described in this chapter. Although lack of responsibility was often discussed as a widespread problem at this time, there was a lack of systematic evidence about the nature and scope of the problem. Two small-scale studies (Walker, 1976; Macintyre, 1981) had confirmed that the level of their responsibility is an important issue for midwives. Robinson and her colleagues had carried out a large-scale postal survey in 1979 of 19% of practising midwives in England and Wales (Robinson, Golden and Bradley, 1983; Robinson, 1989a, 1989b), but no comparable study existed for Scotland.

Our own study, therefore, set out to establish whether the findings of the England and Wales study also applied to midwives' involvement in the Scottish context. The England and Wales study relied mainly on postal questionnaires, followed by interviews with a relatively small number of midwives to explore certain topics in more depth. The findings had raised a number of contradictions in that midwives in many situations appeared satisfied with a level of responsibility which was less than that for which they had trained. Consequently, in the course of our research we sought not only to document midwives' level of responsibility, but also to explore midwives' perceptions and attitudes about their role in more depth than the earlier study. Accordingly, we adopted a different research design.

The aims of the study were:

1. to find out where the midwife's responsibility ended – i.e. where she handed over to another member of the maternity care team;
2. to establish whether the extent of responsibility accorded midwives varied (a) between the separate fields of maternity care provision and (b) between different organizational structures;
3. to determine which areas of work, procedures or decision-making (if any) gave rise to problems when the work of other staff impinged on that of the midwife;
4. to document how potential disagreement or conflict was handled *in situ*;
5. to establish how midwives, themselves, viewed the situation.

METHODS

Choice of research design

The research had two phases: an interview and observation study, followed by a survey using postal questionnaires. Since the study's main aim was to investigate certain features of work practices as well as midwives' perceptions and attitudes towards these practices, it was felt that a combination of observational and interview study would be the most appropriate approach with which to start. An interview study alone would have been quite inadequate to enable us to examine the actual work experience of midwives and how they responded to it within their day-to-day working lives. By going on to interview those who had been observed, however, we were able to link the observers' assessment of the nature of the midwife's responsibility with their own feelings about the situation.

Our resources were limited, and so we knew that the observation and interview phase of the study would have to be very selective. In order to increase generalizability, therefore, a postal questionnaire study of a larger group of midwives was carried out at the end of the first phase.

Phase 1: observation and interview study

Observation and interviews were carried out in nine locations, selected from three broad geographical areas of Scotland and comprising a range of organizational settings (including large and small teaching hospitals, non-teaching hospitals, peripheral maternity units, general practitioner units and health centres). Since the focus of the study was on midwives' involvement in providing care for women with 'normal' pregnancies and experiencing normal childbirth, antenatal wards and special-care baby units were excluded from this part of the study. All the midwives providing direct care in each setting were studied, but student midwives and those whose main job was administration or training were excluded. A total of 93 midwives was observed and then interviewed.

Initial contact with each of the settings selected was by letter to the director of midwifery services, followed by a visit to explain the nature of the study, and how it would be carried out, to the midwives who would be involved. Permission was also obtained from the medical staff, since they too would be observed, although not interviewed. Staff involved in any of the selected settings were, of course, free to withhold permission for the study to be carried out. In fact almost universal co-operation was obtained, apart from one selected unit where staff felt enough research was already in progress. This unit was replaced by another in the same geographical area.

The observation study Observations took place in three different types of environment: hospital wards, clinics and by accompanying midwives on home visits. Fieldwork was preceded by a pilot period involving both researchers, in which we spent several sessions observing the work in a labour ward in a teaching hospital. Through discussions and comparisons of observations we were able to check reliability, as well as to consolidate recording methods and decisions about what was to be observed.

The observational study concentrated on the work of midwives involved in providing care and on the intersection between their work and the work of medical staff on the one hand and support staff on the other. The observations focused on tasks and procedures carried out in each setting and on decision-making, with the aim of answering the following questions:

1. What procedures were routinely performed by (a) midwives, (b) medical staff, (c) support staff?
2. In what circumstances were these routines not adhered to?
3. To what extent, if at all, were tasks carried out by midwives then repeated by doctors, or vice versa?
4. To what extent, if at all, was dissatisfaction expressed, or conflict evident in the carrying out of tasks or procedures?
5. What were the major decision areas? Were decisions made with reference to policies/guidelines taken by midwives or taken by medical staff? Who had the final say?
6. Whom, if anyone, did midwives and medical staff consult before carrying out any aspect of their work, and what was the nature of consultation between midwives, medical staff and support staff?
7. Who deferred to whom, and on what issues, and were there circumstances in which there was overt conflict between midwives and medical staff and between midwives and support staff? If so, how was it handled?
8. Who was regarded as accountable by whom?
9. Was there a difference between midwives' responsibility for the care of normal and abnormal cases, and if so how was the transition negotiated and made?

We used several strategies in the course of the observation study. Sometimes we positioned ourselves in a particular part of the setting and observed what occurred there; sometimes we observed a particular event (such as a ward round); sometimes we spent a period of time with one midwife, and yet on other occasions we moved between several parts of the setting during an observation period. Since the boundaries between midwives' work and doctors' work was a particular focus of the study, much of the time was spent concentrating on interactions between midwives and medical staff. Both day and night duty were observed. Observation was usually concentrated in 2 to 3 hour long sessions, although some observations, notably those at night, entailed a whole shift. All the midwives working in each fieldwork setting during the study period were included in the observation (93 in all). When women, or their family and friends, were observed, their permission was asked for the researcher to be present, and leaflets describing the project were made available for them if they wished.

Field notes were not normally written in the public setting, but in short periods 'off stage' or immediately following an observational session. Items recorded in the field notes were classified and this classification system developed as the fieldwork progressed through the discovery of further relevant items. Numerical coding was applied so that a computerized data retrieval system could be used to facilitate analysis.

The interview study The research design entailed interviewing all the midwives who had been observed, with the aim of obtaining their perceptions of, and reactions to, their role and level of responsibility as already observed by the researchers. Consequently the interviews were carried out towards the end of the fieldwork period in each setting. The interview format was semi-structured since this provided the opportunity to question respondents about experiences which might be influencing their answers, and to probe in order to obtain a more detailed understanding of what their answers meant. The interview schedule covered a range of topics that included:

1. views about the appropriateness of the division of responsibility between midwives and medical staff for undertaking specified tasks and procedures, and for making decisions;
2. satisfaction with the division of responsibility between midwives and medical staff and midwives and support staff;
3. what caused dissatisfaction to midwives, and whether they experienced problems or conflicts in their interaction with other groups of staff; if so, whether they took any action;
4. employment history and experience in midwifery.

All 93 midwives who had been observed agreed to be interviewed, although all were, of course, free to refuse if they wished. The interviews were conducted during working hours, usually on site, although in private. Respondents were encouraged to talk in as much detail as they wished. The interviews were tape recorded and transcribed verbatim by the project secretary. The transcriptions were then coded and, as with the observational field notes, a data retrieval system was employed.

Phase 2: postal survey

The postal survey was carried out in order to follow up some aspects of the observational and interview study and, by using a representative sample, also to make some generalizations about midwives in Scotland. Sample selection was therefore a very important consideration. A sample size of approximately 200 midwives, working in a variety of settings, was deemed sufficient for the type of analysis proposed. In this part of the study information was also sought about midwives' responsibilities in antenatal wards and special care baby units. The sampling frame comprised all midwives working in 14 health board areas – a total of just under three and a half thousand, once those in purely administrative jobs and those who held double or triple duty posts had been excluded. A questionnaire was sent to every thirteenth midwife on this list ($n = 243$) and 77% were returned ($n = 187$). The respondents represented 6% of midwives working in Scotland at the time of the survey.

Issues covered in the questionnaire included the more quantifiable ones and those of good conceptual clarity. Selection and wording of questions were based largely on experience and knowledge gained in the observation and interview study, and the Royal College of Midwives (Scottish Branch) also provided advice. The questions covered the following main areas:

1. who normally carried out a range of tasks and who normally made decisions in the unit in which the midwife worked, and who in the unit she thought should do so;
2. whether midwives felt the division of responsibility between themselves and (a) medical staff and (b) support staff was about right or not;
3. midwives' views about their freedom to practise in their own right;
4. overall feelings of job satisfaction.

The research participants

The clinical areas and settings in which the midwives involved in the observation and interview study worked, and the clinical settings in which the postal survey respondents worked, are shown in Table 3.1. Employment details for participants in both parts of the study showed that they included a wide range in relation to grade of staff, length of time in practice, and full- and part-time working (Askham and Barbour, 1987a).

Analysis of data and presentation of findings

The questionnaire data provided frequencies for events and decisions experienced by midwives within each of the clinical settings and for the sample of midwives as a whole. Some of the observation and interview data were immediately capable of quantitative analysis; in other cases quantification was only possible after careful scrutiny of fieldnotes and interview transcriptions, which allowed for categorization of situations, events or actions. Some categories required extensive qualitative analysis before quantification and some defied categorization altogether. Some of the themes arising from the data were topics that had been defined at the outset; others emerged during the process of analysis.

In relation to each of the main aims of the research, data were drawn from the observation and interview study and from the postal survey; each provided an integral part of the overall picture. In presenting the information we included quotations which we felt were good illustrations of the point under discussion. In this chapter findings are presented on variation in midwives' work content and level of responsibility, on ways in which midwives defined and negotiated responsibility within the various settings studied, and on how midwives viewed the situation. Further findings from the research are available in Askham and Barbour (1987a, 1987b).

Table 3.1 Participants: numbers and locations

Observational and interview study			Postal questionnaire	
Area	*No. of midwives* *(n = 93)*	*Settings*	*Area*	*No. of midwives* *(n = 187*
Antenatal clinics	42	Large non- teaching hospital Small teaching hospital GP surgeries Peripheral clinics	Antenatal clinics	30
Labour ward	52	Large teaching hospital 2 GP units Maternity home	Labour ward	71
Postnatal ward	40	Large teaching hospital Non-teaching hospital	Postnatal ward	79
Community	25	Large teaching hospital GP unit	Community	9
		Health centre	Special care baby units	5
			Antenatal wards	12

1. Figures add up to more than total as some midwives worked in more than one setting or in mixed units.
2. Findings relating to work in special care baby units and antenatal wards are not discussed in this chapter.
3. The postal questionnaire elicited only a handful of replies from community midwives, probably due to the exclusion of double- and triple-duty post-holders.

Source: Compiled by the authors.

FINDINGS

Robinson, Golden and Bradley (1983) had found that 71% of hospital midwives and 74% of community midwives in England and Wales were either completely satisfied or satisfied with most aspects of their work. Our postal survey findings revealed an even higher level of satisfaction amongst midwives in Scotland, with 78% expressing themselves completely satisfied or satisfied with most aspects of their work. However, as Robinson, Golden and Bradley (1983) also discovered, this masked considerable dissatisfaction with regard to particular aspects of their work. The general agreement with regard to satisfaction also belied the huge variation in the extent of the midwife's responsibility and conditions of work in different settings; thus, although satisfaction was generally high, this related to very different situations.

Variation in work content and responsibility in different clinical settings

Antenatal clinics With regard to midwives' involvement at antenatal clinics the scope of their work was partly determined by the presence or absence of medical complications. However, there was a great deal of variation in the midwife's role in examining women with a straightforward pregnancy. In addition, individual midwives experienced vast discrepancies in the amount of responsibility accorded them at the different clinics they attended in the course of their work. Unit policies sometimes restricted the midwife's involvement for specific visits; for example, at all but one of the clinics in which we carried out our observational work, women were seen by members of the medical staff for certain visits, such as the first examination after booking.

The physical layout of clinics played an important part in determining the extent and nature of midwives' involvement. In some clinics doctors moved between adjoining consulting rooms or booths while midwives remained in one room and thus had the opportunity of examining women prior to the doctor's arrival. In the case of one GP clinic the midwife's involvement was confined to having a chat and handing out leaflets. This state of affairs was partly due to her being allocated a room devoid of examining couch or other equipment; moreover, her role was further restricted by the fact that she saw women only after they had been examined by the doctor.

Organizational arrangements and hierarchical distinctions also had an impact on the extent of the individual midwife's involvement. For example, at one consultant clinic only sisters worked alongside medical staff in consulting rooms, while staff midwives serviced the waiting area, taking blood pressure readings and weighing women.

Whether or not midwives' clinics operated depended largely on the attitudes of the consultants involved, although this could be the subject of negotiation (see discussion below). Midwives' clinics were in operation in only two of the settings in which we carried out observations (and involved only part of the midwives' work in these settings). Of the 30 postal questionnaire respondents employed in antenatal clinics seven were involved in midwives' clinics – although even within these clinics the extent of responsibility accorded midwives could vary. This picture appears to have changed little in the intervening years; a large-scale study of antenatal care in Scotland (Howie *et al.*, 1991) confirms that as recently as 1989 only 4% of antenatal visits took place at midwives' clinics (although a slightly higher percentage of antenatal visits (12%) were recorded as having been supervised by a midwife).

Labour wards Much of the concern that has arisen about erosion of the midwife's role relates to the alleged increasing reliance on technology, and our findings confirmed that the degree of technology available and/or utilized in a particular work setting had an important influence on the scope and content of the midwife's work. Within the context of the labour ward Chamberlain *et al.*(1978) provide the following description of the midwife's remit:

> The midwife is qualified to monitor and assess the progress of labour and to conduct normal deliveries under her own responsibility.

However, the range of procedures involved in 'normal deliveries', i.e. those in which there are no medical complications, is subject to continual revision as new technology becomes more widely available. Thus 'normal' labour within the professional remit of the midwives in our study could, and sometimes did, include induced labours with continuous fetal monitoring under epidural analgesia.

Different hospitals, and indeed individual consultants within the same hospital, varied as to the amount of responsibility which they accorded to midwives for carrying out procedures associated with this new technology – such as setting up intravenous infusions, applying scalp electrodes, carrying out artificial rupture of membranes and topping up epidurals. Although midwives might sometimes perform these tasks, in the majority of units covered by the postal questionnaire responsibility was shared between midwives and members of the medical staff. Technology aside, however, the division of responsibility between midwives and medical staff in labour wards was subject to a great deal of variation as other studies have also shown (e.g. Garcia and Garforth, 1991). Even when there were no complications it was very unusual for a labouring woman to be admitted to a teaching hospital labour ward and to be delivered without having been examined at least once by a member of the medical staff; this also applied to night duty, although regulations might be relaxed somewhat. Three-quarters of the teaching hospital midwives responding to our postal questionnaire said that it was unit policy for each woman to be examined on admission by the medical staff. Half the teaching hospital midwives stated that women were examined by a doctor at regular intervals throughout labour, even when progress did not deviate from 'normal'. By contrast, in GP units women were frequently admitted and delivered without being seen by a doctor – this applied to day duty as well as night duty.

One important function of a teaching hospital is obviously to provide instruction and opportunities for 'hands on' experience for a range of staff. In all maternity care settings the training requirements of student nurses, midwives and doctors often took precedence and could restrict the practical, as opposed to supervisory, involvement of the midwife. In GP units doctors were not present for much of the time, leaving midwives, as the only qualified staff, to assume responsibility, although some individual doctors had issued guidelines indicating when midwives should summon them. Our study was carried out during a transitional period for labour ward midwives who were at that time being trained to perform suturing. Both observational work and responses to our postal questionnaire revealed that the most common practice involved giving priority to the training of nursing officers and sisters, with the result that very few staff midwives had yet been certified to carry out this procedure. Of course, this transitional period has long since passed, but this finding is likely to have implications for the introduction of any new procedure requiring certification of already qualified staff.

Postnatal wards Within hospitals, postnatal wards emerged as the area in which doctors spent least time. Moreover, in this setting ward rounds were carried out by registrars or house officers rather than consultants. Significantly this was also the area for which the highest proportion of midwives expressed satisfaction. Community midwives, as the only professionals required to visit mothers and babies in their homes during the first 10 days following delivery (or 14 days in the case of a caesarean section), probably enjoyed the greatest amount of autonomy, deciding when it was appropriate to call in the GP or refer a woman to the hospital. Both within the hospital and community there is wide acceptance that many of the tasks involved in postnatal care are either solely the midwife's province or are her responsibility, but with the assistance of support staff. There was virtually no overlap of responsibilities between midwives and medical staff with regard to helping mothers to establish baby feeding, ensuring that babies were kept clean, warm, dry and adequately fed, informing and advising mothers about how to care for their babies and how to maintain their own health, and providing frequent observation and monitoring of babies in order to detect any signs of abnormality or distress.

Defining and negotiating responsibility

Both in GP units and postnatal wards senior midwives were often dealing with medical staff who had much less experience than they had themselves and this had an impact on the degree to which midwives were able to negotiate with respect to decision-making and allocation of responsibility. Residents or inexperienced GPs tended to be overridden more frequently or to be more overtly negotiated with than were more experienced doctors. In comparison to medical staff in these settings midwives also had much greater and more prolonged contact with labouring women and mothers and babies and could use their superior knowledge to their advantage in influencing decision-making. In the postnatal setting, for example, the midwife was the only professional with responsibility for both mother and baby and could bring her broader knowledge to bear in influencing discharge decisions, as the following excerpt from our fieldnotes illustrates:

Registrar: I think Mrs Brown can probably go home tomorrow.
Sister: Well, we'll see how the feeding is going. It wasn't too good yesterday.
                    (Fieldnotes, teaching hospital postnatal ward)

On the whole the midwives saw themselves as playing a crucial role in the making of discharge decisions, although not all would have put it as strongly as one staff midwife, who commented:

Discharging patients? Well, in the end it comes down to us – we put words into the doctor's mouth and he puts pen to paper to sign.
                    (Interview with teaching hospital postnatal ward midwife)

That midwives played an important role with regard to their informal influence on decision-making in postnatal wards is evidenced by the finding that the majority of midwives working in this setting and replying to our postal questionnaire saw only two decisions as being made by doctors alone: these were the decision to commence phototherapy and the decision to discharge a baby (both of which referred specifically to paediatric staff).

In their work in antenatal clinics, senior midwives might again find themselves paired with relatively inexperienced medical staff; and midwives, in general, tended to be more familiar with the protocols of individual consultants than were their often more transitory medical counterparts. This could be used to the midwife's advantage, in that she could use an individual consultant's alleged preferences to justify making a particular decision or taking a particular course of action. More frequently, however, midwives simply encouraged junior medical staff to follow the guidelines laid down by the consultant in charge. Midwives were skilled exponents of the delicate use of tact – or what Kitzinger, Green and Coupland (1990) have termed 'hierarchy maintenance work'. This involved a whole range of approaches from laying out specific forms or setting out syringes and containers in anticipation of blood samples being taken, to indicating verbally what a consultant's protocol specified. Midwives were thus able to influence the content and outcome of antenatal consultations while allowing junior members of the medical staff ample opportunity for 'face-saving'.

Where such systems of communication broke down midwives could, and sometimes did, resort to appealing directly to the consultant involved. This strategy tended to be confined to the more senior midwives, who indicated that senior medical and midwifery staff held each other in mutual respect, built out of years of working together. According to midwives, the passage of time could make an impact even on doctors who originally had been reluctant to cede more responsibility to midwives – as could continuity in terms of the same midwife regularly attending an antenatal clinic at a particular GP's surgery, since this could place the midwife in a favourable bargaining position:

> Before I was just chatting to patients at one clinic, but now it's reversed. I do the whole thing now. Don't know what changed his mind. There's been a continual turnover of midwives before, but I've gone regularly – it might've been that. He asked if I'd be prepared to do bloods and I said, 'No – only if I was seeing the patient in total'.
>
> (Interview with teaching hospital midwife talking about her involvement at GP clinics)

In practice the rules governing decision-making might be applied with a greater degree of flexibility than is suggested by official regulations. Again, this was dependent on the establishing of relationships based on mutual trust. Thus, for example, midwives might prescribe analgesics for women and get doctors to sign for these drugs at a later stage. This response, however, was largely confined to the more senior midwives or midwives who had worked with doctors for a considerable length of time. Most of the time midwives trod a narrow line between covering themselves legally and risking the displeasure of the doctors involved:

> You get to know what the different doctors are like – for example, some aren't keen on Panadol so you tend not to ask them for that. It seems silly, really, as you can buy that over a counter in a chemist. We used to just give Panadol, iron and vitamins after a delivery but not now. Some doctors are quite good. If you phone them late at night and ask if someone can have a Panadol they may be annoyed. Some you can get to sign afterwards.
>
> (Interview with GP unit midwife)

If medical staff appeared to midwives to be overly rigid with regard to the issue of prescribing analgesics they could, and sometimes did, contrive to call doctors in the middle of the night to have these orders confirmed; again this related mostly to junior members of the medical staff, who usually responded by relaxing arrangements to enable them to have an unbroken sleep.

Overt differences of opinion were relatively rare and much more commonly there was evidence of agreement about which course of action should be pursued, with midwives frequently anticipating doctors' decisions. In practice, the way in which decisions were reached was often less clear cut than formal job descriptions would suggest, with non-verbal communication playing an important part in this process. Thus midwives were observed, for example, to fetch a trolley for a forceps delivery or to go ahead and get theatre set up without having been explicitly instructed, or, indeed, without anything more than a glance being exchanged between midwife and doctor.

Defining and negotiating responsibility within GP units was a particularly complex process, depending – perhaps more fully than in other work settings – on the combination of personalities involved and the length of service of different members of staff. For the midwife working in these units it took some time to find her feet and to determine which strategies to use with which GPs. According to midwives' reports GPs could often be perverse:

> You have to watch with GPs. Some of them if you say black they'll say white just to spite you. If you want someone transferred, for example, you've to let on that it doesn't matter really.
>
> (Interview with GP unit midwife)

However, doctors who wished to attend deliveries had to rely, for the most part, on midwives to summon them once a woman entered second-stage labour. If the GP in question was defined by the midwife in attendance as being likely to 'interfere' she could, and sometimes did, delay making the relevant telephone call:

> You get fly to those GPs who'll take a delivery from you and you just make sure you tell them at the last minute.
>
> (Interview with GP unit midwife)

Occasionally senior midwives were observed to coach less experienced midwives with regard to strategies for circumventing medical staff when it was felt that inappropriate decisions had been made. In the example which follows, one of the senior midwives in the large teaching hospital labour ward was providing advice for her more junior colleagues as to how they could use the gender imbalance between medical staff and midwives to their advantage when dealing with disagreements – in this case a disagreement over the decision to perform a forceps delivery. The senior midwife commented:

> Of course, you can't say anything in front of the patient, but, provided it's a male doctor, he can't even examine her without you there to chaperone, so you can just go and wait outside the delivery room and ask if you can have a word with him.
>
> (Fieldnotes, teaching hospital labour ward)

In the example given above it is interesting to note that the midwife appears to view her own responsibility as extending beyond the official definition, since clearly the registrar would have been the person answerable for the decision in question. Although midwives seldom became involved in overt conflict with medical staff, their concerns about medical staff's decisions frequently reflect this wider definition of a midwife's responsibility. Commenting on a spirited disagreement between a midwifery sister-in-charge of a teaching hospital antenatal clinic and a registrar who had sent a woman home with a high blood pressure reading, another more junior midwife said:

> Had that lady been in my room I would have questioned it. There's no way I would leave anything that I thought was as important as that ... you wouldn't have it on your own conscience.
>
> (Interview with teaching hospital midwife)

Comparing her involvement at midwives' clinics with that at other clinics where responsibility was shared with a doctor, one midwife concluded:

> You do anyway go to exhaustive lengths to look after a woman, because if something does go wrong you tend to blame yourself even though you maybe didn't play much part in it. I would rather have the (formal) responsibility. There's more in favour of it than against.
>
> (Interview with health centre midwife – text in parentheses added by researcher)

Although doctors might be the members of the maternity care team legally accountable for particular decisions or courses of action, midwives often viewed their responsibility as extending beyond the formal definitions:

> We do have the back-up of the consultants. We can phone a doctor at the consultant unit and the GPs don't really mind us going over their heads if the mother and baby are in danger. I don't feel it's going over their heads because it's two lives you're thinking of. You've to bear that in mind always.
>
> (Interview with GP unit midwife)

> Some of the older school GPs would VE even if a patient was bleeding. One said, 'Get me a pair of gloves and I'll VE her. I said, 'You really mean you're going to VE her? Not when I'm on duty. I'll call the Nursing Officer and you can do it with her.' He sent her to the consultant unit. I think some of the midwives here would've gone ahead, thinking, 'Oh, well, it's his responsibility', but I think it's everybody's.
>
> (Interview with GP unit midwife)

Defining her role more widely might persuade a midwife to carry out extra work, as in the example below:

> With the doctor present (at antenatal clinics) it's sometimes a barrier. If I feel a patient has a problem then I'll write her name down and go and visit her antentally as soon as possible after and just find out if there are any problems. I've found out quite a few worries which they wouldn't speak to the doctor about – mainly social problems.
>
> (Interview with teaching hospital midwife)

The above example also suggests the somewhat different relationship which midwives enjoy with women. This was by virtue of the fact that midwives share a bond with them as other women and are more likely to be perceived as equals, since they do not occupy the same exalted position as doctors. According to midwives, one of the implications of this was that women were more likely to confide in midwives:

There's a rapport with the midwife and the patient. The patient will tell the midwife rather than tell the doctor – even if it's quite a pressing problem. The fact that we're female probably makes the difference.

(Interview with teaching hospital midwife)

Our observational work established that midwives did frequently assume the role of 'go-between', both encouraging women to air their concerns and reinterpreting for women information given by medical staff:

I had observed a midwife at an antenatal clinic talking at some length with a patient prior to the arrival of the consultant. A large part of this conversation had been devoted to discussing a vaginal discharge which the woman had been experiencing. When the consultant arrived he asked the woman, 'And how have you been?', to which she replied, 'Oh, fine, thanks.' Here the midwife laughingly interrupted and said, 'Now, that's not what you've been telling me, is it?' The woman then went on to raise the topic of her discharge with the doctor.

(Fieldnotes, teaching hospital antenatal clinic)

You often clarify things the doctor has said when you leave a room with a patient ... An awful lot of doctors garble out the word 'amniocentesis' and 'little injection' and the mothers are petrified, you know.

(Interview with teaching hospital midwife)

One of the doctors this morning couldn't find a fetal heart. Then he said it was faint. That, I think, is the wrong thing to say to a mum, because they immediately think the fetal heart (itself) is faint. I would (usually) wait until she was out of the room and I would say, 'Don't worry about that.'

(Interview with teaching hospital midwife)

Although outside midwives' clinics midwives had sole responsibility neither for abdominal palpation nor for counselling women, our findings suggest that they were able to derive considerable professional satisfaction from their input and that they were able to maximize their involvement by creative use of their role in preparing women for doctors' examinations and chaperoning women between consulting rooms.

This special woman-to-woman relationship was evident in all areas of maternity care and particularly in the labour ward (Barbour, 1990). Robinson (1989b) argues that midwifery care in labour has advantages over medical care in terms of providing advice and emotional support. Some midwives suggested that having had children oneself was an important - factor:

> The midwife is more at a personal level with her patient because she's a woman and knows her needs more than the doctor, who seems to be on a pedestal to the patient ... It's to do with being a woman as well, but it makes a difference once you've had children yourself – you understand what they're going through, you have more compassion.
>
> (Interview with teaching hospital midwife)

The midwives whom we observed might also, on occasion, use their status as mothers to their advantage in dealing with those junior members of the medical staff perceived by midwives as 'stepping out of line':

> House officer (to patient): You'll just have to keep on trying. You'll find the most comfortable position (for sleeping) yourself.
>
> Staff midwife (laughing): ... says the man who's never been pregnant. When you've had children you realize there is no comfortable position once you get to this stage (of pregnancy).
>
> (Fieldnotes, teaching hospital antenatal clinic)

Midwives' views

Midwives' views of the other professionals who form part of the maternity care team also illuminated the way in which they perceived themselves and their role within this team.

The group most often singled out for criticism by midwives was GPs. As our observations in GP units revealed, this was the area in which individual personalities played the most important role in defining and negotiating responsibility, so it is perhaps not surprising that it was in this context that disagreements were experienced in a particularly immediate way. As generalists, GPs sometimes had considerably less obstetric knowledge and skill than had the midwives working alongside them – either at clinics, in the labour room or in the postnatal ward. However, according to the midwives in our study, GPs did not always give midwives the recognition they felt they deserved:

> An awful lot of the midwife's talents are wasted. If GPs knew what training midwives go through I think they would use midwives as midwives and not just as nurses ... I don't think they regard you as anything more than a pair of helping hands. It would be nice to be used as a midwife rather than someone who is there in the background.
>
> (Interview with health centre midwife)

This lack of appreciation by GPs was by no means universal and one midwife cited with satisfaction the following incident:

> Doctors do rely on us quite a bit. There was one incident when a very competent doctor asked me, 'What do you think?' You're the ultimate authority, really. The doctors are seeing a lot of other things, but you're doing all the midwifery.
>
> (Interview with health centre midwife)

Midwives sometimes criticized GPs in terms of their lack of skill in obstetrics and their departures from the practice of consultant units as experienced by the midwives either in their current jobs or in previous posts:

> GPs sit on patients who should be transferred ... doing inductions on unfavourable cervices; their technique in delivery may not be good ... forceps deliveries. Sometimes it's really frightening. They should be up to date and have done some in a training school within a certain length of time. Quite often their technique at suturing is just desperate ... Another GP tried to remove a placenta manually without a general anaesthetic.
>
> (Interview with GP unit midwife)

Unlike the situation in teaching hospitals where the midwife often had a direct line of communication with senior medical staff, and where the less experienced doctors were overseen by the medical hierarchy, midwives in GP units often perceived themselves as the only other members of staff responsible for ensuring high standards of care. As one nursing officer commented of the midwife's involvement in working with GPs:

> The midwife knows what is good obstetrics and can only push the GP.
>
> (Interview with nursing officer)

It is perhaps because of this heightened perception amongst midwives in GP units of their own responsibility that they appeared more critical of doctors' expertise. Perhaps also because of the immediacy of the situation in which midwives saw themselves as being the only individuals charged with the responsibility of ensuring that safety standards were maintained, they were more likely to recall dramatic incidents. Certainly the midwife quoted above, who was very critical of the expertise of some other GPs with whom she worked, was quick to add:

> But some of the others are really good. I feel bad about saying that.
>
> (Interview with GP unit midwife)

However, some of the teaching hospital midwives in our study were also critical of the expertise of some of the medical staff involved and questioned the desirability of 'flinging' junior members of the medical staff 'in at the deep end':

Residents with very little experience of obstetrics or midwifery are expected to be the first point of referral for analgesia prescription, VE, abnormal fetal heart tracing, etc. I feel it is unrealistic to expect them to deal effectively with such problems ... I'd like to see them in more of a learning capacity.

(Interview with midwife in teaching hospital labour ward)

In some situations midwives felt that safety standards were being compromised due to this approach and, again, might attempt to intervene:

The resident phoned the registrar regarding manual removal of the placenta. The registrar said she should have carried on. The next time she didn't phone and I advised her to. When he told her to carry on I was very nearly screaming.

(Interview with midwife in teaching hospital labour ward).

One of the researchers had been present when this exchange took place and had recorded in her fieldnotes the following comments from the midwife involved:

I'm much more experienced and I can't do a manual removal of a placenta. How could that wee lassie? She can't even manage third stage.

(Fieldnotes, teaching hospital labour ward)

None of the midwives studied, either in the observational study or the postal questionnaire, complained about their involvement in carrying out tasks such as taking blood pressure readings, weighing women or testing urine samples. That is, they did not object to such tasks *per se*. Where their role was confined to such tasks, however, midwives were usually very critical; particularly if they also worked at other clinics where the midwife was granted greater responsibility. This applied to all areas of maternity care; generally, it appeared to be exposure to situations affording the midwives greater responsibility which determined midwives' attitudes, rather than age or length of experience.

Despite the fact that repetition by doctors of midwives' examinations was observed to occur in most settings, most particularly in antenatal clinics (with both doctors and midwives performing abdominal palpation and examining for oedema), this situation aroused surprisingly little adverse comment from midwives. In this respect our findings mirrored those of Robinson, Golden and Bradley (1983). One possible explanation is the very different way in which midwives viewed the performance of these tasks. Great importance was attached by midwives to maintaining their skills and thus their examinations were prized for the opportunity they afforded of gaining practice. Within this context it was irrelevant whether abdominal palpations were repeated by other categories of staff. Midwives went to considerable lengths to ensure that they got experience in palpating:

> A staff midwife was palpating a woman in the consulting room while waiting for the senior house officer to arrive. A second midwife entered the room to borrow a sonic aid, which startled the first midwife, who responded, 'Oh ... as long as it's only you! I'm trying to get my palpations in before the doctor comes and I thought it was him coming in.
>
> (Fieldnotes, teaching hospital antenatal clinic)

Midwives might also perceive their own input as being qualitatively distinct from that of doctors:

> Maybe the patient wants to know. I'll tell her where the baby's lying ... the doctor would just say, 'everything's fine.'
>
> (Interview with midwife at teaching hospital antenatal clinic)

Midwives strove to maximize their involvement in abdominal palpation and counselling, these being seen as important components of their work. It is, of course, possible that midwives used their involvement in counselling women to justify their lack of responsibility for other procedures at antenatal clinics. However, our observational work established that midwives also sought to maximize opportunities for counselling at midwives' clinics, where they had much greater responsibility for carrying out other procedures and making decisions. Our findings showed that midwives tended to view their responsibilities as extending beyond those formally accorded them, and, indeed, some midwives saw themselves as overseeing the input of junior medical staff. Thus the midwife in charge of one teaching hospital clinic explained:

> If a midwife had a junior doctor (in with her at a clinic) she would automatically palpate a patient again, after him, to satisfy herself.
>
> (Interview with teaching hospital midwife)

Several midwives working at peripheral maternity units also appeared to be appealing to this wider notion of responsibility when they stressed their eagerness to gain instruction in how to intubate babies:

> We should be taught how to intubate a baby at birth ... I don't know why they concentrated on doing suturing of episiotomies rather than that. It's a life or death situation.
>
> (Interview with GP unit midwife)

Midwives' enthusiasm for extending their repertoire to include intubating babies reflects their concern to improve overall safety standards rather than a desire to enhance the professional standing of the midwife by expanding her job description – although, of course, these goals are not necessarily usually exclusive.

Midwives' response to the then recent extension of their role to encompass the suturing of episiotomies was interesting. One might expect midwives wholeheartedly to embrace such an extension, which would appear to acknowledge the primacy of the midwife in attending 'normal' deliveries. Midwives, however, were often reluctant to suture. Like abdominal palpation, suturing was a skill which, according to midwives, could be lost through lack of practice. In marked contrast to their attempts to maximize opportunities for palpating, however, midwives were often slow to assert themselves as the appropriate members of staff to carry out suturing. Although opportunities for suturing were undoubtedly limited by factors such as staff shortages, the number of forceps deliveries or caesarean sections, and, of course, intact perineums, our findings show that midwives were not suturing as often as they could have done. Even in the teaching hospital, where two-thirds of the midwives had been trained to suture, it was still fairly common practice for medical staff to suture after episiotomies performed by midwives. Teaching hospital midwives replying to our postal questionnaire confirmed that, even where midwives had undergone training, the responsibility for suturing after episiotomies was still shared between midwives and medical staff; only half of these midwives were dissatisfied with this arrangement. Our findings suggest that midwives were applying their own standards of competence which went above and beyond the requirements of their training course:

> Even though I'll have my certificate soon I still won't do any without supervision for a while until I feel competent to do it on my own.
> (Interview with teaching hospital midwife)

Midwives were often concerned about the long-term effects on women of badly repaired perineums and hence were sometimes reluctant to take on this responsibility. Fear of litigation should anything go wrong may also have influenced their behaviour with regard to suturing, although midwives tended to talk about the prospect of litigation in more general terms, without referring to specific procedures. That this may have been a factor is suggested by a comment made in the course of our fieldwork by a registrar. Although this individual, perhaps, does exaggerate the likelihood of such a turn of events, the comment, nonetheless, does also serve to confirm that midwives were passing up opportunities to suture:

> Another thing that bugs me is that midwives won't suture. I mean – they have the certificates – but when it comes down to it they won't do it … It's partly because of the comeback. If I repair a perineum and it breaks down I get my leg pulled about it for ages, but if a midwife does it, there's an enquiry and she ends up out of a job. So you can understand their reluctance a bit.
> (Fieldnotes, teaching hospital labour ward – registrar)

Although midwives did not seek to explain their own reluctance to suture in terms of the implications for litigation, this was, nevertheless, a concern which was at the back of their minds throughout their work. Midwives in all settings were preoccupied with 'writing things down' and more experienced midwives were observed to advise junior midwifery staff to ensure that they did this. In those situations when midwives obtained a doctor's consent over the phone, midwives were careful to have instructions (particularly those relating to prescribing analgesics) confirmed in writing. This was seen as affording the midwife protection:

> If you don't have things in writing they'll agree black is white orally and then turn round and say they didn't, so you have to be careful.
> (Interview with GP unit midwife)

These recordings did not merely detail the midwife's actions, but might also allude to perceived shortcomings on the part of the medical staff:

> I always cover myself ... I'd put – I have done – 'Dr M. informed but most reluctant to come and see the patient'.
> (Interview with GP unit midwife)

Again, this highlights midwives' broader definition of their role as ensuring that the highest standards of care are provided by the maternity care team as a whole. Midwives in a variety of settings were particularly critical of what they saw as illogical restrictions on their involvement. The tasks most often concerned were the carrying out of venepuncture for routine haemoglobin tests on postnatal wards and the prescribing and administering of analgesics on the labour ward and postnatal ward:

> We're not allowed to do the haemoglobin bloods. I have done it occasionally and then been told off. I think it's crazy. If midwives can take blood for one reason why can't they take it for another?
> (Interview with midwife on teaching hospital postnatal ward)

Two-thirds of the postnatal ward midwives responding to our postal questionnaire stated that doctors usually performed venepuncture for this purpose and two-thirds of those in this situation were dissatisfied with the exclusion of midwives.

A frequent grouse on the part of midwives centred around the fact that while they were now required to suture perineums, which they viewed as a complex surgical procedure, they were not being trusted to prescribe two Panadols (which could be bought over the counter at a chemist's). This was a popular parallel alluded to in all settings.

As with most of the other decisions over which midwives expressed some dissatisfaction with the present pattern, midwives were not advocating that they should take over formal responsibility for making this decision. Where midwives expressed a desire for change what they generally wanted was for medical staff to pay more attention to their opinions:

> But the doctors know better sometimes than the midwife who's been with the patient all the time. They don't know what her contractions are like or see her pushing for a while.
>
>   (Interview with teaching hospital labour ward midwife)

> The doctors tend to go by the monitors, sometimes, rather than the midwife.
>
>   (Interview with teaching hospital labour ward midwife)

A vocal minority of midwives working in a variety of labour ward settings were critical of what they saw as the over-involvement of doctors in care of women with 'normal' labours. They felt that the midwife was better equipped to make certain decisions by virtue of the insights afforded by her role as labour attendant:

> I'd like to see changes about the type of pain relief and when you would require it because patients put on a brave smile when they see the medical staff, but, having sat with the patient, the midwife is aware of the patient's needs. The decision as to when a patient should start pushing is one which should be left to the person who has sat with the patient and who is going to deliver her. It annoys me when the medical staff interfere.
>
>   (Interview with GP unit midwife)

Where midwives considered that technology was used too often, their dissatisfaction always related to the implications which this had for the involvement of doctors in 'normal' deliveries to the exclusion of midwives. Where midwives had been accorded additional responsibilities in dealing with the new technology of the labour ward they performed these tasks (such as applying scalp electrodes, setting up intravenous infusions, and topping up of epidurals) without complaint. However, there was little enthusiasm, either amongst the midwives we interviewed or those replying to our postal questionnaire, for making such tasks the sole prerogative of the midwife. Likewise, midwives were almost unanimous in stating that they did not wish their role to be extended to include performing amniotomies and forceps deliveries.

Midwives' satisfaction with their role

We found that midwives in all settings expressed a high degree of satisfaction with their role and the extent of their responsibilities. Given, however, that there were areas in which the ownership of responsibility appeared to be uncertain, problematic or subject to debate, one might ask why there is not more overall dissatisfaction or even militancy amongst midwives. Our study suggests several answers.

Many aspects of work are almost universally accepted as the midwife's sphere. Moreover, these are likely to be the very aspects of the work from which midwives derive the greatest satisfaction.

Midwives were shown to have a great deal of scope in informally influencing decisions. In many ways midwives were in an ideal situation, being able to exert their influence without carrying the formal responsibility or laying themselves open to the possibility of litigation. Some midwives were doubtful as to whether their own professional body, although keen formally to extend the midwife's role, would actually support the individual midwife if something were to 'go wrong'.

Due to the range of situations (each affording different levels of responsibility) which are covered in the course of an individual midwife's work, it is unlikely that she will have to endure at all times a division of responsibility which she finds unsatisfactory.

Our data suggest that there may be an element of self-selection, with the individual midwife gravitating towards those areas of midwifery practice or work settings which afford that precise degree of responsibility with which she herself is comfortable or which afford the opportunity to pursue her own interests. Thus there was a tendency for midwives in all settings to view their own situation favourably in contrast to that of midwives employed elsewhere:

> I think we have a lot of freedom in managing patients' labours, deciding about pain relief in comparison with other places, doing VEs, putting on scalp electrodes, carrying out ARMS.
> > (Interview with midwife in teaching hospital labour ward)

> There seems to be a lot of scope here – chair deliveries, research which we are taking part in.
> > (Interview with midwife in teaching hospital labour ward)

> Community's very different from the wards because you're out there on your own. Nobody else is seeing the mother and baby, so it's up to you to take a note of things ... Community's a challenge and you don't know what you're going on to ... In hospital, there's always paediatric staff, sometimes the responsibility's greater than in labour ward because there's only you.
> > (Interview with community midwife)

Our study also documented the ways in which a midwife might define her responsibilities more widely than does her official job description, which is an inadequate measure of her actual involvement. Such an appraisal of their role could lead to midwives having a broader appreciation of their work and go some way towards explaining the apparent inconsistency in some settings with low levels of formal responsibility being associated with high levels of satisfaction. Official job remits are inadequate tools for understanding the midwife's work situation, her responsibilities and her satisfactions and dissatisfactions.

Finally, there is an aspect of the midwife's work which is often overlooked in evaluations of her role and responsibilities. This is the sheer enjoyment which she may derive from the work, which may render some dissatisfactions irrelevant – at least for part of the time. The sense of fulfilment is evident in the following quotes from midwives in a range of settings:

> I don't think of it as a temporary relationship with the patient. You're teaching them things you know will maybe last a lifetime and be passed on to their children.
>
> (Interview with community midwife)

> Oh, it makes me quite tearful myself. What a lovely couple – I wish all deliveries were like that. You could see they were so fond of each other and it's just lovely to deliver a baby to a couple like that … If only all couples were as happy … that's the sort of thing that makes your job worthwhile, having nice deliveries.
>
> (Fieldnotes, GP unit)

> The part I enjoy most is showing the mothers what to do with their babies, bathing their babies, feeding – I just enjoy talking to the mothers about the babies – I just enjoy working with patients in general.
>
> (Interview with midwife in teaching hospital postnatal ward)

CONCLUSION

The data reported in this chapter were collected in the mid-1980s, but nonetheless remain relevant to maternity care in the mid-1990s in Scotland and in England and Wales. The study was one of the earliest large-scale investigations of the role of the midwife and the first to take place in Scotland.

Since the mid-1980s onwards many schemes have been initiated by which midwives have sought to restore their role (Robinson, 1990). At the same time, however, a succession of studies has demonstrated that aspects of the midwife's role and responsibilities in many clinical settings remain restricted, primarily by medical involvement in normal maternity care; these studies include Garcia and Garforth (1991), Green, Kitzinger and Coupland (1986, 1994) for England and Howie *et al.* (1991) for Scotland.

Moves to restore the midwife's role have recently received government backing in England and Wales with the publication of *Changing Childbirth* (Department of Health, 1993), and in Scotland with the publication of *Provision of Maternity Services in Scotland* (Scottish Home and Health Department, 1993). A continuing programme of research, of the kind reported here, is required to assess the extent to which these recommendations are translated into practice.

By means of observation and interview this study demonstrated strategies used by midwives to negotiate a role in the maternity team which enabled them to achieve job satisfaction and to ensure care was provided to the standard they perceived as desirable. This process of negotiating a role within the team has been the subject of subsequent research; most notably by Green, Kitzinger and Coupland (1986, 1994) and Kirkham (1989). This too will be a fruitful area of research on both sides of the border as midwives seek to define their changing role in the maternity services of today.

ACKNOWLEDGEMENTS

We would like to thank the Chief Scientist's Office of the Scottish Home and Health Department for the grant to carry out this project; the Royal College of Midwives (Scottish Board) for their support, and for help in drawing our samples; the Department of Obstetrics and Gynaecology in Aberdeen, to which we were attached; the midwives and other members of the maternity teams who took part in the study; and the women and men who so willingly put up with our presence while they were preparing for or having their babies.

REFERENCES

Askham, J. and Barbour, R.S. (1987a) The role and responsibilities of the midwife in Scotland: the final report of a research project. Unpublished report presented to SHHD, Department of Obstetrics and Gynaecology, University of Aberdeen.

Askham, J. and Barbour, R.S. (1987b) The role and responsibilities of the midwife in Scotland. *Health Bulletin*, **45**(3), 153–9.

Barbour, R.S. (1990) Fathers: the emergence of a new consumer group. In Garcia, J., Kilpatrick, R. and Richards, M. (eds), *The Politics of Maternity Care*. Clarendon Press, Oxford, pp. 202–16.

Barnet, Z. (1979) The changing pattern of maternity care and the future role of the midwife. *Midwives Chronicle and Nursing Notes*, **92**(1102), 381–4.

Bent, E. (1978) The future role of the midwife: the midwife's viewpoint. *Midwives Chronicle and Nursing Notes*, **91**(1082), 51–4.

Brain, M. (1979) *Observations by a Midwife*. In report of a conference on the reduction of perinatal mortality and morbidity. DHSS, London.

Central Midwives' Board for Scotland, Northern Ireland Council for Nurses and Midwives an Bord Altranais, Central Midwives' Board (1983) *The Role of the Midwife*. Hymns Ancient and Modern, Suffolk.

Chamberlain, G., Philipp, E., Howlett, B. and Master, K. (1978) *British Births 1970. Vol. 2: Obstetric Care*. Heinemann Medical Books, London.

Department of Health (1993) *Changing Childbirth* (2 parts). HMSO, London.

Garcia, J. and Garforth, S. (1991) Midwifery policies and policy-making. In Robinson, S. and Thomson, A.M. (eds), *Midwives, Research and Childbirth*, Vol. II. Chapman & Hall, London, pp. 16–47.

Green, J., Kitzinger, J. and Coupland, V. (1986) The division of labour: implications of medical staffing structures for midwives and doctors on the labour ward. Unpublished report, Centre for Family Research, University of Cambridge.

Green, J., Kitzinger, J. and Coupland, V. (1994) Midwives' responsibilities, medical staffing structures and women's choice in childbirth. In Robinson, S. and Thomson, A.M. (eds), *Midwives, Research and Childbirth*, Vol. III. Chapman & Hall, London, pp. 5–29.

Howie, P.W., McIlwaine, G., Duflorey, C. and Tucker, J. (1991) *What is Antenatal Care in Scotland?* Final Report. University of Dundee.

Kirkham, M. (1989) Midwives and information-giving in labour. In Robinson, S. and Thomson, A.M. (eds), *Midwives, Research and Childbirth*, Vol. I. Chapman & Hall, London, pp. 117–38.

Kitzinger, J., Green, J. and Coupland, V. (1990) Labour relations: midwives and doctors on the labour ward. In Garcia, J., Kilpatrick, R. and Richards, M. (eds), *The Politics of Maternity Care*. Clarendon Press, Oxford, pp. 149–62.

MacIntyre, S. (1981) Personal communication.

MacLean, G. (1980) Where have all the midwives gone? *Midwives Chronicle*, **93**(1108), 158–9.

Maternity Services Advisory Committee (1982) *Maternity Care in Action: Part 1 – Antenatal Care*. HMSO, London.

Robinson, S. (1989a) Caring for childbearing women: the interrelationship between midwifery and medical responsibilities. In Robinson, S. and Thomson, A. (eds), *Midwives, Research and Childbirth*, Vol. I. Chapman & Hall, London, pp. 8–41.

Robinson, S. (1989b) The role of the midwife: opportunities and constraints. In Chalmers, I., Enkin, M. and Keirse, M. (eds) *Effective Care in Pregnancy and Childbirth*. Oxford University Press, Oxford, pp. 162–80.

Robinson, S. (1990) Maintaining the independence of the midwifery profession: a continuing struggle. In Garcia, J., Kilpatrick, K. and Richard, M. (eds), *The Politics of Maternity Care*. Clarendon Press, Oxford, pp. 61–91.

Robinson, S., Golden, J. and Bradley, S. (1983) *A Study of the Role and Responsibilities of the Midwife*. NERU Report No 1, King's College, London University.

Royal College of Obstetricians and Gynaecologists (1982) *Report of a Working Party on Antenatal and Intrapartum Care*. RCOG, London.

Scottish Home and Health Department (1993) *Provision of Maternity Services in Scotland: A Policy Review*. Scottish Office, Edinburgh.

Social Services Committee – House of Commons (1980) *Report on Perinatal and Neonatal Mortality* (Chairman R. Short). HMSO, London.

Thomson, A.M. (1980) Planned or unplanned? Are midwives ready for the 1980s?*Midwives Chronicle*, **93**(1106), 68–72.

Walker, J. (1976) Midwife or obstetric nurse? Some perceptions of midwives and - obstetricians of the role of the midwife. *Journal of Advanced Nursing*, **1**(2), 129–38.

CHAPTER FOUR

Choice or chance? The selection of student midwives

Robyn Phillips

INTRODUCTION

The task of selecting potential midwifery recruits is a routine responsibility undertaken with regularity by midwife teachers, yet is one that may have important implications for subsequent midwifery practice. Entrance to the profession of midwifery is largely determined by being selected to undertake a midwifery course, since once selected, as Dellar (1981) highlights in relation to health visiting, few students fail the course. Similarly with midwifery, choosing prospective midwifery students determines future midwives and hence has implications for the quality and provision of midwifery care. Competition for a place on a course is often keen, despite the intention of many applicants not to pursue a career in midwifery after qualification (Mander, 1987). Statistics have long indicated, however, that less than one-fifth of qualified midwives in the UK are practising midwifery (e.g. Royal College of Midwives, 1985). The process of selecting students for midwifery may well contribute to such statistics, given that 20% of those selected to enter a course have no intention of practising as a midwife upon completion (Robinson, 1986a). The implications arising from what appear at face value to be simple selection decisions may therefore be far reaching.

The subject of this chapter is an exploratory study that aimed to describe the key criteria and processes used in the selection of potential student midwives. The rationale for the study arose from the aforementioned concerns, particularly in view of personal involvement as a midwife teacher in the selection process. Observation of the progress of student midwives during the 18-month course, their subsequent retention or otherwise in midwifery practice on qualification and registration as a midwife, and the career pathways of those who remained, stimulated a nagging doubt that there may well have been few concrete criteria upon which selection decisions were made. Preliminary discussions with colleagues from midwifery schools throughout England and Wales revealed a diversity of selection methods and criteria in operation, in addition to similar concerns and interest in student midwife selection.

The study was undertaken in my own time, while employed full-time as a midwife teacher. The completed dissertation which described the research was submitted in September 1989 in partial fulfilment of the requirements for the degree of Master in Education of the University of Wales. An Iolanthe Trust Fund award is gratefully acknowledged for full funding of the study, in addition to providing the fees for the initial two taught years of the Masters course.

BACKGROUND TO THE RESEARCH

Despite the apparent interest in this aspect of midwifery education no research specifically related to selection of student midwives in England and Wales, nor indeed elsewhere, was identified in a literature search. Several studies, however, had investigated varying issues in the selection of students for other health care occupations.

White (1985) traces the historical background to educational requirements for entry to nurse training and argues that ensuring quantity rather than quality of applicants was the predominant factor in setting minimum educational standards for entry. Grahame (1985) takes issue with the prerequisite academic requirements for nurse training, advocating that applicants should possess at least two 'A' levels, not merely the minimum of five 'O' level subjects traditionally accepted by many nursing schools.The validity of specifying five 'O' level passes as a requirement for entry to district nurse training was investigated by Jarvis and Gibson (1981) in a study that compared the applicants' educational qualifications prior to selection with their subsequent achievement, both practical and theoretical, during the course. No evidence was found to indicate that students with five 'O' level passes coped better with the district nursing course than those less academically qualified. Indeed, Jarvis and Gibson (1981) suggest:

> Possession of this number of GCSE passes may merely be a social selection mechanism that if incorporated into district nursing, or any other semi-professional occupation such as health visiting, midwifery, etc., may deprive it of effective practitioners.

Ray (1979) reviewed the processes influencing selection of students for a course in health visiting. Apart from the obligatory Registered General Nurse qualification, Ray identified the following elements in the selection process for intending health visitor students; the letter of enquiry, the application form, the interview, references and tests to establish level of intelligence and/or personality traits. The selection procedures for prospective health visitor students were similarly analysed by Dellar (1981), who found that an entire day was utilized for the process. The total procedure included informal measures aimed at becoming acquainted with applicants and allowing them to relax, in addition to more formal processes such as the administration of written tests and a 30-minute interview.

The use of written tests in the selection of potential health visitors (Fader, 1976; Dellar, 1981) and district nurses (Lopez and Radford, 1985) has been investigated. Fader (1976) found that most training institutions conducting health visitor courses applied a written entrance test for each applicant, regardless of educational qualifications. Such tests varied, but the essay was one format used frequently. Other research regarding selection of health visitor students (Hack, 1973) has concentrated upon the relationship between scores obtained on written entrance tests and both the subsequent performance of students during the course and eventual practice as a health visitor. The use of written tests in the selection of students for general nursing is also described in the literature, for example, 'trainability tests' (Belbin and Toye, 1978) and tests for psychological assessment (Jordan, 1987). Lewis (1980) postulates from the findings of her study into the personality profiles of qualified nurses that it may indeed be possible to develop criteria based on personality assessment that would indicate suitability for nursing.

Despite criticism of the reliability and validity of the employment interview (Arvey and Campion, 1982) it is often central to the process of selection of students for many of the health care professions, for example general nursing (Reeve, 1978; Borrill, 1987), psychiatric nursing (Leach, 1988; Jones, 1985), medicine (Richards, McManus and Maitlis, 1988) and health visiting (Dellar, 1981). In Arvy and Campion's (1982) comprehensive review of research relating to the employment interview, they highlight the relatively low reliability (different judgements of the same candidate by different interviewers) and low validity (assessment of potential at interview matches poorly with job performance) cited in past literature. Arvy and Campion do, however, note that later research demonstrates that reliability and validity of the interview process can be improved with the use of a panel of interviewers and interview questions based directly on an analysis of the job to be undertaken. Indeed, a study by Richards, McManus and Maitlis (1988) showed that using panels of interviewers for selection of potential medical students could be a reliable measure, since the overall recommendations of the interview panels were very similar to each other.

Lopez and Radford (1985) describe some pertinent findings from their survey regarding recruitment and selection of applicants for district nurse training. There was little advertising of the courses by the institutions concerned and only one-quarter of students were recruited from health authorities other than the one in which the institution was located. McManus and Richards (1984) identified favourable factors in candidates for medical school. 'A' level examination results were found to be the prime factor in determining shortlisting for interview whereas other factors, such as early application and parents with a medical background, played a much smaller part in the selection process. This study drew on literature relating to selection of students in health care professions other than midwifery, in order to explore the issues surrounding student midwife selection. Rules relating to admission of a person to undertake training for Part 10 of the UKCC Professional Registrar are clearly laid out (UKCC, 1991). Rules relating to criteria for entry to a midwifery programme nevertheless do not address the issue of how potential midwives should be selected, nor do they stipulate other attributes that may be relevant beyond the basics of minimum age and educational attainment. Currently it is the prerogative of each individual school to decide their own additional entry criteria and the processes to be used in the selection of student midwives. The generally agreed purpose, however, of the overall selection procedure is to select the most suitable recruits to the midwifery profession.

The implications of selection decisions on the delivery of health care have been raised in the literature. The *Lancet* (1984) highlights the difficult responsibility bestowed on those in medical education of selecting a potential 'product' or quality deserved by the public, i.e. 'good' doctors. Lazarus and Van Niekerk (1986) also equate selection of medical students with appropriate academic potential and personal qualities with the quality of subsequent medical care – qualities they suggest cannot be instilled through a programme of education. Equally, women deserve high-quality midwifery care and 'good' midwives. The implications of selection decisions made in midwifery education are thus as profound as those professed for medical education. Consequently, an attempt was made in this study to explore the criteria and characteristics believed to be important in midwifery recruits and to describe the means by which aspiring students are chosen. The study design, data collection and analysis are described first, followed by discussion of selected findings and their implications for midwifery.

METHODS

Overview of study design

The aim of the study was to gain a total view of how and why student midwives in England and Wales were selected. The method chosen for data collection was therefore a survey by postal questionnaire sent to all senior midwife teachers in England and Wales responsible for a school approved by the respective national Board to provide an 18-month course in midwifery, following registration as a general nurse.

Preliminary data collection began in August 1987 with observation of a programmed discussion group held as a component part of a statutory refresher course for midwife teachers. This was followed in September and October of the same year by observation of selection procedures in two midwifery schools with which I was unfamiliar. The purpose of the initial qualitative work was to elicit a broader perspective on selection beyond personal knowledge and experience. Together with the literature review, the preliminary observation sessions enabled key issues in selection decisions to be identified for inclusion in the questionnaire, thus making it relevant to the frame of reference of all those to be involved in the subsequent survey. The questionnaire was distributed in July 1988.

Qualitative design work

Field and Morse (1985) state that qualitative and quantitative research methods are different but complementary approaches towards the same goal and outline means by which both approaches may be used in the same study to strengthen the research.This can include using the two approaches simultaneously, i.e. 'triangulation' (Smith, 1981) or, alternatively, undertaking initial qualitative work which then leads into a broader study using quantitative techniques.

In designing the survey, it was essential to ensure that the research topic was of interest and relevance to participants and that each question addressed an important issue concerning selection of potential midwifery recruits. The response options offered in each question had to enable individual senior midwife teachers to give an answer that realistically reflected their true beliefs and practice. Morton-Williams (1978) advocates using initial small-scale qualitative work to highlight issues and ranges of behaviour, thus avoiding respondents being forced into indicating responses inappropriate to their own viewpoint or situation. Consequently, preliminary design work was undertaken that included observing a formal discussion regarding the topic of student midwife selection, and observing selection procedures used by two midwifery schools. The questionnaire was subsequently compiled on the basis of issues identified from the literature review, from itemizing and categorizing data from the preliminary observation sessions as described by Akinsanya (1988), in addition to personal knowledge of processes involved in selection of potential students of midwifery.

The initial qualitative work began with observation of a discussion session which was a planned component of a statutory refresher course of which I was a participant. All 12 members of the discussion group were midwife teachers. Each worked in a different midwifery school and hence had knowledge and experience of varying notions of selection of potential student midwives. I was anxious not to participate in the discussion nor chair the group, wishing only to observe and note issues raised by colleagues. To be given permission to be a 'passive participant' was therefore important (Spradley, 1980, p. 59). Had the observations been made in a covert manner,

I would not have been contributing to the group activities as expected. No problems with my declaration of interest and intent appeared to be perceived and my request was granted. The broad remit of the group was to discuss recruitment and selection of student midwives. Throughout the session I sat quietly but attentively, unobtrusively jotting down the issues raised. This was also done during the subsequent plenary session encompassing the total course cohort. While recognizing that these observations did not amount to a full ethnographic record, what Spradley (1980, p. 70) has called an 'expanded account' was made from the field notes the same evening. From the field notes and expanded account, it was possible to identify issues that midwife teacher colleagues had highlighted as being important in the selection of student midwives. The issues raised were diverse and included the following: 'communication skills; academic ability; the Board's criteria; past experience; handwriting; age; 'gut' feeling at interview; references; personality; appearance; no 'baby lovers'; the opinion of the midwifery school secretary; rapport; sickness/absence record; and the opinion of other students'. The remarks made in summary at the conclusion of the discussion demonstrated general agreement that there were few concrete criteria upon which to base decisions regarding an applicant's suitability for midwifery. Some aspects in particular were open to subjective appraisal, for example 'personality', 'appearance' or 'rapport'. Individual teachers agreed that in the final analysis they relied heavily on 'gut' feelings when deciding whether to select or reject an applicant for a place on a midwifery course.

The discussion during the plenary session reiterated the ideas of the group, particularly the notion of intuition and 'gut' reaction. The view was expressed that midwifery needed to address some key questions, similar to those posed by Ray (1979) in relation to health visiting.What makes a good midwife? Who sets the criteria? What criteria does one choose in order to predict success? How can the 'correct' personality be measured?

The second stage of the preliminary design work involved visiting two schools of midwifery in order to observe the selection procedures and glean information from staff by observation and informal dialogue as opportunities arose. The two schools were located in different health authorities and their policies and procedures regarding selection of midwifery students were unknown to me. This was a key factor in choosing schools, together with ease of access.

Field and Morse (1985) describe how informal contacts can be valuable when obtaining information regarding access to an organization or institution. In this case, the senior midwife teacher was both the informal contact and what Lofland and Lofland (1984) have called the prime gatekeeper. Lofland and Lofland (1984) advise the use of 'connections' such as these to facilitate access for research. Although the policies and organizations of these two schools were unfamiliar, I had met the two senior midwife teachers on several occasions previously. Therefore it was possible to approach them directly on informal, first-name terms and to use formal gatekeepers as if they were informal sponsors, thus minimizing the difficulties sometimes encountered in negotiating access (Hammersley and Atkinson, 1983). There was no difficulty in obtaining permission to visit and observe selection procedures for student midwives in either school.

The same format for data collection was used in each school. Informal discussions relating to selection of midwifery recruits were held with available teachers and, in one instance, a clinical manager. Having already identified several issues that appeared important to midwife teachers regarding 'selection' during the first stage of the design work, these issues were introduced to respondents and their responses noted. The processes through which applicants passed in order to gain selection, including the selection interviews themselves, were then observed and recorded for each school. Unobtrusive field notes were taken throughout the observation period and methodically recorded as advocated by Robertson and Boyle (1984). Though conscious of the simple, unsophisticated nature of the information gathering, an 'expanded account' (Spradley, 1980, p. 70) was made from the field notes at the conclusion of each visit.

Spradley (1979, p. 103) describes the steps in a 'preliminary domain search' and, using his meticulous format of analysis as a guide, it was possible to highlight both formal and informal criteria which seemed to be important in these two particular midwifery schools. There were many similarities between them in the criteria identified, e.g. 'academic ability' and 'personality'. At both schools staff also indicated that they accepted candidates unless a definite reason to reject was evident, rather than accepting only those they believed would be ideal. There were also some areas over which the schools differed, for example the personnel who were responsible for shortlisting applicants; 'the school secretary's reaction to the candidate' was noted in one school only and 'preference for teaching/learning methods' was considered in the other.

The questionnaire

Having now identified a range of numerous issues relevant to selection of student midwives, the next stage was to design a questionnaire in which these were reflected.

De Vaus (1986, p.70) describes four preliminary considerations in the design of a questionnaire, namely: identifying the important issues involved in the study; the way in which these issues may be explored in the questionnaire; intuition concerning links and relationships between variables; and the way in which the questionnaire is to be administered. Analysis of the resultant data is another vital preliminary consideration prior to construction of a questionnaire. Paying due regard to all these considerations, it was then necessary to identify precisely which issues were the most important to include (Selltiz, Wrightman and Cook, 1965), the format of each question (Sweeney and Olivieri, 1981), the wording of each question (Hughes, 1976), question sequence (Oppenheim, 1966) and the total layout and appearance of the proposed questionnaire (Adams and Schvaneveldt, 1985).

In the course of the preliminary design work, some 35 issues were identified as being relevant to selection of student midwives in one or more schools of midwifery. Clearly it was not feasible to address each of these areas, while at the same time creating a questionnaire of acceptable length. The researcher is strongly advised to avoid the temptation of including any question or topic of only vague interest, in the greater cause of brevity, relevance and ultimately an improved response rate (e.g. Youngman, 1979). The initial fieldwork indicated that the process by which potential midwifery recruits were selected varied between schools. The data were therefore categorized (Selltiz, Wrightman and Cook, 1965) in order to identify themes that could then be translated into questionnaire items. The frequency with which a particular issue (e.g. 'academic background') appeared in the preliminary data influenced the extent to which it was included in the final draft questionnaire.

In deciding the format of questions, consideration had to be given to ease of completion for respondents who had busy work schedules, the proposed coding and analysis of the responses, the nature of the information required and the desire to interest and motivate respondents to complete the questionnaire. The advantages and disadvantages of closed and open-ended questions, which are well documented (Oppenheim, 1966; Cannell and Kahn, 1968; Hughes, 1976; Selltiz, Wrightman and Cook, 1976; Smith, 1981) were also important considerations in determining the format of questions. Smith (1981) indicates that it is usual for a questionnaire to contain various formats of both closed and open-ended questions. The questionnaire was designed, therefore, with a predominance of closed questions, using a limited range of formats for ease of answering and subsequent analysis, with some open-ended questions to allow respondents the freedom to reply in the manner described by Oppenheim (1966, p. 41). The closed questions also required careful consideration to ensure that the response options given were mutually exclusive and enabled respondents to give an unbiased answer that accurately reflected their true opinion.

From the first draft of the questionnaire it became obvious that despite initial focusing and identification of themes, it was too lengthy and in some instances more than one question was used to elicit the same information. Applying Selltiz, Wrightman and Cook's questions 'Is this question necessary? Just how will it be useful?' was a salutary lesson and enabled the questionnaire to be condensed considerably without apparent loss of information (Selltiz, Wrightman and Cook, 1976, p. 552).

The sample

I wished to describe as comprehensively as possible the selection of student midwives in England and Wales. I was particularly interested in the less tangible elements that individual senior midwife teachers felt were important to identify in applicants for midwifery, in addition to the pragmatics of the selection procedure. The sample thus identified for the purpose of the survey was in fact a total population sample of all of the 153 senior midwife teachers in England and Wales in 1988. Each of these teachers was responsible for a midwifery school approved by the relevant National Board for Nursing, Midwifery and Health Visiting, to conduct an 18-month course in midwifery for those on Part 1 of the UKCC Professional Register.

The decision to survey the total population, rather than a sample, was made after careful consideration of various practical issues identified by Rogers (1988): for example, resources available and ease of contact of all the proposed participants; the need to minimize bias that might arise with sampling error (Williamson, 1981) and sample size (Cohen and Manion, 1985).

The total population sample of 153 senior midwife teachers in separate schools of midwifery was current at the time of the survey. The questionnaire was distributed to each senior midwife teacher in July 1988. If this study were to be replicated today then the number of teachers would be smaller, given the current climate of amalgamation and merger of 'schools' of midwifery with each other and with schools of nursing and other health-related occupations to form colleges or institutes, together with the various stages of merger and links with higher education. Although the target population for such a study might well have to be reconsidered in view of these changes, the issues to be explored would, nonetheless, be very similar.

Ethical considerations

Ethical considerations in this research centred, in particular, on informed consent and confidentiality. In relation to observation of the peer discussion group, verbal consent for notes to be taken was granted from group members.

Access to the two midwifery schools was gained through personal contact with each senior midwife teacher as previously described. Teachers within each of the schools were made aware of the purposes of my visit by their senior midwife teacher and the welcome given in each demonstrated their consent and willingness to be of assistance. When meeting them personally, it was again stressed that neither they nor the midwifery school would be identified in the final report (Field and Morse, 1985). It was also vital that prospective students presenting for selection were not disadvantaged by the presence of an observer. In each school, therefore, the teacher responsible for the selection process spoke to each applicant when they arrived and requested their permission for me to observe the interview. The explanation given to them was that the purpose was to record the manner of selection in that particular school and not to observe or judge them personally. Consent was readily given in each case, but I was conscious of a 'captive audience' (Treece and Treece, 1986). Applicants for a place on the course would be anxious to please and make a good impression of themselves. They may, therefore, have felt that a refusal of my presence would have prejudiced their chances of selection. To minimize any disadvantage to candidates created by my presence and note-taking during their interview, I sat out of view and took no part in the proceedings.

Regarding the questionnaires, it was desirable that those which were not returned could be identified so that reminder letters to maximize the response rate could be sent only to those senior midwife teachers who had not responded (Brook, 1978). This meant numbering each questionnaire and assigning a corresponding number to each respondent, hence anonymity could not be promised. Accordingly, respect of confidentiality was stressed in the covering letter accompanying each questionnaire and an assurance given that no individual or school of midwifery would be identified in the findings.

Pilot study

Many of the difficulties associated with survey research using a postal questionnaire as the tool for data collection can be identified in the course of a pilot study and hence minimized in the full study (Moser and Kalton, 1979). Selltiz, Wrightman and Cook (1976) stress the importance of ensuring that the sample population and conditions used in the pilot are aligned as closely as possible to the participants in the full study. However, as the proposed full-scale research was targeted at a total population sample of senior midwife teachers, it was not possible to use senior midwife teachers in the pilot group. The questionnaire was tested therefore with a small number of midwife teachers who were chosen in respect of their long experience of midwifery education, akin to that of a senior midwife teacher.

All the factors listed by Moser and Kalton (1979) in relation to the questionnaire were tested by the pilot study; these included the layout, ease and correctness of completion, clarity of the instructions and the question wording, and interpretation of the questions. The pilot study highlighted some important areas in the questionnaire that required amendment; for example, there were areas of redundancy with more than one question seeking the same information. This repetition was easily identified by respondents in the pilot study. There did not appear to be any difficulty with the instructions given nor in interpretation of the questions. The initial length of the questionnaire was of some concern so this was an important aspect to test. Respondents taking part in the pilot study were asked to record their commencement and completion times, in order to gauge the length of time required to complete the questionnaire and hence the commitment being asked of busy personnel. Most of the midwife teachers who tested the questionnaire found that they required from one to one and a half hours for its completion, but stated that they did not notice the time factor while absorbed in this task. This was taken as an encouraging sign!

With some amendments and reduction in length, the final version was printed and distributed.

Response rate

The response rate in surveys has important implications for the validity of findings. Mailed questionnaires are often assumed to have a notoriously low rate of return (Williamson, 1981). Brook (1978) argues that this need not necessarily be so, commenting that the covering letter, the interest created by the questionnaire and particularly the reminder letter to follow up non-returned questionnaires can all contribute towards a healthy response rate. In this study, the initial response of 88% (134/153) showed that these measures had been effective, but is also a testament to the interest and generosity of the respondents in taking time to complete a relatively time-consuming questionnaire. Only one reminder letter was thought to be warranted in view of the initial high response rate. A response rate of 95% (145/153) was ultimately achieved.

Coding and analysis

Preliminary coding of the question responses was undertaken, using the completed pilot questionnaires to assist in determining categories for the open-ended questions.The preliminary coding categories which had been determined from the pilot questionnaires were tested for range and grouping of responses against 20 questionnaires returned from the full study in the manner described by Walker (1978, p. 159), albeit on a much smaller scale. Some additions to the categories in the open-response questions were made following this exercise, prior to the determination of the final coding frame.

FINDINGS

The findings of this survey demonstrated that while the methods of selection appeared to be fairly uniform across the majority of midwifery schools, the criteria believed to be important in applicants for midwifery varied, as did the rationale for such criteria. In this chapter only the key findings from the study are presented, together with discussion of their implications. A full account of the study is available elsewhere (Phillips, 1989).

Criteria: what are we looking for?

General attributes

Respondents were asked to indicate, from a given range of options, the qualities/attributes they believed to be of value in a student entering a midwifery course. By far the most popular attribute indicated was 'an ability to express an opinion verbally', with 92% (134) agreeing that this was important. This was followed by 'an interest in current affairs', 72% (104). 'Assertiveness' was also a popular attribute, perhaps surprisingly so given the fairly traditional nature of midwifery education up to the time of the study. Sixty-one per cent (89) of respondents cited assertiveness to be a valuable quality in a student entering midwifery, thus reflecting a welcome trend towards a more andro-gogical approach to education in midwifery.

The notion of choosing applicants who will not 'rock the boat' is fascinating. Forty per cent (58) of senior midwife teachers stated that 'fitting in' with the clinical midwifery staff was a quality/attribute they believed to be valuable in a prospective student midwife, while 25% (36) felt that this was important in relation to the midwifery teaching staff. Although the type of personality envisaged is not described and is therefore open to conjecture and individual interpretation, midwifery has a long history of a conformist image and it would appear that some would prefer to keep it that way.

Communication skills The responses to several items throughout the questionnaire indicated that nearly all senior midwife teachers looked for evidence of skills in communication in applicants for midwifery.

Motivation/commitment/knowledge of midwifery Being widely read regarding midwifery and having an understanding of the prospective course indicated to 34% (50) of senior midwife teachers that an applicant 'demonstrated commitment' to midwifery and this was seen to be an important attribute. Indeed, poor knowledge of midwifery and, by implication, poor motivation was cited by 49% (71) respondents as a factor that would lead them to doubt the suitability of the applicant for the course. Despite this, only 22% (32) would not accept a prospective midwifery student who had little knowledge of the sphere of practice of a midwife.

Academic background It is of interest to observe that when given the opportunity to choose the ideal academic background of a prospective midwife, 30% (44) of senior midwife teachers were satisfied with the minimum requirements, while a further 8% (12) had no preference. Other respondents, however, described a wide variety of academic achievement and experience as desirable; for example, 'one or more "A" levels' (26), 'evidence of ongoing learning' (21), 'a degree' (16), and 'RGN qualification at the first attempt' (12).

In response to a separate question, however, only 41 of the respondents who desired an academic background from applicants beyond just registration as a nurse indicated that in reality they would aim to select applicants with a higher and/or broader academic basis.

At the time of this study it seemed, therefore, that the majority of midwifery schools did not state particular academic entry criteria beyond the statutory minimum. However, it may be an advantage for potential student midwives applying to some schools to have a broader academic background than those stipulated by statutory requirements.

Health   Nearly all senior midwife teachers stated that there were factors relating to an applicant's health record that they considered as relevant to their decision to select an applicant for a career in midwifery. Specific conditions/illnesses, for example epilepsy and deafness, echoed the National Board guidelines, while others listed included dermatitis and back problems. The most commonly cited aspect of an applicant's health record that would cause concern to respondents, however, was an unexplained history of frequent short periods of sick leave; this, in particular, would militate against an applicant's chance of selection, despite a health clearance from the Occupational Health Department.

Past work experience   The most commonly cited desired work experience prior to entering a midwifery course was a period of six months or longer working as a staff nurse – 33% (48). This raises interesting implications regarding the difficulties that may occur when adapting to midwifery practice after prior socialization as a nurse. Davies (1988 and Chapter 5 in this volume) identified role conflicts experienced by student midwives during the initial days of their midwifery course that were associated with their prior socialization into a nursing role. This, in turn, may have implications for subsequent attrition from midwifery practice, if the adaptation from an illness to a health model of care and the associated change in the role of the practitioner is difficult or impossible to make. Indeed, this study also showed that in the experience of 25% (36) of senior midwife teachers the most common problem encountered by student midwives was the change from registered nurse to student midwife, while a further 12% (17) cited the change from an illness to a health model of care to be the most common problem that midwifery students encountered. Golden (1980) found that many midwives returned to nursing because they preferred to nurse ill patients than care for those who were well.

Project 2000 programmes of nurse preparation have a greater emphasis on health than traditional nurse training. It will be interesting, therefore, to observe in due course the socialization and role change required to become a competent midwife of those with a background in nurse education through a Project 2000 programme.

Future intentions   The fact that many applicants for midwifery do not intend to practise as midwives on qualification is well known (Robinson, 1986a). Moreover, as Mander (1987) demonstrated, a midwifery qualification is often used as a means to an end other than midwifery practice. It is perhaps surprising, therefore, that 32% (47) of respondents in this study were prepared to accept an applicant as a student midwife even if the stated long-term goal was health visiting.

'Wishful thinking' may play a part in accepting an applicant as a student midwife in these circumstances, for example:

> I never intended to do midwifery myself ... if I think they would make a good midwife I would train them and hope they would decide to stay.
> (Respondent 117)

It would appear that some senior midwife teachers are prepared to take a chance and that stating a wish to be a health visitor does not necessarily preclude an applicant being offered a midwifery course place if otherwise suitable. Several respondents stated that they believed a midwifery qualification was essential to a career in health visiting.

The local girl   Respondents were asked to say how they would choose between two applicants of similar background and equal potential, when the only difference was their locality of residence. Almost half the senior midwife teachers 44% (64) chose the local applicant, stating the rationale for their choice, as either local policy beyond their control, or that they believed a 'local' applicant provided better potential for subsequent retention in midwifery practice in the sponsoring health authority upon qualification and registration. Costs involved and difficulty with providing residential accommodation were also stated to be influencing factors in the choice. Only 7% (10) of respondents chose the opposite candidate, while the remainder 38% (55) did not have a preference – or perhaps a need for one? In nearly half the midwifery schools, therefore, it appeared that applicants who live locally would have an enhanced chance of selection, provided equality of criteria.

Age   The age of a student commencing an 18-month course in midwifery appeared to be unimportant to the majority of senior midwife teachers. Of the minority particularly preferring younger applicants, 12 respondents stated 21–25 as the ideal age and 7 favoured 26–30 years.

Gender   Midwifery is traditionally a female occupation. Although men have been able to train and practise as midwives on equal terms with women since 1 September 1983, they remain very much in the minority. Eighty-four per cent (122) of respondents stated that there had been no male students in the immediate past three cohorts in their school. An earlier study in 1987 by Lewis found that 82% of midwifery schools in the UK as a whole had not had a male student (Lewis, 1991). Respondents were invited to state if they had a preference for female rather than male applicants and, perhaps surprisingly, half indicated that they did not. This is an interesting observation in relation to an issue that can be emotive and maybe reflected a small change in attitude towards men in midwifery. Forty-four per cent (64) of senior midwife teachers did state a preference for female students; it is assumed, however, that this factor would not necessarily preclude a male applicant from being accepted for a place in these schools.

Appearance Only one-quarter of respondents (37) reported that an applicant's dress would have no bearing on their decision to select. A smart appearance, however, would give a favourable impression of the applicant to 57% (83) senior midwife teachers, with 23% (34) going so far as to indicate that they might be adversely influenced by an applicant's casual appearance.

Definitions of appropriate dress, and what is regarded as casual or fashionable, may be difficult, particularly if there is a generation difference in age between interviewer and interviewee. A slightly unconventional appearance may lead to assumptions being made about aspects of personality (Lee, 1985; Salvage, 1989). Prospective student midwives would therefore be wise to attend for interview in 'smart' rather than casual attire, in order to create a favourable first impression of themselves.

This survey set out to explore the main qualities, attributes and characteristics that senior midwife teachers in England and Wales believe to be important in aspiring student midwives, and hence the criteria they use when making selection decisions. The study also explored the processes used to identify whether applicants met these criteria. In doing so, some of the less obvious attributes that are taken into consideration became apparent.

Processes: methods for determining whether applicants meet the criteria

Letters and application forms The process of selection or rejection of potential student midwives commences with receipt of their initial letter requesting an application form. Fifty-five per cent (80) of respondents had in fact rejected applicants on the basis of the initial letter, since in their perception it indicated limited ability in written communication skills; for example:

> Illegible or very untidy writing (e.g. lots of crossings out, blots, etc.) militate against the applicant.
>
> (Respondent 115)

The application form itself is a vital component of the process of selection since it plays a subtle part in the early introduction and presentation of the prospective student midwife to her selectors. There is, reputedly, a general notion that presenting a completed application form in typescript gives a good impression since it demonstrates motivation and willingness to pay attention to detail. However, 35% (51) of respondents preferred application forms to be completed in the potential student's own handwriting. Some examples of commonly cited reasons for this preference range from interest in the applicant's academic capabilities (although how this was assessed on handwriting as opposed to typescript was not made explicit), to concern regarding the prospective midwife's record-keeping in her future midwifery practice. Some respondents stated that they preferred handwritten application forms to reassure themselves that the form had been completed by the applicant herself and not by a third party. Handwriting was also quoted as giving useful clues to an applicant's personality and ability to communicate.

The majority of senior midwife teachers – 62% (90) – however, had no preference for mode of completion, but accuracy was viewed as important by all. The most important points for aspiring student midwives to note, therefore, is to ensure that their application form is completed legibly and accurately in order to give a good impression of themselves to their selectors.

References Consideration of references is a routine part of the selection process, but it appeared that midwifery schools had interestingly different notions of the usefulness or otherwise of 'outstanding' references and 'poor' references. References were viewed prior to shortlisting an applicant for interview in the majority of schools.

Half (72) of the senior midwife teachers stated that they would be 'guided favourably by outstanding references', but as many as 28% (40) indicated that outstanding references would be taken with 'a pinch of salt'. For these respondents, then, glowing references do not necessarily indicate a glowing applicant!

Regarding poor references, 25% (36) of senior midwife teachers considered these to be sufficient evidence to reject an applicant outright. On the other hand, 13% (19) viewed poor references 'with a pinch of salt'. In these circumstances, the value of obtaining references at all is questionable, if unfavourable references are not considered to be highly significant. The greatest proportion of senior midwife teachers 60% (87) stated that they would seek further information about an applicant with poor references. It would have been useful to identify the nature of such information required and the manner in which that gleaned from the initial two referees failed to meet the requirements of the selectors.

The written exercise There was a fairly even division of opinion between midwifery schools on the use of a short written exercise as part of the selection process. While no respondent cited the 'written exercise' as being the single stage of the selection process to which they attached most importance, 48% (70) indicated that a short written exercise formed part of their process of selection of students. Marginally more senior midwife teachers 52% (75), however, stated that they did not use this technique as a selection tool and questioned its value.

Those who did use a written exercise in their selection procedure described its value as enabling assessment of a candidate's skills in written expression, and assessment of less tangible attributes of the applicant, such as communication skills, attitudes and motivation.

The informal visit Though not part of the selection procedures *per se*, informal visits were encouraged in over half of the midwifery schools. The prime value ascribed to such visits was that it enabled applicants to sample the school and maternity unit in an informal way, in order to make an informed decision regarding their own requirements. Ensuring that prospective students have an opportunity to choose a midwifery school that would suit their individual needs was said to be an important element in reducing subsequent wastage. On the other hand, 30% (43) of senior midwife teachers stated that they did not encourage such informal visits, citing constraints of time, finance and/ or staff resources as prime reasons. The overall impression gained, however, was that even when it was stated that informal visits were not encouraged, arrangements would be made to comply with an applicant's specific request to visit the school prior to interview. Informal visits were seen by most respondents as benefiting the student more directly than the school.

The interview Applicants for places on midwifery courses were always interviewed as an integral part of the selection procedure in 133 of the schools, with a further 8 schools interviewing applicants 'sometimes'. The interview was generally viewed as a key aspect of the process of selection, since it afforded face-to-face interaction and personal assessment of the applicant. While 37% (53) of senior midwife teachers stated that they believed interviews could be used objectively to assess the suitability of applicants for midwifery, a little over half recognized the subjectivity of an interview assessment, but nevertheless believed to be an invaluable tool for selecting midwifery recruits.

Responsibility for shortlisting prospective student midwives for interview varied between midwifery schools. Selection for interview always involved midwife teachers, except in one school alone in which selection for interview for a place was sometimes decided solely by a service colleague. In 57 midwifery schools candidates for interview were always shortlisted by joint consultation between education and midwifery service. In approximately one-third of schools, however, midwifery teachers only selected for interview, with the senior midwife teacher 'always' taking sole responsibility for such decisions in 22 schools.

The prime reason stated for conducting a selection interview was by far 'to confirm suitability/motivation/interest' (73% (106) of respondents). A little over half the schools (76) used a predetermined interview schedule, with a further 35 doing so 'sometimes'. A vast range of topics/areas was covered collectively by the schedules, some of which were discussed explicitly with the applicant, while others were impressions gained by the interviewers of the applicant's personal qualities.

In many midwifery schools it appeared, therefore, that all applicants who were interviewed for that particular school were at least appraised on the same core of topics or areas, although this varied on occasions. Twenty-one per cent (30) of senior midwife teachers, however, indicated that predetermined interview schedules were not used in their school. It could be postulated, therefore, that in midwifery schools where prospective student midwives were interviewed without using an agreed interview schedule, competing applicants may be measured against differing criteria on an *ad hoc* basis, dependent upon the preference or bias of the interviewers, thus confirming why interviews are sometimes criticized as being unreliable selection techniques (Borrill, 1987). Given that the prime reason stated for the selection interview was 'to confirm suitability, motivation and interest', then following the recommendations of Arvey and Campion (1982) it is suggested that a consensus should be determined regarding the core areas and topics that are pertinent to achieving that aim.

In the majority of schools (125) interviews were usually conducted by representatives from both midwifery education and service. In 53 schools the education representative was normally the senior midwife teacher. There were, however, some variations. For example, 17 did not have a representative from midwifery service to interview prospective student midwives and one senior midwife teacher usually interviewed prospective students on her own. The prospective course teacher for the cohort in question was specifically involved in the selection interviews in 15 schools. It was pointed out by some senior midwife teachers that 'availability of personnel' determined who actually conducted the selection interviews.

Borrill (1987) strongly suggests paying attention to recruitment and preselection in order to streamline the selection process. Borrill also recommends determining clear selection criteria and using other techniques as well as the interview in order to improve the reliability and validity of the selection process. Richards, McManus and Maitlis (1988) advocate a panel approach to improve the reliability of the interview as a selection tool. Given that some midwifery schools have well in excess of 100 applications per annum and many others have only a small pool of teachers, the staff resources and time implications of interviewing each applicant by a minimum of two busy senior personnel are important considerations. Borrill's recommendations, in relation to recruitment and pre-selection, are very relevant to future debates by those involved in the selection of student midwives.

Subtle processes It has been shown that those involved in the selection of student midwives in England and Wales used a number of well-established formal processes to determine the characteristics and criteria they were seeking in recruits to midwifery. However, it would also appear that there were some more subtle processes involved in some schools, and that these were used to enhance the total picture of an applicant upon which decisions to select or reject could be taken with relative confidence.

Prior knowledge Knowledge of a potential student midwife gained by the selectors during the applicant's previous maternity care experience during their nurse training may or may not be to the applicant's advantage. There was a fairly even division of opinion regarding the value of knowledge gained in this manner. Forty-one per cent (59) of senior midwife teachers felt this information was not helpful, whereas 47% (68) believed that it was. Perhaps the rationale for both viewpoints is best summed up by one respondent who did not mark either response option but stated:

Not necessarily – if they were good YES!

(Respondent 114)

Applicants who demonstrated high 'interest and aptitude' (respondent 141) for midwifery when student nurses may well maximize their chance of selection if they apply to the same midwifery school in which they gained their maternity care experience and 'if they are remembered personally' (respondent 052).

The secretary Another of the more subtle processes involved in determining the characteristics and attitudes of potential student midwives was by seeking the secretary's opinion of the applicant. Although the secretary did not have direct contact with applicants in one-quarter of the schools and 25% (36) of senior midwife teachers disagreed that the secretary's opinion of an applicant was valuable, there were other respondents who did include their secretary in the selection process. Thirty-six per cent (52) of senior midwife teachers indicated that they sometimes sought the secretary's opinion of an applicant, while an additional 13 always did so.

It is not suggested that student midwives are chosen by the secretary to the midwifery teaching department, nor indeed that she may have a major influence on the selection decision. However, an applicant's presentation, and her/his interaction and communication with the secretary, may play some small part in the ultimate chance of being selected for a place in some of the midwifery schools in England and Wales.

Other student midwives The notion of using current student midwives in the selection of future students is an innovative and potentially controversial one. There were indications that a few midwifery schools used students to assist in gathering information about a prospective recruit, albeit in a casual manner, but occasionally in a structured way.

Two concrete examples were described. In both these schools, students were actively involved in the selection of future students and, in one case, the final decision. The ethics of this innovation would provoke an interesting and lively debate amongst midwife teachers.

Intuition/'gut' feeling The other tacit process that many senior midwife teachers relied upon when making select or reject decisions regarding applicants was 'intuition'. Seventy-eight per cent (113) of respondents stated that they sometimes knew intuitively when an applicant would make a suitable midwife. However, when asked if they were able to describe the basis of their intuition, over half indicated that they were unable to do so, therefore implying that their intuition was a 'gut' feeling about a potential student midwife. Those who did describe the basis of their intuitive feelings about an applicant for midwifery did so on the strengths of their personal experience as midwife teachers and acquired knowledge of people which enabled them to assess an applicant's presentation of her/himself.

Similarly, when asked if they were able to know intuitively when an applicant was unsuitable to become a midwife, 74% (108) of senior midwife teachers felt able to do so on some occasions and an additional 6% (9) 'always'. Again, a minority only were able to describe the basis of their intuitive feelings towards an unsuitable applicant for a midwifery place and did so in terms of the potential student's personality or attitude. Respondents varied, however, in the absolute use they made of their 'gut' feelings about an applicant, with only one-quarter rejecting an applicant 'on instinct'.

No criticism is intended in describing this use of intuition. In the absence of evidence to the contrary, intuition and 'gut' reaction may well have an equally valid part to play in the selection of potential midwives as the formal processes described. Indeed, it has been postulated that intuitive thinking is valuable and those involved in nurse education should therefore appreciate and use such personal judgements based on intuition (Beckman Blomquist, 1985).

'Jumping the queue' At 107 of the 145 midwifery schools applications were received on an *ad hoc* basis and after formal selection suitable recruits were subsequently placed on a waiting list for a course place. This was usually of less than 12 months duration (in 61 midwifery schools), but could be up to two years or longer. In 63 schools it was often possible for applicants to be offered a place on an earlier course than that originally promised. Circumstances whereby this situation arose usually centred around last-minute cancellations of confirmed places by applicants and the ready availability of others to take their place at short notice. This might not be the first person on the waiting list.

Only a minority of senior midwife teachers (14% – 21) indicated that they had insufficient applicants to require a waiting-list facility. Alternatively, respondents from 13 midwifery schools stated that they formally advertised each course at a relevant period in time, prior to the specified course commencement date. Selection therefore was for a designated course only, with no waiting-list provision.

Thus there was a marked difference in supply and demand of applicants for courses and keen applicants may do well to shop around. Given that many applicants who accept a place do not intend to practise as a midwife (Robinson, 1986b), then perhaps selection of students for a specified intake may facilitate the identification of currently suitable and motivated applicants who have greater intentions of practising midwifery on qualification and registration.

DISCUSSION AND RECOMMENDATIONS

A wealth of data regarding the criteria and processes used in the selection of student midwives in England and Wales was obtained in the course of this descriptive study. In this concluding section, the main methodological issues are reviewed and the implications of the findings considered. The importance of careful preparation and planning of the survey in general, and the questionnaire in particular, was discussed in some depth. The various factors to be taken into account in such planning were observed as far as possible in the design of this survey, and a small pilot study was undertaken. Only minor difficulties, associated with a small number of questions, were evident in the full survey. There were some questions in which a minority of respondents found difficulty in restricting themselves to the response options offered and therefore added their own comments. This was valuable additional data to the overall picture.

The length of the questionnaire, and hence the length of time required for its completion, was always of some concern, and was carefully tested in the pilot study. In the full study, a few respondents commented particularly on the length of the questionnaire. However, 145 senior midwife teachers (95%) returned the questionnaire, for the most part completed comprehensively, demonstrating the interest that the subject generated as well as the motivation and commitment of the population.

The open-ended questions, in particular, provided valuable information, but were time consuming to code and analyse. The time and effort spent, however, were well rewarded by the amount and nature of description obtained.

The study demonstrated that while methods used to select aspiring student midwives are relatively informed throughout England and Wales, the criteria believed to be important varied, as did the rationale for their use. The overt methods used in the selection process included scrutiny of the initial letter of application and the application form itself, consideration of references, setting a written exercise and the applicant's self-presentation at interview. More subtle processes of information gathering were also demonstrated; for example, eliciting the secretary's impression of the candidate. The extent to which more covert processes were used, however, varied between different midwifery schools. Factors that appeared to be consistently important in potential midwifery recruits included 'motivation', 'communication skills' and 'commitment to midwifery', although the manner in which these attributes were identified varied. Other criteria desired in applicants for midwifery and the rationale for their inclusion were similarly diverse.

There are many issues arising from this study, which are worthy of consideration by those concerned with student midwife selection, namely:

1. the cost effectiveness of the current methods of selection, which require considerable resources in terms of time and personnel;
2. the subjectivity of desired criteria and attributes of potential midwives, for example 'communication skills', 'attitudes', 'personality';
3. the diversity of criteria which may exist between one midwifery school and another, and between one midwife teacher and her colleagues;
4. the validity of the overt processes used in selection, for example the interview, but particularly the more subtle methods such as intuition and 'gut' reaction;
5. 'What is actually associated with success of particular qualities which we desire in our candidates?' (Edis and Gilligan, 1988, p. 51);
6. the element of choice, which may be minimal for midwifery schools with small numbers of applicants;
7. the element of chance, which may determine an applicant's ultimate selection or rejection for a place on a midwifery course.

This study has described several aspects of the selection of student midwives in England and Wales and raised many more questions than perhaps it has answered. The total picture of selection of students for a midwifery place appears to be a vast information-gathering exercise, followed by a decision based on relatively subjective criteria and processes, the validity of which remain questionable.

Little appears to have changed in the intervening years since this study took place. Land (1993) reviewed the methods of selecting potential students in nurse education and addresses similar issues to those raised in previous literature reviews and papers on 'selection' (Arvey and Campion, 1982; Borrill, 1987). Colleges of midwifery appear to be continuing to use similar techniques for selection of student midwives to those used previously, although at the time of writing there has been no published work in this area. Until midwifery educationalists address the issues raised by this study, it could be argued that selection of future practitioners of midwifery will remain more a matter of chance than choice.

REFERENCES

Adams, G. and Schvaneveldt, J. (1985) *Understanding Research Methods*. Longman, New York.

Akinsanya, J. (1988) Complementary approaches. *Senior Nurse*, **8**(5), 20–2.

Arvey, R. and Campion, J. (1982) The employment interview: a summary and review of recent research. *Personnel Psychology*, **35**(2), 281–322.

Beckman Blomquist, K. (1985) Evaluation of students: intuition is important. *Nurse Educator*, **10**(6), 8–11.

Belbin, R. and Toye, J. (1978) Trainability tests and the recruitment of student nurses. *Journal of Advanced Nursing*, **3**(3), 227–85.

Borrill, C. (1987) The chosen ones. *Nursing Times*, **83**(40), 52–3.

Brook, L. (1978) Postal survey procedures. In Hoinville, G., Jowell, R. and associates, (eds), *Survey Research Practice*. Heinemann Educational, London, Ch. 7, pp. 124–43.

Cannell, C. and Kahn, R. (1968) Interviewing. In Lindzey, G. and Aronson, E. (eds), *The Handbook of Social Psychology: Vol. 2 – Research Methods*. Addison, Wesley, New York.

Cohen, L. and Manion, L. (1985) *Research Methods in Education* (2nd edn). Croom Helm, London.

Davies, R. (1988) 'The happy end of nursing': an ethnographic study of initial encounters in a midwifery school. Unpublished MSc thesis, University College, Cardiff.

Dellar, C. (1981) The selection of students for health visitors training courses. *Journal of Advanced Nursing*, **6**(2), 111–15.

De Vaus, D. (1986) *Surveys in Social Research*. George Allen & Unwin, London.

Edis, M. and Gilligan, H. (1989) Supplements to the interview. *Nursing Times*, **85**(34) 51–3.

Fader, W. (1976) *Qualifying Procedures for Health Visitors*. National Federation for Educational Research, Slough.

Field, P. and Morse, J. (1985) *Nursing Research: The Application of Qualitative Approaches*. Croom Helm, London.

Golden, J. (1980) Midwifery training: the views of newly qualified midwives. *Midwives' Chronicle and Nursing Notes,* **93**(1109), 190–4.

Grahame, C. (1985) Killed by kindness? *Nursing Times*, **81**(26), 52.

Hack, K. (1973) Predictors of success in health visiting. Occasional papers. *Nursing Times*, **69**(14), 57–60.

Hammersley, M. and Atkinson, P. (1983) *Ethnography: Principles in Practice*. Tavistock, London.

Hughes, J. (1976) *Sociological Analysis: Methods of Discovery.* Nelson, Sunbury-on-Thames.

Jarvis, P. and Gibson, S. (1981) An investigation into the validity of specifying 5 'O' levels in the General Certificate of Education as an entry requirement for the education and training of district nurses. *Journal of Advanced Nursing*, **6**(6) 471–82.

Jones, S. (1985) How should we choose? *Nursing Mirror*, **161**(5), 16–17.

Jordan, M. (1987) Safe selection. *Nursing Times*, **83**(43), 40–1.

Lancet (1984) Medical student selection in the UK. **24** 1190–1.

Land, L. (1993) Selecting potential nurses: a review of the methods. *Nurse Education Today*, **13**(1), 30–9.

Lazarus, J. and Van Niekerk, J. (1986) Selecting medical students: a rational approach. *Medical Teacher*, 8(4), 343–57.

Leach, R. (1988) Student nurse selection: an experiential approach. *Nurse Education Today*, 8(6), 359–63.

Lee, D. (1985) A process of elimination. *Nursing Mirror*, 160(7), 42–3.

Lewis, B. (1980) Personality profiles for qualified nurses: possible implications for recruitment and selection of trainee nurses. *International Journal of Nursing Studies*, 17(4), 221–34.

Lewis, P. (1991) Men in midwifery: their experiences as students and as practitioners. In Robinson, S. and Thomson, A.M. (eds), *Midwives, Research and Childbirth*, Vol. 2. Chapman & Hall, London, pp. 271–301.

Lofland, J. and Lofland, L. (1984) *Analyzing Social Settings: A Guide to Qualitative Observation and Analysis* (2nd edn). Wadsworth, Belmont.

Lopez, M. and Radford, N. (1985) District nurse training: a pilot survey of demand, provision and students. *Journal of Advanced Nursing*, 10, 361–7.

Mander, R. (1987) Why choose midwifery? *Nursing Times*, 83(27), 54–6.

McManus, I. and Richards, P. (1984) Audit of admission to medical school. *British Medical Journal*, 289, 1201–4, 1288–90, 1365–7.

Morton-Williams, J. (1978) Unstructured design work. In Hoinville, G. and Jowell, R. and associates (eds) *Survey Research Practice* Heinemann Educational, London, Ch. 2, pp. 9–25.

Moser, C. and Kalton, G. (979) *Survey Methods in Social Investigation* (2nd edn). Heinemann Educational, London.

Oppenheim, A. (1966) *Questionnaire Design and Attitude Measurement*. Heinemann Educational, London.

Phillips, R. (1989) Choice or chance? An exploratory study describing the criteria and processes used to select midwifery students. Unpublished MEd thesis, University College, Cardiff.

Ray, G. (1979) Health visitor selection: a review of the processes influencing the selection of potential students in the United Kingdom. *Journal of Advanced Nursing*, 4(5), 513–29.

Reeve, P. (1978) The selection interview in the assessment of suitability for nurse training. *Journal of Advanced Nursing*, 3, 167–179.

Richards, P., McManus, I. and Maitlis, S. (1988) Reliability of interviewing in medical student selection. *British Medical Journal*, 296, 1520–1.

Robertson, M. and Boyle, J. (1984) Ethnography: contributions to nursing research. *Journal of Advanced Nursing*, 9(1), 43–9.

Robinson, S. (1986a) Career intentions of newly qualified midwives. *Midwifery*, 2(1), 25–36.

Robinson, S. (1986b) The 18-month training: what difference has it made? *Midwives Chronicle*, 99(1177), 22–8.

Royal College of Midwives (1985) Evidence to the Review body for Nursing Staff, Midwives, Health Visitors and Professions Allied to Medicine. *MIDIRS Information Pack No. 1*. MIDIRS, Bristol.

Salvage, J. (1989) The select few. *Nursing Times*, 85(2), 24.

Selltiz, C., Wrightman, L. and Cook, S. (1965) *Research Methods in Social Relations*. Methuen, London.

Selltiz, C., Wrightman, L. and Cook, S. (1976) *Research Methods in Social Relations* (3rd edn). Holt, Rinehart & Winston, New York.

Smith, H. (1981) *Strategies of Social Research* (2nd edn). Prentice Hall, Englewood Cliffs, NJ.

Spradley, J. (1979) *The Ethnographic Interview.* Holt, Rinehart & Winston, New York.

Spradley, J. (1980) *Participant Observation.* Holt, Rinehart & Winston. New York.

Sweeney, M. and Olivieri, P. (1981) *An Introduction to Nursing Research.* Lippincott, Philadelphia.

Treece, E. and Treece, J. (1986) *Elements of Research in Nursing* (4th edn). Mosby, St Louis.

United Kingdom Central Council for Nursing, Midwifery and Health Visiting (1991) *Midwives Rules.* UKCC. London.

Walker, D. (1978) Data preparation. In Hoinville, G. Jowell, R. and associates (1978) *Research Practice.* Heinemann Educational, London, pp. 144–63.

White, R. (1985) Educational entry requirements for nurse registration: an historical perspective. *Journal of Advanced Nursing*, **10**(6), 583–90.

Williamson, Y. (1981) *Research Methodology and its Application to Nursing.* Wiley, New York.

Youngman, M. (1979) *Analysing Social and Educational Research Data.* McGraw-Hill, London.

CHAPTER FIVE

'Practitioners in their own right': an ethnographic study of the perceptions of student midwives

Ruth M. Davies

This chapter is concerned with a study of the perceptions of student midwives during their initial encounters in a school of midwifery. Each of the students in the study had qualified as a nurse prior to entry into another distinctive occupation – that of midwifery. The research arose from a personal belief that there are fundamental differences in the two allied occupations of midwifery and nursing, and a desire to understand the complexities surrounding the socialization of midwives who begin their preparation for midwifery as registered nurses. These students, entering midwifery courses with a sickness orientation, are required to undergo a fairly rapid metamorphosis in order to become competent health-orientated midwives.

The idea for a study of this process was conceived while I was working as a senior midwife teacher. At that time I also wished to pursue the opportunity to develop a curriculum for pre-registration midwifery. I could, however, find no research evidence to show the advantages of a three-year programme for initial registration as a midwife compared with the 18-month course available for those already registered as nurses. These two interests culminated in the research described in this chapter. The study was undertaken in my own time, while newly employed as the Professional Officer (midwifery) at the Welsh National Board for Nursing, Midwifery and Health Visiting, and was submitted as a dissertation in partial fulfilment of the requirements for the award of MSc (Econ) at the University of Wales (Davies, 1988).

The research method chosen was an ethnographic study of one set of students during the first part of their course. The findings provided insights into the 'folk' culture which unfolded during the first 18 weeks of status passage from nurse to midwife, and show how this new social position created anxieties for the students as their concepts of their routinized world of nursing were challenged.

The first section provides a discussion of the differences between the occupations of midwifery and nursing as a contextual background for the study. The reason for adopting an ethnographic approach is described, and the processes through which the novice ethnographer passes are discussed in some detail.A selection of findings, relating to one of the major themes to emerge from the study, is then presented.

MIDWIFERY AND NURSING: PROFESSIONS WITH A DIFFERENCE?

From my involvement in midwifery education I have always been convinced that major change is required of a nurse early on in her midwifery course if knowledge and skills appropriate to midwifery are to be demonstrated following registration as a midwife. Nurses entering midwifery courses are required to reappraise their attitudes and beliefs regarding the health status of a different 'consumer' group. My belief that there are fundamental differences between midwifery and nursing is the view proclaimed by most practising midwives, some nurses and certain members of the lay public (Rankin, 1980; Boyd and Sellers, 1982; Towler and Bramwell, 1986). Rankin (1980) asserts that nurses are motivated by the challenge of the ill patient. She suggests that such a challenge does not exist in midwifery and states that 'nurses must overcome this hurdle before rising to the very different challenge of midwifery'.

Health, as defined by the World Health Organization, is 'a state of complete physical, psychological and social well-being and not merely the absence of disease or infirmity' (WHO, 1948). The realization of all that this health status implies, in the form of self-reliance, self-discipline, self-determination and accountability for one's actions and decisions, must impinge upon the 'would-be' midwife in a way which determines her attitude towards relatively healthy pregnant women. The skill of a midwife may be measured by the degree of sensitivity with which she meets individual needs as determined by consumers. There is an adjustment to be made in her behaviour when dealing with women who may not require, or want, her nursing skills.

The midwife's role, particularly in many of the sociopsychological aspects of childbearing, is complementary to that of the doctor. In the areas of clinical/technical skills, however, there is often overlap of roles between the two professions (Central Midwives Board, 1983); the extent to which this is the case has been demonstrated in research from the mid-1970s onwards (e.g. Walker, 1976; Robinson, Golden and Bradley, 1983; Robinson, 1985; Garcia and Garforth, 1991; Green, Kitzinger and Coupland, 1994; Robinson and Owen, 1994). Midwifery has similarities with the 'preventive health' aspects of many occupational groups, for example health visitors and social workers. It encompasses those aspects of the nurse's role that require resuscitation in circumstances in which pathological conditions such as haemorrhage or eclampsia develop in pregnancy, during labour or following delivery. The limited prescribing rights of the midwife can be equated with aspects of medical practice, along with her essential skill in diagnosis of disease onset in childbearing women and newborn babies.

It is during illness or disability that the skills of a nurse are generally sought by the public. In comparison, the majority of pregnant women in the UK require a midwife only to monitor progress, provide reassurance and appropriate information and assist the family through that which is often seen as the climax of the process – the labour and delivery of the baby. Finally, and most often quoted by midwives as an essential difference between themselves and nurses, is that on registration the qualified midwife becomes a practitioner of normal midwifery, entitled to practise in the National Health Service, or in the private sector, or to be self-employed as an independent practitioner. In the case of the latter, no such legal 'right' exists in the field of nursing.

White (1987) postulates that 'nursing recruits have been processed and socialized by general (sickness) nurses training and have been imbued with a way of thinking, values and attitudes to which all student nurses are subjected' (White, 1987). Whether these values and attitudes are entirely modified or simply reinforced within a midwifery school remains to be demonstrated in subsequent research, which falls outside the scope of this chapter. It remains for the reader to judge the extent to which either may be true of the initial socializing processes investigated in this study.

In a survey of newly qualified midwives' view of their training, Golden (1980) provided evidence that some nurses do not enjoy midwifery, preferring to look after sick people, whom they perceive 'really need them'. Golden suggested that this 'noticeable' comparison between nursing and midwifery was associated with the view that midwifery training might be more beneficial if undertaken without a previous nurse training that has concentrated upon the care of the sick. A report published in 1986 by the United Kingdom Central Council for Nursing, Midwifery and Health Visiting indicated these role differences:

The role of the midwife can be said to be substantially different from that of the nurse in that a midwife potentially has a greater professional independence as the level of decision making is of a different order. The midwife is expected to have diagnostic skills relating to both mother and baby that are at one level similar to the obstetrician and indeed there is an overlap of skills between the two. Midwives also have a limited responsibility to prescribe certain scheduled drugs and the right to referral and discharge from hospital within limitations. All this together with a need for manual dexterity and to develop the confidence to function in this way, point to a potentially special and different preparation for midwifery. We are also aware there is considerable support for direct entry into midwifery.

(United Kingdom Central Council, 1986a, 6.33)

Since the early 1980s the view that the differences between nursing and midwifery necessitate separate educational provision has gained momentum (Radford and Thompson, 1994). It is these differences between nursing and midwifery that provided the framework within which this study was designed.

METHODS

Choice of research design

The aims of the study were to examine the differences and similarities between nursing and midwifery through the eyes of a set of student midwives, and to understand ways in which they attempted to 'make sense' of their new world. A qualitative approach, using the ethnographic tradition, was chosen as the most appropriate method to understand these phenomena. Ethnography is concerned with understanding cultural perspectives; its aims are thus to identify participants' understanding of the situation, their assumptions, values, beliefs and intentions and the way that these influence the actions within the setting. Ethnographers employ a range of qualitative techniques, in particular observational methods in national settings (Hedges and Ritchie, 1987).

The study began with a short period of participant observation in a school of midwifery within a district general hospital in the UK. The focus of the study was a set of nine student midwives in the first 18 weeks of their course. In addition to fieldwork observation, data were gathered by means of solicited and unsolicited accounts of events using ethnographic interviews with each of the students concerned. Their personal written accounts of daily events within clinical settings, in the form of diaries, constituted additional data. The senior midwife teacher made available the students' biographical details and handouts of learning materials were also provided. Data from all these sources were drawn on in constructing the student's experiences and responses – a process of 'triangulation' of complementary data sources (Denzin, 1978; Fielding and Fielding, 1986).

A review of the literature revealed a paucity of ethnographic research into the education of student midwives upon which I could draw in the design of this study. As shown in Chapter 7 of this volume midwifery education generally has received much less research attention than midwifery practice, and that which has been undertaken has tended to use quantitative rather than qualitative methods. The only study using fieldwork methods found in the literature at the time the research was being planned was that undertaken by Reid (1986) of the apprenticeship of lay midwives in America, for which an interactionist approach was adopted. There are, however, few if any similarities between midwifery education in Britain, which is strictly regularized, and the apprenticeship system of lay midwifery observed by Reid. Lay midwifery is also considered illegal in the USA. Reid observes:

> Precisely what is being taught at the bedside and how a student midwife develops her art is seldom the focus of research and investigation.
>
> (Reid, 1986, p. 127)

She notes, however, that the student midwife does gradually develop her clinical acumen to the extent that she can practise without supervision. Given this dearth of relevant data the study drew on ethnographic research in the field of nursing and health visiting education (Olesen and Whittaker, 1968; Dingwall, 1977; Melia, 1987) and of medical education (Becker et al., 1961; Atkinson, 1981a).

The research tradition

The approach adopted for the study drew upon the tradition of Weber and others in which the social sciences are held to be distinct from the natural sciences, and therefore require different research strategies. The subjective aspect of human motivation is held to be of considerable importance; hence steps were taken to analyse the students' 'actions', to explore their language in order to gain knowledge of their conceptual frameworks and describe their perceptions of 'reality'. My intention therefore was to enter the students' world of purpose, meaning and beliefs in the Weberian tradition of *verstehen*.

In Parson's translation of Weber's work the following extract explains this interpretative tradition more clearly:

> a system of sociological categories couched in terms of the subjective point of view, that is of the meaning of persons, things, ideas, normative patterns and motives from the point of view of the persons whose action is being studied.
>
> (Weber, trans. Henderson and Parsons, 1947, p. 8, cited by Melia, 1987)

More specifically, the research was located within the interactionist tradition whereby occupational socialization is seen as the situational adaptation to organizational and professional demands and it drew upon these symbolic interactionist approach in particular (Rose, 1962). Students' active construction of their identities and understandings was stressed, and the symbolic interactionist approach showed how student midwives in maternity wards actively constructed and reconstructed their world, based upon their interpretations of events and the meanings they attributed to their environment. The concern in this study has been with locating the processes by which the informants made sense of their world. It called for rigorous analysis of their definitions of the situation using the same approach to that used, for example, by Melia (1987) in a study of students' experiences of becoming nurses and by Atkinson (1981) in a study of medical students.

Olesen and Whittaker (1968) describe their version of the symbolic interactionist approach as:

> a position that permits analysis of the students' existential encounters in which the students defined, chose, and acted on their choices.
>
> (Olesen and Whittaker, 1968, p. 15)

This approach, then, called for intensive fieldwork in which the actors' everyday actions and perspectives were explored. It emphasized the situational aspects of socialization. Such a perspective inevitably created a wide range of interpretations and meanings that could be imputed to the behaviours observed. These in turn, however, could simply serve to show how the differences, in this case of the midwife from the nurse, could be contingent upon the specific circumstances of the social situation under investigation (Cuff and Payne, 1979). As noted earlier, a disproportionate emphasis on quantitative research methodologies still exists in nursing and midwifery research (Duffy, 1985). Although these lay claim to objectivity they often ignore the interviewer as a source of influence. Yet it is an 'existential fact that the researcher is part of the social world being studied and one should recognize it and be constantly reminded of it' (Hammersley and Atkinson, 1983). I determined therefore that I would need to master this notion of reflexivity, in order to study student midwives' accounts of their initial training, while at the same time their reactivity to me, the researcher, would also be a valuable source of data. As Melia (1982) puts it:

> By the very nature of the (qualitative) method the researcher and the data are inextricably bound up.
>
> (Melia, 1982, p. 329)

A range of techniques typically used in ethnographic research became possible during the fieldwork; these included observation, interview, analysis of diaries kept by respondents and of other documents. An eclectic approach was adopted in an attempt to gather the 'richest data possible' (Lofland, 1971). Before discussing these in detail, the process of gaining access to the research site is described.

Gaining access to Oldville

The study was undertaken at Oldville School of Midwifery and could be described as opportunistic, since it was with relative ease that I was able to gain access to the social setting in my capacity as a professional officer. I was able to use people with authority to grant me access, described by Lofland and Lofland (1984) as formal gatekeepers, as if they were informal sponsors. This ensured that the potentially problematic negotiation of access to the chosen school was completed in a short time and with few difficulties.

The senior midwife teacher was first approached during one of our relatively frequent meetings in relation to official school business. My research was briefly mentioned in an attempt to assess her response. She showed interest and, although guarded at first, agreed that in view of the good rapport which extended between us Oldville could be studied. I stressed from the start that anonymity of the informants would be observed. Confidentiality was also emphasized.

My formal request to undertake the research was addressed to the chief administrative nursing officer, who transferred the request for access to a key person of whom I had no previous knowledge. This newly appointed research nurse requested further information as to the detail of the proposed study. I perceived a reluctance to accept that little detail of the study could be provided at this early stage – a recurrent problem in negotiations to undertake ethnographic research, as I have since discovered. She seemed disconcerted by the fact that I could not show her a questionnaire nor indicate the sample size in advance. I did offer to visit her to explain the method I had chosen but my offer was not taken up.

The ethical implications of the study were considered and discussed with another key person within the nursing hierarchy who was enlisted from within the informal social network. No further communication was received from the research nurse but permission was given by the director of nursing services.

As no direct contact or observation of patients was intended during the study those whom I approached felt it was not necessary to apply to the District Ethics Committee for permission to carry out the research. It seemed that the teaching team may have been influenced by the prime 'gate-keeper', who showed interest in the chosen method, which was one of which they had little prior knowledge. The non-judgemental attitude to be adopted by the researcher was especially emphasized, as was the decision to specifically observe student encounters rather than teachers. I was conscious of Spradley's (1979) warning that ethnographic research represents a powerful tool for invading other people's way of life.

Negotiation of access continued even when I was in the field, as each informant was approached and each lecturer introduced by Mrs R, the main 'gatekeeper'. It was interesting that one member of the teaching team, absent during the researcher's initial explanations of the research design, was the only one unwilling to permit observation of her teaching sessions. For my benefit she was therefore 'excused' from any classroom teaching commitment during the students' initial week of study.

The pilot study

In an attempt to test my own ability to make strange those things that were to some degree familiar, I undertook a 'pilot' observation in the study school. Permission for this was given by the senior teacher and, taking along my research supervisor, I began a short period of participant observation, as well as informal opportunistic interviews with one group of student midwives attending a study day. A different group of students became my informants during the later study. I tape recorded the lectures during that day in order to judge student reactivity to its use and my ability to operate it in an unobtrusive fashion. This introduction to 'doing research' proved an enlightening and sobering experience, particularly when I compared my field notes with those of my expert companion. I wrote up these field notes into an expanded account later that day. The amount of data generated from the transcribed tapes, together with my jottings of observed phenomena, gave me insight into the necessity for a thoroughly systematic organization of data, filing and coding of what appeared to be vast quantities of data, even at this stage.

Some time later I began the longer period of concentrated fieldwork in which the specific focus was upon the early days of the course. It is that early period which Beynon and others suggest is crucial in the forming of students' perspectives:

> Initial encounters are a complex process of semiosis, with teachers and pupils as highly skilled coders and encoders of messages through signs by means of which status, allegiances, activities, rules demands and rejections are signalled and interpreted.
>
> (Beynon, 1985, p. 226)

In the field

My first day in the field with the students who were to become my informants in the major part of the study was for them the first day of their course. I had been careful to choose something relatively unobtrusive from my wardrobe of formal and informal clothing. A simple blouse and skirt and warm sweater seemed to me to be most appropriate for 'fitting in' with the students and not the 'uniform' associated with the 'establishment' (I normally wore a smart suit and blouse when visiting as a professional officer).

I carried only a small shorthand notebook, which fitted easily into my large cloth handbag, as did the tape recorder. The teachers had been most accommodating and had fitted up an extension lead from the back of the classroom in order that I could use the equipment quietly and easily from my seat at the end of the semi-circle of desk chairs. I kept a detailed record of my activities, also in a fieldwork journal or 'diary', which I then used in an attempt to capture the part I played in the social world being studied. Each entry was dated so that I could recapture the doubts, fears and personal biases and my mistakes. I later returned home to analyse and code these data as soon as possible.

I had chosen to introduce myself by using my first name. I explained briefly that I had been a nurse and a midwife but was currently following a course at the university. There were nods of interest as I explained that my aim was to learn from them what it was like to be a student midwife at Oldville Hospital in 1987. With their agreement I was therefore joining them as a fellow student for their first week of classroom-based instruction. I mentioned that I had been given permission to use a tape recorder for the lectures but would refrain from using it if they so wished. I saw no sign of dissent. I asked them if they would also allow me to learn their views on certain aspects of midwifery, by means of informal interviews. I was also allowed to tape record these to facilitate ease of conversation and accuracy.

At this early stage, the students' possible reaction to discovering the full professional identity of their researcher 'friend' was held to be an important factor that might inhibit rapport. This degree of detail was therefore simply omitted from the introductions. I learned much later that in any event it would have had no significance for them had they been told I was a 'Board Officer'. However, the qualified staff painted this picture of my officialdom as soon as the students entered the wards. Nevertheless, my early participation in the students' world allowed me to be included, *inter alia*, in the boring introductory form-filling and in that which seemed to me to be the more fascinating activity, of collecting throat swabs during the first morning of the course.

An extract from the field journal reassured me that I was beginning to grasp the notion of 'making the familiar strange':

First day 2nd March 1987
Mrs Grey having introduced herself to the assembled class starts to explain: 'horrible things, these throat and nasal swabs that have to be done. There's a toilet opposite' (she does not say why she has mentioned that). She instructs us how to fill in the 'path forms' providing detail on the blackboard: 'name in full; commenced training; today's date; you're obviously females, so sex – we won't have any trouble with that' – slight titter – 'I'll tell you your hospital number in a minute'. She continues to write on the board and students copy as

instructed and in silence. She continues, 'Culture and sensitivity – it's a bit of an insult really, you know that, it's routine. I'll collect them and check them.'

Now I feel irritated but the students seem compliant and unconcerned. Students leave the room in ones and twos and enter the door opposite which can be seen from the classroom. I need to ask them why they do so and not make assumptions. Later one student offers the explanation: 'It's easier to take the swabs using a mirror'. I remembered this swab ritual from my past experience and am surprised to know it is still in use. Trying to see things as a sociologist and not as a midwifery teacher, I ask Mrs R. why they are taken. I must not allow my considerable 'translation competence' to cloud my observations, my ability to 'see' with fresh eyes.

In total I was a participant observer for 32 hours during the first week of the course, accompanying the students during coffee and lunch breaks as well as visits to the library and during classroom and clinical teaching sessions. I participated in the learning environment to the degree described by Burgess (1984) as an 'involved observer'. An example from my fieldwork journal demonstrates the notion of 'involvement' as participant observer. Blodwen, being the most chatty student in the group at the outset, sat next to me on the first morning of the course and responded with enthusiasm to all the activities, chattering away about the form-filling and asking questions in her apparent anxiety to 'do well'.

Hello, I'm Blod. I'll sit next to you, OK?

I was continually treated as a fellow student and during the first week invited along with others in the group to look at Sian's room in the nurse's residence. On discovering from comments, made by clinical staff some while later, that her fellow student had also some considerable influence in the unit and was, in fact, the dreaded professional officer from the Board, Blod was overheard reflecting on her first meeting with her classmate:

I thought to myself at the time, there's a mature student!

At this stage I had not yet announced that I was there in the capacity of a university student undertaking research by joining them as a midwifery student.

I also took the role of a 'passive participant' standing around the coffee lounge etc., listening intently to the conversations of students and those between teachers and students. I alternated between the insider/outsider position described by Spradley (1979, 1980), experiencing the frustrations and emotions of a student while also being an outsider and viewing the lesson, the other students and myself as 'objects'. It was not possible to identify the use of a single theoretical typology of participation, as I moved somewhere within the centre field of roles described by Gold (1958) and Junker (1960). Within the continuum ranging from the complete participant to the complete observer I often took the role of observer-as-participant, particularly during the informal sessions. This role entailed entering into the conversation, but taking care not to influence it or miss any of the talk going on in peripheral groups during coffee breaks etc.

I kept detailed field notes, which was relatively easy to accomplish in an unobtrusive fashion during classroom activities, but less so during the coffee and lunch breaks and clinical sessions. I recorded the unsolicited interviews as soon after the event as possible. Sometimes I even made notes quickly in the toilet, until I discovered Sian and Denise often waited for me, chatting at the washbasins before leaving. Alicia, whom I sat next to in class, became so curious about my note-taking on one occasion that I was alerted to adopt a more relaxed attitude, using opportunities to write only when the students were taking lecture notes, for fear that my scribbling might inhibit their 'natural' behaviour and jeopardize my attempts to build an easy rapport with them.

Interviews and diaries

I undertook taped ethnographic interviews with each of the nine students on two separate occasions, each of approximately one hour in length. Group discussion/interviews were also undertaken after one, four and 18 weeks of their course programme, in order to pursue emerging themes. A course diary was written by each student, detailing their perceptions of daily experiences in clinical settings.

The interviews were conducted in conversational style, allowing for flexibility, while loosely following my agenda. This agenda was, however, to be ultimately determined by the responses of the students. The ideas raised by them, often spontaneously, were 'tested' at later interviews which were held in a quiet, comfortable room. Few notes were taken during these interviews, apart from the occasional comment which I feared may not be picked up on tape and which I felt worthy of verbatim recording.

Schatzman and Strauss (973) indicate that while the informal interview should be sufficiently flexible to accommodate new themes there should, nevertheless, be a clear aim in the researcher's mind at the outset. In view of this, I defined my goal and had the possible agenda visible during each interview. The topics which I wished the informant to address usually began around the question of what was the student's notion of 'midwife' and how it related to her concept of a 'nurse'. Other items on the agenda included the following:

1. Describe previous work experiences
2. Reasons for entering midwifery training

3. Sources of knowledge of midwifery
4. Expectations of the course
5. Feelings about experiences during the first week – first impressions of people and things.
6. How it feels to be a student again.

At 'follow-up' interviews I pursued many of the concepts which were briefly addressed at initial interview and several additional issues which were written about in their 'diaries'. The diaries produced an abundance of data, the students being very eager to 'talk' by this later stage in the relationship with the researcher and following intensive exposure to the clinical environment.

Advantages and some problems of becoming an insider researcher

Some of my informants responded with some amusement and others with concern, to the discovery that their 'friend and student researcher' was a person who, according to the midwives, 'had the power to close us down'. This 'semi-covert' phase of the research posed problems faced by many ethnographers; that of deciding how much self-disclosure is necessary to meet ethical acceptability, yet to provide data that are less affected by reactivity to the presence of the researcher.

It was during participant observation that I had the unique experience of being 'told off' by a fellow student for walking through a ward when being totally disorientated with the geography of the hospital. The personal journal entry following this incident reveals something of the feelings of a novice ethnographer:

> Today I felt peeved being told off by Ceridwen for walking through C Ward. She chastised me: 'You can't have every Tom, Dick or Harry walking through wards when there are women around breast feeding and half naked, you know.' I felt ashamed but somewhat ambivalent, pleased about being treated as one of 'them' and yet strangely uncomfortable – after all, I would be escorted to enter any department in my capacity as midwifery officer.
>
> (Extract: Fieldwork Journal, Thursday 6.3.87)

An insider researcher has the advantage of escaping the time-consuming process of 'learning the ropes' and the 'routines' of the organization. I was familiar with the 'jargon' of the occupational group under study. I recognized, however, that this could be a two-edged sword and consequently reminded myself of the warning by Spradley (1979) to avoid 'going native'. This familiarity, know as translation competence, with which I entered the field, was a factor I needed constantly to bear in mind. However, my relative unfamiliarity with this particular school made the task of attaining strangeness a little less difficult. Defining the conflict of my professional values, I took comfort in the fact that it is not an uncommon phenomenon amongst ethnographers.

While Beynon found it necessary to intervene as a teacher when his schoolboy informants' pranks were of a dangerous nature, I had problems of a different, yet equally disturbing nature. An extract from my 'reflexive' journal illustrates the point further:

> *Confessions of a novice researcher. 5.3.87.*
> Today incorrect statements were being made by the teacher, which are potentially dangerous. Also there was a tendency to offer dubious advice which was unsubstantiated; at this point I 'blew it' and could not restrain myself! I spoke up as calmly as I could, stating that in my view the (suggested action) could be very traumatic for the newborn child. I am now being a teacher *not* a researcher!! I shall have to watch that.

Similar experiences are recounted by others who have undertaken research into midwifery by means of observation (e.g. Kirkham, 1989).

Sampling procedures and analysis of data

Sampling is an issue with which the 'positivist' researcher is associated and in that context means a predefined statistical sample of research subjects or respondents. Glaser and Strauss (1967) distinguished differences between statistical and theoretical sampling, the latter being used in ethnographic studies. Theoretical sampling, which was used in this study, requires equally complex procedures and rigour as that used in statistical sampling.

Categories of theoretical concepts are identified when the ethnographer becomes immersed in data analysis, during as well as after the data collection is completed. These conceptual categories lead the researcher to undertake further data collection which is progressively focused until each category becomes saturated; that is, nothing new emerges from field data which fit into a particular theme. An acknowledged weakness of this study was the inability within the time constraints, to reach such theoretical saturation of every theme. Nevertheless, several analytical themes were developed, following the 'grounded theory' approach advocated by Glaser and Strauss (1967). The sampling in this case entailed a fairly lengthy, in-depth study of a cohort of student midwives within the context of the natural setting in which the events were taking place – an activity which Hammersley and Atkinson (1983) refer to as providing 'ecological validity'. A situation was not 'set up' especially for the research purpose as in experimental research design.

Organizing and analysing data

In due course the written data I had collected were organized under several headings and placed in separate piles. I was fortunate to be able to employ an audio-typist to transcribe at least some of the tapes – a lengthy procedure, as I soon discovered. I chose to have the interview data typed verbatim while later on I still needed to listen to major sections of each one, having read and re-read the transcripts, using highlighter pens for ease of identification later. Sometimes the inflexion in a voice or a hesitation was significant in the context of the conversation, yet could not have been captured in type. This brought back vivid memories of the students' interesting statements and spontaneous comments. One such example was when Denise referred to a brief period she had spent as a staff nurse in a postnatal ward; she implied by her facial expression and tone of voice, as much as the language used, that she was acting 'illegally' as a midwife and was not wanting to broadcast the fact. During a later conversation, I was able to follow up this statement and discover the meanings she attached to this concept of the legal status of the midwife.

I waded through the observational field notes, the journal and my analytical memos in the same rigorous fashion. Biographical details of the students, lesson handouts I had collected as a participant 'student' and finally the students' diaries all made fascinating reading and what seemed enormous amounts of data to analyse. In organizing these data I chose an alphabetical index with which to label the emerging themes. There seemed to be hundreds of them initially. Having exhausted the letters of the alphabet, I continued with AA and BB etc. until I had identified 39 categories, which were then placed into large box files.

I extracted the verbatim passages from typed transcripts and from handwritten notes which I had highlighted and photocopied. I usually remembered to file all the references to read, also in alphabetical order in yet another box file. These categorized data I then 'cut and pasted' to form cards using treasury tags or staples for fear of loss or disruption by unintentional 'do gooders' tidying up the study. I leaned heavily for guidance on Lofland and Lofland (1984), Burgess (1984) and Hammersley and Atkinson (1983) during this experience. Another brief extract from my journal illustrates my feelings at the time:

> Midnight again! What a mess, cards and bits of paper everywhere, all of which seem to be useful data. I must lock the door. Imagine having to sort it out again if Kate decides to tidy up!

Emergence of themes

Gradually, but not before many moments of doubt and frustration, this time-consuming activity began to bring its own rewards; the major themes began to emerge and the chapter headings were pinned to my notice board.

The first theme concerned the notion of the midwife as a practitioner in her own right. Despite the students' initial belief that midwives are 'practitioners in their own right', in most instances it appeared to them to be a myth. Conflict and ambiguity in the transition from the role of 'competent nurse' to student midwife constituted a second theme, and was a source of much anxiety for those participating in the study. This was closely associated with a third theme to emerge: namely the wide range of strategies which students learnt very early on as a means of coping with their anxieties. One of these strategies was a focus on ritualized and routine aspects of work, many of which were a continuation of nursing experience. Some students perceived midwifery as a 'respected part of nursing', contrasting in particular with chronic geriatric nursing. One student coined the phrase 'the happy end of nursing' to describe her idea of midwifery, a concept which implies an occupational link between nursing and midwifery that 'socialized' midwives deny.

A theme that recurred throughout the study was that of a compromise between the provision of service and the education of the student. Experience on the wards was often a matter of unsupervised trial and error, and the aspirations of the ward staff were perceived as different from the teaching staff's idealized version of midwifery practice.

A full account of these themes and supporting data is available in Davies (1988). Findings on the ritualized aspects of midwifery have been published (Davies and Atkinson, 1991). This chapter focuses on the findings on the notion of the midwife as independent practitioner.

PRACTITIONER STATUS: RHETORIC OR REALITY?

The notion of the midwife as 'practitioner in her own right' was initially perceived by the students to exist; in fact, it was one of the attractions of gaining entry to membership of the profession. This may not seem worthy of comment, were it not for considerable evidence to the contrary perceived by the informants while they moved through their early clinical placements.

The rhetoric

During the students' initial encounters in the classroom they were constantly exposed to the rhetoric that the professional status and power of the midwife are equal to that of the obstetrician. The 'education side' or the 'teaching department' promulgated the notion of the midwife taking decisions independently of medical staff. Midwife teachers' beliefs and values distinguish them from the 'service side' in ways similar to those described by Bucher and Strauss (1961) in the classic literature on 'segmentation' within professions. Midwives who give direct care to childbearing women are generally referred to by maternity personnel as the 'service side'. This implies a separateness which legitimizes the notion of segmentation. It was clear from the findings of my study that the liturgy which emanated from the education segment during the early socialization period of potential midwives was the version of midwives giving total, individualized care based upon a 'needs' model. In order to demonstrate the ritualistic manner in which images of the midwife were developed by the group of students, extracts from field notes and early tape-recorded lectures are provided:

Field note extract. 3.3.87
Jackie Wild, in poetic style, pronounces her portrayal of the role of the midwife. There is a quiet reverence in the tone of her voice. One can hear a pin drop while each student appears mesmerized by the expert reciting the 'articles of faith' of the midwifery profession. Almost in a whisper as if concluding a sermon she says:
A midwife is a practitioner, she has the responsibility, the knowledge and the expertise to practise in her own right. Whether you take this responsibility is up to you as individuals. You can be practitioners in your own right, where you can prescribe care, you can give care, or you can refer to a doctor if necessary. We are concerned with normal aspects of midwifery, of pregnancy, of childbirth and of the postnatal period. That doesn't mean to say we won't become involved with abnormal things. I envy you in many ways the fact that you are starting, it's so exciting in my opinion to be able to act like this.'

This monologue clearly painted a picture of midwifery as the teacher would have the student see it. She seemed to imply that she envied them, regretting her missed opportunities to practise the idealized version of midwifery.
Later during the introductory week of classroom-based teaching, Jackie introduced the subject of antenatal care when these constructs were challenged, albeit in a non-assertive manner, by one of the more mature students:

Teacher: Yes, the GP will confirm the pregnancy and then will refer her to the booking clinic at the hospital – if the woman so wishes and the GP so agrees ... It might be that she finds her own independent midwife and has some home care from the midwife.

Student: How many women know that you can actually do that?'

Teacher: Very few I would suggest. I think women are becoming more aware of things, but it is a possibility. There is a cost involved and that's not to say that we can't change things within the health service to make care far more individual and far more personalized than it is at present. We've come a long way in the last few years ... Is it best for women? Do they know what they want?

This dialogue suggests that the practitioner status of the midwife appeared to be a myth. The student, herself a mother of four, raised the issue in an attempt to explore the reason why so few women avail themselves of the facility to employ an independent midwife. The teacher pointed out that the cost factor is a possible deterrent, while her rhetorical questions implied that women have no opinions on the matter. She may have been hedging her bets in the knowledge of the 'reality' of the situation in practice. There were no independent midwives in practice within the health authority in which the student was gaining her experience – a factor yet to impinge upon her on entering the clinical field.

The service segment, however, directed the student in a different manner which promoted routinized activity in order to get through the work. Very much as Melia described the nurses' 'workload approach' involving performance of tasks and routines (Melia, 1987), so student midwives at Oldville described their work as repetitious and routinized.

Denise, one of the informants, described her memories of ward work:

> We had antenatal and postnatals on the ward. You start at one end of the ward with the trolley and do all the antenatals ... I felt it was really task oriented. I didn't really enjoy that ward experience.

The students' reality

Prior to their commencement of clinical experience the students talked openly about their perception of the midwife as a different professional from the nurse.

Ceridwen explained her view of these differences during the hour-long ethnographic interview undertaken prior to her 'ward work':

> *Ceridwen*: I know that the view of midwives and midwifery in general was that they are very different from nursing ... they hold themselves very much aloof ... the impression was that midwives always think that they are a bit better than anybody else, that sort of thing. It's an overall impression and I don't know perhaps by the time we've finished this course and examined one hundred babies, examined one hundred mothers and delivered however many hundreds ... [laughter] ... perhaps you do feel – well, I mean it's a terrific training. I'm seeing what's involved this week. I am more than ever amazed at the fact that you get no extra pay for it. No financial recognition that you've taken something extra, that you've done all that work and become a practitioner in your own right, that's the way I look at it.

> *RD*: Do you see nurses as practitioners?

Ceridwen: No, no I don't think I do, a lot of it you are governed so much by what the doctor wants and, hum, his instructions ... Which, you know as a midwife, I mean I'm talking about the ideal situation, but that woman is your responsibility, you make the decisions with her about what's right and wrong for her. Well I've certainly seen that a lot more clearly this week. I found out that in fact midwives can themselves say that lady is ready to go home.

Another account, however, this time from Lorraine, illustrates the confusion faced by these students when exposed to the clinical situation. The following extract is from the diary of this student written contemporaneously while gaining ward experience during the first three months of the course:

The school will tell you one thing and the books will say it, but the staff on the ward will say that's not the way you do it, you do it this way, for example a palpation: we were taught to take the fundal height then lateral palpation, then pelvic, whereas on labour ward you were taught to do fundal, pelvic and then lateral.

In the antenatal clinic Lorraine identified more tensions, this time between doctors and midwives competing for status recognition while again providing insights into the 'reality' of the practitioner midwife's role:

Everyone says we are practitioners in our own right when we qualify. From what I understand the midwife will do a proper palpation and always listen to the fetal heart. We start clinic about nine to half past nine, they do the urines, their weight, bloods, BP, and, you know the things that the midwife does; then they (the patients) wait outside for about an hour. You are lucky to see a doctor before ten. She's got to wait until the doctor comes, just to be seen by the doctor who says, hello Mrs Jones how are you? He may do a vague abdominal palpation, he might see if the head is engaged. It has been said, 'is that what I've been waiting for?' They wait for an hour for a two-minute consultation.

I don't see the need for a doctor in a lot of these cases ... The midwife knows more than SHOs ... yet they are not allowed to go until the doctor sees them. The midwives are allowed to do it by law but it's the consultants in this hospital who won't let it happen. The consultants like the doctor to see the patient. I suppose they are more so (practitioners) on labour wards, they have more control of the situation on labour wards by night ... not so much by day. You usually see a doctor poking his nose in, not actually doing anything. Everyone seems to be geared towards – you must cover yourself to avoid being sued.

This power and control of the clinic at Oldville was not unlike that which existed in other institutions in which medical dominance prevailed over nurses. Melia provides a clear picture of the ways in which student nurses perceived the claims of the profession. She describes various themes pervading the students' accounts, which point to the complexity of this notion of profession. Of relevance here is her third theme, that of 'the idea that nursing is influenced to some extent by medical dominance'. In her exploration of the usage of the term 'profession' Melia argues that it is used in several different ways by what she also calls 'segments of nursing' (Melia, 1987):

> In broad terms we can say that there are different ideas canvassed within nursing, ideas which concern what nursing should look like and what status the occupation should ideally have. First we have the service segment, where the predominant ethos is to get the work done and the way of achieving this is to appeal to the notion of 'profession' with its connotations of duty and compliance. Second we have an academic group from higher education, within the education segment. ... There is a problem for nursing if it is to lay a successful claim to 'profession'. The claim is essentially problematic because nursing work is not autonomous, by virtue of the fact that part of nursing's work is dictated by medicine.
>
> (Melia, 1987, p. 166)

Oldville students' theories of practitioner status seemed to be determined through the invocation of their own notion of social reality. They attributed the inability of midwives to work as practitioners to the controlling influence of medical staff. This explanation was crystallized in several accounts of students' experiences while undertaking night duty. Here is Ceridwen's account of 'working on nights':

> Nights are less frantic somehow. You are obstetric nurses on days, but midwives on nights – yes – you are practising on nights. The aim on nights is to have a lovely normal delivery, anything to avoid the doctors. They (the midwives) were telling the doctors what to do – 'doctor come and do so and so, or, I want to give pethidine one fifty – she is telling him while pretending to ask. The midwife was protesting to the students by saying, 'It's ridiculous, I'm a practitioner in my own right and I have to wake him up' – stupid when she knows she is competent to give it.

These indirect negotiations with doctors may appear to the novice to be strategies for managing the powerful and controlling influence of doctors. However, Simpson found student nurses were attracted to the 'doctor–nurse' relationship [which] is publicly stereotyped as a handmaiden relationship with the nurse a helper of the doctor and subordinate to him' (Simpson, 1979, p. 89).

Dingwall (1977) asserts that midwives are encouraged in training and by official theories of their occupation to define themselves as 'professionals' and consequently on a par with doctors. Yet this notion appeared to cause considerable confusion for the students in this study. Having been fed the 'received wisdom', they had to deal with what they perceived as the contrary situation in practice.

These student midwives' accounts of their educational programme undoubtedly raised the question of the appropriateness of that particular course for their future practice as midwives. The rhetoric to which they were exposed, and the reality of practice they experienced, may adversely affect their desire to remain in midwifery, even though most students complete the course and qualify as midwives. This should be of concern to managers of the maternity services since it is a waste of an expensive resource. It could be argued that failure to practise at the end of the course is attributable to several factors which may exist universally and some of which were demonstrated at Oldville. The most notable factor was the conflict between the role of the midwife previously anticipated and portrayed in the classroom, and that which emerged in the student's 'reality'. The socialization process in midwifery may take a little longer than the time allowed within the post-registration course, especially since the socialization into nursing has previously taken a minimum of three years.

CONCLUSION

The data obtained in this ethnographic study by means of observation, from interviews and from students' diary accounts can only be said to represent one group of informants in one midwifery school. From subjective experience and a substantial volume of research, it can, however, be argued that the school and the students studied are unlikely to differ from midwifery schools and student midwives in England and Wales as a whole. Certainly informal feedback from midwives who have listened to the presentation of the research findings indicate an identification with very similar situations in their own experience. It seems therefore that the conclusions of the research are relevant to midwifery educationists generally.

The study was conceived within the framework of the transition from nurse to midwife; the themes that emerged concerning the two professions have relevance to the maternity services today. This is particularly so with regard to the theme discussed in this chapter: the concept of the independent practitioner in midwifery. The study provided data which belie the education segment's pronouncements of the 'articles of faith' of the profession, showing it as a myth for those in the study site embarking upon their road to socialization into midwifery. Competition between the doctor and midwife for role and status further highlights the existence of the myth.

The way in which midwifery has been managed and practised in some districts has not been conducive to the promotion of independent practice on entry to Part 10 of the professional register. Since the completion of the research described in this chapter two major developments have occurred in midwifery: first the introduction of new pre-registration midwifery programmes; and second, the publication of *Changing Childbirth*, advocating considerable autonomy of practice for the qualified midwife (Department of Health, 1993). If these recent opportunities for midwives to develop autonomy and innovative practice are to remain available to them at the turn of the century, then it is essential that midwifery is not regarded or practised as merely 'the happy ending of nursing'. If it is so regarded then this will facilitate the push by some for genericism of the caring professions, and this in turn may put at risk that which many overseas midwives covet most in British midwifery.

The extent to which these recent developments have an impact on midwifery education and practice must be monitored and assessed by a continuous programme of research. This chapter has shown that the ethnographic tradition, employed somewhat infrequently in the history of midwifery research, should be an important component of such a programme. The strength of ethnography is the facility it affords of understanding various ways in which student midwives and qualified staff absorb and make sense of their environment, and how this in turn influences the practice of midwifery within particular settings.

REFERENCES

Atkinson, P. (1981) The Clinical Experience: *The Construction and Reconstruction of Medical Reality*. Gower, Farnborough.

Becker, H., Geer, B., Hughes, E.C. and Strauss, A.L. (1961) *Boys in White*. University of Chicago Press, Chicago.

Beynon, J. (1985) *Initial Encounters in the Secondary School*. Falmer Press, London.

Boyd, C. and Sellers, L. (1982) *The British Way of Birth*. Pan Books, London.

Bucher, R. and Strauss, A. (1961) Professions in process. *American Journal of Sociology*, **66**, 325–34.

Burgess, R. (1984) *In the Field: An Introduction to Field Research*. Allen & Unwin, London.

Central Midwives Board (1983) *The Role of the Midwife*. CMB, London.

Cuff, E. and Payne, G. (eds) (1979) *Perspectives in Sociology*. Allen & Unwin, London.

Davies, R.M. (1988) The happy end of nursing: an ethnographic study of initial encounters in a midwifery school. Unpublished MSc dissertation, University of Wales, Cardiff.

Davies, R.M. and Atkinson, P. (1991) Students of midwifery: 'doing the obs' and other coping strategies. *Midwifery*, **7**(3), 113–21.

Denzin N, (1978) *The Research Act* (2nd edn). McGraw-Hill, New York.

Department of Health (1993) *Changing Childbirth*, Vols I and II. HMSO, London.

Dingwall, R. (1977) *The Social Organisation of Health Visitor Training*. Croom Helm, London.

Duffy, M. (1985) Designing nursing research: the qualitative–quantitative debate. *Journal of Advanced Nursing*, **10**, 225–32.

Fielding, N. and Fielding, J. (1986) *Linking Data*. Sage, Beverly Hills, CA.

Garcia, J. and Garforth, S. (1991) Midwifery policies and policy-making. In Robinson, S. and Thomson, A.M. (eds), *Midwives, Research and Childbirth*, Vol. II. Chapman & Hall, London, pp. 16–47.

Glaser, B. and Strauss, A. (1967) *The Discovery of Grounded Theory: Strategies for Qualitative Research*. Aldine, Chicago.

Gold, R. (1958) Roles in sociological field observations. *Social Forces*, **36**, 217–23.

Golden, J. (1980) Midwifery training: the views of newly qualified midwives. *Midwives Chronicle*, **93**(1109), 190–94.

Green, J., Kitzinger, J. and Coupland, V. (1994) Midwives' responsibilities, medical staffing structures and women's choice in childbirth. In Robinson, S. and Thomson, A.M. (eds), *Midwives, Research and Childbirth*, Vol. III. Chapman & Hall, London, pp. 5–29.

Hammersley, M. and Atkinson, P. (1983) *Ethnography: Principles in Practice*. Tavistock, London.

Hedges, B. and Ritchie, J. (1987) *Research and Policy: the Choice of Appropriate Research Methods*. Social and Community Planning Research, London.

Junker, B. (1960) *Fieldwork: An Introduction to the Social Sciences*. Cases in Fieldwork. University of Chicago Press, Chicago.

Kirkham, M. (1989) Midwives and information-giving during labour. In Robinson, S. and Thomson, A.M. (eds), *Midwives, Research and Childbirth*, Vol. I. Chapman & Hall, London, pp. 117–38.

Lofland, J. (1971) *Analysing Social Settings: A Guide to Qualitative Observation and Analysis*. Wadsworth, Belmont, CA.

Lofland, L. and Lofland, J. (1984) *Analysing Social Settings: A Guide to Qualitative Observation and Analysis* (2nd edn). Wadsworth, Belmont, CA.

Melia, K. (1982) 'Tell it as it is'. Qualitative methodology and nursing research: understanding the student nurse's world. *Journal of Advanced Nursing*, **7**(4), 327–35.

Melia, K. (1987) *Learning and Working: The Occupational Socialisation of Nurses*. Tavistock, London.

Olesen, V. and Whittaker, E. (1968) *The Silent Dialogue: A Study of the Social Psychology of Professional Socialisation*. Jossey Bros, San Francisco.

Radford, N. and Thompson, A. (1994) A study of issues concerning the implementation of direct entry midwifery education. In Robinson, S. and Thomson, A.M. (eds), *Midwives, Research and Childbirth*, Vol. III. Chapman & Hall, London.

Rankin, S. (1980) Midwives first – nurses second? *Nursing Mirror*, **151**(24), 22–3.

Reid, M. (1986) Apprenticeship into midwifery: an American example *Midwifery*, **2**(3), 126–34.

Robinson, S. (1985) Midwives, obstetricians and general practitioners: the need for role clarification. *Midwifery*, **1**(2), 102–13.

Robinson, S. and Owen, H. (1994) Retention in midwifery: findings from a longitudinal study of midwives' careers. In Robinson, S. and Thomson, A.M. (eds), *Midwives, Research and Childbirth*, Vol III. Chapman & Hall, pp. 175–32.

Robinson, S. Golden, J. and Bradley, S. (1983) *A Study of the Role and Responsibilities of the Midwife*. Nursing Research Unit, King's College, London.

Rose, A.M. (1962) A systematic summary of symbolic interaction theory. In Rose, A.M. (ed.) *Human Behaviour and Social Processes: an Interactionist Approach*. Routledge & Kegan Paul, London.

Schatzman, L. and Strauss, A. (1973) *Field Research: Strategies for a Natural Sociology.* Prentice-Hall, Englewood Cliffs, NJ.

Simpson, I. (1979) *From Student to Nurse: A Longitudinal Study of Socialisation.* Cambridge University Press, Cambridge.

Spradley, J. (1979) *The Ethnographic Interview.* Holt, Rhinehart & Winston, New York.

Spradley, J. (1980) *Participant Observation.* Holt, Rhinehart & Winston, New York.

Towler, J. and Bramwell, J. (1986) *Midwives in History and Society.* Croom Helm, London.

United Kingdom Central Council for Nursing, Midwifery and Health Visiting (1986) *Project 2000: A New Preparation for Practice.* UKCC, London.

Walker, J. (1976) Midwife or obstetric nurse? Some perceptions of midwives and obstetricians of the role of the midwife. *Journal of Advanced Nursing,* **1**(2), 129–38.

White, R. (1987) Health visitors: the willing horses. *Health Visitor,* **60**, 163–8.

World Health Organization (1948) *The Constitution: Declaration.* Alma Ata. Geneva.

CHAPTER SIX

The clinical education of
student midwives

Marie Chamberlain

This chapter is concerned with learning opportunities for student midwives in the clinical environment and is based on a study of the subject undertaken at the end of the 1980s. Feelings of professional competence are often engendered and maintained during the student midwife's experiences in the clinical environment; consequently, the learning opportunities that it affords constitute an important component of the confidence which the newly qualified midwife will hopefully bring to her practice.

It is in the clinical environment that students are exposed to, and learn from, the role fulfilled by midwives. The study was undertaken at a time when, in many hospitals, this role was the subject of considerable concern; in particular from the medicalization of childbirth and the advent of a wide range of technological developments that replaced traditional midwifery skills. Student midwives often found that the role of the midwife they were taught in the classroom did not match that practised in the clinical setting. Moreover, if they had entered midwifery with the expectation of a career that would provide them with more autonomy than nursing, then many were subsequently to be disappointed.

Taking a broad historical perspective the role of the midwife has changed from one based in the community providing continuity of care throughout pregnancy, labour and the puerperium, to one based in hospital working on one aspect of care, with concomitant loss of continuity for both midwives and women. For midwives this move has been accompanied by increasing loss of autonomy in decision-making concerning the management of care. The main events in this long and complex history have been elucidated, in differing degrees of detail, by a number of authors and so are not discussed here (e.g. Donnison, 1977, 1988; Cowell and Wainwright, 1981; Bent, 1982; Towler and Brammall, 1986; Oakley, 1986; Robinson, 1990). Recent years, however, have witnessed moves to restore not only the midwife's responsibilities for the care of those women who experience a normal pregnancy, labour and puerperium, but also the continuity with which this care is provided (Robinson, 1990). This trend has recently received government backing in the form of a report (*Changing Childbirth*) based on the deliberations of a Parliamentary Select Committee (House of Commons, 1992). These developments have profound implications for the clinical education of student midwives. Newly qualified members of the profession will only be able to respond to the challenge of practising in the ways recommended if they are confident in the clinical skills developed in the course of their own education. Consequently the issues raised by the research discussed in this chapter are as relevant to the mid-1990s as to the late 1980s.

BACKGROUND TO THE RESEARCH

This study was conducted as part of the requirements for a doctorate in an English university and was unfunded. My initial interest in pursuing the subject of clinical education was the proposed legislation of midwifery as a health profession in Ontario, Canada. After training and working as a nurse and midwife in England, Wales and Australia, I moved to Canada. I found it difficult to work in maternity units in Canada because of the lack of responsibility accorded nurses for women in labour and the fact that at the end of caring for these women a doctor would arrive for the delivery. I moved north to the Canadian Arctic, where I enjoyed two and a half years of being responsible for only myself and the Inuit (Eskimo) people for whom I cared. The nearest hospital and general practitioner were four hours away by plane. I only left because I decided to return to university to further my education.

The topic of my study reflects a long interest in midwifery education, particularly in the clinical area. As a clinically based person who had spent time in Australia, as well as Canada, it was clear to me on my return to England that the role of the midwife had been seriously eroded. Many aspects of the role of the midwife now being reintroduced in Britain were common practices when I undertook my training in 1968. Midwives ran the antenatal clinics and women were only seen by medical staff when referred by midwives. Home births were still a reality, although a decreasing one, and I obtained my 10 home births within the three months community period of my training. Many of the changes that led to constraints in the midwife's role in the 1970s and 1980s were, however, already being introduced in the late 1960s (Robinson, 1990). Nonetheless, it was still with a great deal of shock and some disbelief that I read the findings of a national survey of the role of the midwife prior to my return to Britain (Robinson, Golden and Bradley, 1983; Robinson, 1985).

When I first began my studies I intended to conduct research into midwifery but was not clear upon which aspect to focus. I had already determined to embark upon a refresher course in order to continue my midwifery practice and to bring me up to date on recent changes, since I felt that both were a prerequisite for research into midwifery. It was the 'refresher' course which allowed me useful insights into the education of student midwives in England and led me to formulate the focus of my study as an exploration of the teaching and learning of midwifery skills in the clinical environment. From the 'refresher' course I also obtained information which, after analysis, provided themes to explore and direct my future research. Consequently, this course became the 'exploratory phase' of the study.

When I reviewed the literature for information on research into the clinical education of student midwives I found very little upon which to build (see Chapter 7). As others have commented, the emphasis in midwifery research has been primarily on practice and on the organization of care (Robinson, Thomson and Tickner, 1989; Murphy-Black, 1991).

AIMS AND METHODS

Choice of research design

The paucity of previous research, together with the recognition that a study such as the one I proposed required insights into interactions within the clinical environment, led to my decision to adopt a qualitative approach. A qualitative study would enable me to identify those factors important in clinical education in midwifery and assess how they interacted and affected the student's competency in clinical skills. Only a qualitative approach could provide the depth and type of knowledge required to answer these questions.

Qualitative research encourages the investigator to choose as topics for research start situations with which one is currently familiar or has been in the past. The overall goal of qualitative research is to collect the richest and most diverse data as possible over a relatively prolonged period of time. The qualitative researcher seeks to observe people directly in the real world, in order to gain an understanding of how they interact with their environment – an approach sometimes described as naturalism (Hammersley and Atkinson, 1983). With this philosophy the preferred method for gathering data is through face-to-face contact and a prolonged immersion in the same environment as the subject (Lofland and Lofland, 1984).

One type of qualitative approach used increasingly by health researchers is that of ethnography, usually defined as an approach towards developing concepts with which to understand human behaviour from the point of view of the subject. An ethnographic study can readily encompass the use of symbolic interactionism, a theory created for the study of human interactions (Rose, 1962). For this investigation I used an ethnographic approach to identify the concepts and values that guided student midwives' attempts to gain clinical competence in midwifery, and then to develop a theoretical analysis that was grounded in my data in the manner advocated by Glaser and Strauss (1967). This approach has been used in a number of midwifery research projects, for example Kirkham's study of information-giving in labour (Kirkham, 1989) and Davies's study of the early experiences of student midwives (Davies 1988 and Chapter 5 in this volume).

The most usual methods of data collection for an ethnographic study are observation and interview. Observation, whether participant or non-participant, requires the selection of small samples and relatively few informants. For increased reliability and validity it is usually accompanied by unstructured interviewing and a review of documents; data from sources are then combined in the course of descriptive analysis. Such were the methods used in this study.

Research site and time scale

Gaining access to a research site can pose difficulties if one is not already known to some of the site personnel. I chose to conduct my study on the site on which I was based for my 'refresher' course, since this provided me with ready access to personnel. Permission to undertake the study was given by the heads of the midwifery service and midwifery education. This site was an urban maternity hospital with a long-established midwifery training school. It had a high-technology approach to maternity care which I felt at that time would approximate the conditions under which midwifery in Canada would take place. However, this assumption proved to be erroneous because it has been decided that midwifery in Ontario will be community based and the midwife will only enter the hospital if her client wishes to have her delivery there. The hospital in which I undertook the research had a 24-hour coverage by obstetric staff, paediatric staff and anaesthetists. At the time of the study the hospital had just over 4000 deliveries a year and 3000 new bookings. Just over 1000 community antenatal visits were made, there were some 2500 postnatal visits and about a dozen deliveries took place at home.

The fieldwork was undertaken between April 1988 and March 1989; it entailed eight months' observation and informal interviewing, followed by a three-month period of more structured interviewing. I undertook most of the subsequent analysis and writing up part-time while holding a full-time lectureship, first in England and then in Canada.

Sample selection and analysis

The goal of the qualitative researcher is to identify patterns and commonalities by inference from specific ideas to more generalized ideas. This process should result in the identification of concepts and potential relationships between concepts (Field and Morse, 1985). This type of research does not require a sample to be statistically representative of the population but does require that the characteristics to be investigated by the researcher are represented among the sample.

Five intakes of students of post-registration midwifery courses were selected to represent students at different points in an 18-month period. Two intakes (sets D and E) were observed from the beginning of their course, one intake at the completion of their course (set A) and two intakes (sets B and C) between these two extremes. As a result the project took the form of a cross-sectional study of learning opportunities in the clinical environment with respect to student midwives in different phases of their training experience. From each intake 5 students were selected, to make a total of 25 students in all. When describing the experiences of the students, and the midwife teachers and service staff, the generic term of 'she' is used, since there were no males in the sample and only one in the wards. Names used in anecdotal statements have been altered to protect the anonymity of participants.

The composition of the sample was based on the researcher's judgement of the range of people best able to provide the comprehensive information needed for the study (Wilson, 1985). Approximately 60% of the students in each set volunteered to participate in the study. As such the sample was non-random and one of convenience. An attempt was made to select randomly from among the students who had volunteered to participate by using one of the oldest techniques for random sampling: namely, putting names in a hat and drawing out five.

Students were contacted through their teachers, who then provided me with the time to speak to students about the objectives of the study and to request their voluntary participation. In addition to being observed students were interviewed on a formal and informal basis. Midwifery staff were informed by their managers after I had attended a midwifery managers' meeting in which details of the study were provided and co-operation sought. Eight midwife teachers and 18 midwives and midwife managers were formally interviewed at least once over a period of 15 months.

Non-participant observation

Non-participant observation entails a process whereby an investigator establishes and sustains a relatively long-term relationship with another person in that person's natural setting (Lofland and Lofland, 1984). I observed midwifery students in this manner over an eight-month period. Behavioural skills were chosen for observation, since it was anticipated that these would demonstrate that learning had occurred. The observations took place in all clinical areas, with greater emphasis on the labour ward and antenatal clinics than on the community and special-care baby unit. Clinical areas to which access was easiest were the labour ward, the postnatal wards, antenatal ward and the antenatal clinic. The community was difficult for observation because the presence of another person in addition to that of the student and midwife was awkward when visiting most homes and could be intimidating for some families. As a result the community midwife usually chose the families she felt were best able to accommodate an observer such as myself.

The special-care baby unit was also an area difficult to access because of the small size of the premises and the many sick babies. It seemed that every time an observation was arranged with a student, there would be an influx of sick babies, promptly followed by a large number of medical staff, and this left little room for myself. Less time was spent in the antenatal ward than the postnatal wards because the students did not work there until towards the end of their course.

Initial observations were fairly unfocused, despite the earlier exploratory phase which had provided the opportunity to observe in some areas. With time and experience, however, my observations became more specific and gradually began to include the documentation of verbal exchanges thought to add richness, and another dimension, to the observational data. Observation was a skill which had to be developed and did not come as easily as I had expected for someone who had been a nurse and midwife and supposedly skilled in this respect. It took a little time for me to realize that observing someone's condition required a different set of skills from those needed for the observation of an interaction.

In the early stages of the study I decided to observe students only when they were actively involved in performing a skill. This was to ensure that I did not waste time observing students when there was little happening. It was one of the main reasons for the large numbers of observations in the labour ward and the antenatal clinics, as they were not places subject to 'quiet moments'. I also decided that the entire process of performing a skill would be observed rather than just observing for a fixed amount of time. This was in order to observe the interactions around the skill, or to obtain a complete picture of the more complex extended skills that were performed. Examples of such types of observation were booking a new client in the antenatal clinic, which took approximately one hour, or the care of a woman in labour, through to the delivery and immediate postpartum care, which often took several hours.

Observations, when possible, were transcribed immediately after the event. Most researchers suggest this course of action so that details of the event, which may not have been written down, are still remembered (Chenitz and Swanson, 1986; Strauss and Corbin, 1990). This was excellent advice since I found that information was lost when it was not followed. The aim of my observation was to find out how students learned their skills and what factors affected their learning; an initial analysis to this effect was made for each observation once it was written up. As noted previously, behavioural skills were chosen for observation as a means of demonstrating that learning had occurred and this perception was then validated through formal and informal interviews.

During the eight-month period of fieldwork students were observed for a total of 344 hours; this figure comprise 158.5 hours in the labour ward, 49.5 hours in postnatal wards, 28 hours in antenatal wards, 62.5 hours in the antenatal clinic, 36.5 hours in the community and 9 hours in the special care baby unit.

Interviews

Interviews were used initially to validate informally the observer's perceptions of the social interactions taking place in the setting. Later on they were used to validate themes arising from an analysis of the data. Whenever possible initial informal interviews were carried out after a student had completed a procedure or demonstrated a behaviour that suggested learning had taken place. Such questioning occurred whenever and wherever it was convenient for the student: sometimes when weighing a placenta in the sluice, on the way up or down in the lift after discharging a woman to the postnatal ward, or during coffee and mealtimes.

Initially, the questions that students were asked followed the format of 'Why did you perform the skill in that way?' and later gave way to questions such as 'What do you find helpful when you are learning skills?' The latter type of questions were asked during the formal interviews, which took place in a quiet, private place in the unit or the education department. Midwife teachers were interviewed at the beginning of the study and in the final phase. Other midwives were interviewed after several analyses of the observational data, the majority some six months after the observational phase had been completed. The information gained from interviews, which were tape recorded, was also transcribed in the fashion described above. These formal interviews were utilized to validate themes that were emerging from the observation and informal interviews.

Additional methods of validation were sought through the presentation of findings to midwives attending research study days and to midwives at conferences such as the Research and the Midwife conference held in Manchester in 1991 (Chamberlain, 1992). The purpose of such presentations was to obtain feedback from the 'experts' attending and from the midwives themselves, in order to ensure that my concepts provided a rational and logical explanation of learning in the clinical environment.

Data analysis

This was conducted along the principles outlined by Glaser and Strauss (1967) for the development of grounded theory. Data were gathered, transcribed and analysed for themes and words that would provide insight into student learning. Once identified, these words and themes became the focus of further data collection. This process of data collection, transcription and analysis was repeated several times until it was clear that no new ideas were emerging from the data. These ideas then became the starting point of developing a category. Categories were fully identified after constant comparative latent analysis of the data had been completed. The data were not computerized and the analysis was undertaken by hand.

FINDINGS ON THE LEARNING PROCESS IN THE CLINICAL ENVIRONMENT

This chapter presents some of the main findings to emerge from this research on the learning process in the clinical environment; teaching methods are considered first, followed by factors that assist or constrain student learning.

Boud, Keogh and Walker (1985) remind us that only learners themselves can learn and only if they can reflect on their experiences. While the learner determines what she is able to learn she has, however, only a limited control over her learning opportunities. In institutional settings, like the hospital in which this research was undertaken, the learning environment was controlled by others such as the medical and administrative staff, closely followed by senior midwives, and this is reflected in the findings that follow.

Teaching methods

Observation The first method used for teaching new students in the clinical area was observation. Students were placed with midwives whom they followed around for several days, watching what they did and the procedures they performed. This type of teaching was confined to the first few days of the students' programme and was usually terminated by the eagerness of the student to move into a more active role or the midwife to initiate her into a more active participation. Some students were surprised to find that after a few days of observation they were unable to replicate many of the procedures carried out by the midwife. Some of the midwives, however, did not appear aware of this as a problem.

'Show and tell' This was the next phase of most student teaching and consisted of the student being shown a skill once or twice and then being expected to perform it with some degree of expertise. Many midwives made a conscious attempt to provide demonstrations for students, but these were often limited by a shortage of staff and heavy workload and occasionally by a lack of motivation on the part of the midwife. Some midwives were very conscientious in demonstrating skills until the student felt confident enough to function on her own. A few, however, believed in the minimal number of demonstrations and often did not wait to assess the student's ability and confidence in performing the skill. There were numerous complaints from students about this style of teaching, usually because they felt they were not provided with enough demonstrations or supervision. Peggy, a senior student, describes her experiences.

> It's ages since I was supervised. Usually you get supervised for the first one or two (antenatal assessments) and then you're on your own.
>
> (Peggy, 15 months into course)

A certain amount of learning was achieved indirectly through unconscious role-modelling by the midwife or the medical staff. When the doctor or the midwife stopped to explain situations and terms to women the students would stand close by and listen. Many felt that they learned more this way because the 'show and tell' opportunities were so few.

Tutorial teaching Midwifery teaching staff were not much in evidence in the clinical area during the time that the observations were made. As one student pointed out, sometimes promises were made which were not kept:

> In general there is a need for more clinical tutoring. I had no tutor come up while I was here (labour ward) and I'm finished here at the end of the week. Been up here ... let me see ... six weeks plus nights ... about 14 weeks altogether. Tutors said they would get up as much as possible but I've seen no one.
>
> (Janet, Set B, 10 months into course)

The midwife teachers did not appear very often in the clinical areas, but both the midwives and the students expected to receive more input from them than was forthcoming. Midwives said that the educational staff should have a more active role, in order to ensure continuity of teaching for the students when they themselves were busy. In addition, midwives felt the teachers' presence would be beneficial in that it would help clinical staff become current with the latest research. The students wanted the educators present as a means of improving upon what they themselves perceived as insufficient teaching by the midwives. Students also felt that the presence of the educational staff would help to emphasize their role as students and to enhance their status with the service staff.

'Trial and error' Vollman (1989) defines clinical learning experience as the totality of directed activity in which a student engages with a patient. In her definition the emphasis is on the 'directed' (supervised) nature of the activity, with an assumption that this direction will be provided by someone 'expert' in the area. For the majority of students in this study, however, there was little directed activity and the chief teaching strategy of the midwives was learning by 'trial and error'. For some midwives this was an extension of the belief that in order to learn you first have 'to do'. Many failed to recognize, however, that learning cannot occur in isolation without teaching demonstrations, supervision and feedback. Three forms of 'trial and error' teaching strategies were identified in this study.

'Thrown in'   The most common form of 'trial and error' learning was what I refer to as 'thrown in'. In this situation not only did the student not experience supervised or directed learning activity but was left on her own to determine her own learning opportunities. In a typical scenario the student would arrive in the postnatal ward and receive the ward report on all the women present. She would then be sent to 'care' for one six-bedded room with no instruction or evaluation of her skills. The midwife would tell her to 'call if you need me' and she would disappear into the next room to care for her group of women. A similar situation was often present in the labour ward, where fairly junior students would be placed with women in labour with little or no instruction other than to call the midwife in the next room if needed. Students became extremely anxious in these circumstances and the most graphic descriptions given by students were those which related to their experiences in the labour ward. The majority used words such as 'imprisoned, 'isolated' and 'confined' to describe how they felt when left alone with a woman in labour.

Preview   This approach tended to be used the most with fairly junior students who had little clinical knowledge but could be used with senior students entering a clinical area for the first time. A skill would be demonstrated once to the student, with the expectation that she could now continue on her own:

> We were shown when they came from labour ward ... once. They tend to say 'best way to do it is do it by yourself and if you have problems ...
> (Jackie, Set E, 10 months into course)

For most students this was the strategy used most consistently in the clinical area. Some students received even less instruction than that defined above. When Myrtle asked the ward sister about doing a CTG (cardiotocograph) she was told to 'go and do it and then I will come and check'. Myrtle had not undertaken one since her labour ward experience some three months ago and felt very unsure of her skill in this area. She felt compelled to ask a more senior student for assistance. This student informed her that she should not do a CTG until she had first done an abdominal assessment, but she forbore to assist her with this task. Myrtle solved her own dilemma by taking the woman's temperature instead.

A common complaint made by students was that if the midwife was asked to come because of a problem with a client she was often too busy to respond immediately. When she eventually came, the student had either solved the problem herself or moved onto someone else in her effort and anxiety to get her work done. This meant that although students were exposed to many learning opportunities, their learning was limited because they received so little information on how the solution to a problem could be achieved.

The numbers game Many students and midwives subscribed to the belief that having performed a number of skills automatically conferred an expertise upon them. One of the senior students discussed the number of abdominal palpations she had done but did not address the amount of confidence she felt when performing this skill:

> I have 160 palpations. I need to get a lot signed but no one has checked them for me. I was offered some supervision this week but I didn't need it.
>
> (Peggy, Set A, 15 months into course)

Observation of this student revealed her as still unsure of her abdominal palpations when performed on women in their second trimester, women who were obese or had excess amniotic fluid. Despite this she saw no need for someone to supervise her in this area because of the number she had completed. Another senior student felt that having performed vaginal examinations on 24 women she should not be feeling as unsure as she was:

> Once it gets to 6 centimetres – well, even 4 – I have trouble even though I've done 24.
>
> (Bronwen, Set B, 11 months into course)

Other senior students became very concerned that staff expected them to teach students when they themselves had only just completed their programme. They felt that their own skills were too uncertain for them to be expected to take responsibility for students. Some concern was also expressed that the institution had prepared students only to the extent of being able to work in that environment. The high-technology approach had left them feeling deprived of midwifery skills which might be required if they were to work elsewhere.

Factors assisting student learning

Many factors assisted students in their learning and with their opportunities to learn: the personality of the student, the motivation of the midwife for teaching and the time and opportunity to learn. The factors discussed in detail in this chapter are those which appeared from the data to have had most impact, namely teaching strategies of midwives, learning style of students and the nature of the learning climate in the institution.

Teaching strategies Generally midwives took an interest in teaching students and some felt a responsibility for what the students learned. This sense of responsibility was further increased with the introduction of mentorship. Unfortunately, in the hospital in which this study was undertaken, mentorship was not introduced in a manner that obtained the full acceptance of the senior midwives. This resulted in only the more conscientious midwives feeling the need to address the learning requirements of their mentees, who were often placed on different shifts from themselves. These midwives had to go out of their way to identify strategies that would aid the students in their learning during periods when they themselves were not present.

When faced with teaching skills that could not be seen, such as vaginal examinations or abdominal palpations, midwives were quite creative in their attempts to reproduce visually those parts of the skills the student was attempting to learn. The depiction of the birth canal as the S-bend under the sink or a banana, the thinning of the cervix as pulling a polo-necked jumper over your head with the neck gradually thinning and opening as it was pulled down, were strategies used to identify the non-visual component of the skill. Some midwives would draw pictures of what the student was feeling or sensing to aid her comprehension of the situation. Whatever method was used those midwives interested in teaching appeared to recognize the need for creative methods, despite the fact that very few had any education in teaching skills.

Students found that the most helpful procedure in learning skills with no visual component was to have the midwife perform the skill first and then guide and assess the student's performance. All students recognized the need for the midwife to evaluate them on their procedures and if the findings were not congruent to explain why this was so. Unfortunately, many midwives did not fully evaluate the student and, if they did, often failed to explain why the fetal position or rate of cervical dilation was different from that identified by the student. In these cases a learning opportunity was lost because the student, while recognizing she had made an error, rarely found out the cause.

Many students found the midwife 'talking through' skills to be very helpful, particularly in the early stages of the course. Some midwives did not do so because they felt too unsure of their own skills. Most students were aware of this insecurity, despite strategies used by the midwife to hide it. Students were helped more by the midwives' interest in teaching them than in how knowledgeable they were themselves. The type of midwife deemed most helpful to student learning was the one who felt comfortable with students and was responsive to their needs. A midwife did not have to be perceived as an expert practitioner, but did have to be responsive to a student's need for information, particularly with regard to learning how to make decisions about a woman's care. As may be expected, however, the midwives who were most comfortable with teaching students were those who were competent in their own skills.

Learning styles   The characteristics and motivation of a learner are important in any learning process. The learner's response to new experiences is determined by her experiences in the past; if the latter were successful then she will enter more fully into a new context and obtain more from the exposure (Boud, Keogh and Walker, 1985). These authors similarly suggest that negative experiences can create feelings of discomfort in the student when faced with a similar situation. Feelings of discomfort can interfere with learning if the student becomes preoccupied with emotional responses invoked by the memory of a negative experience.

The majority of student midwives come from a nursing background. As already identified by other researchers, learner nurses have not always had positive learning experiences (Orton, 1981; Jacka and Lewin, 1987; Ogier, 1989). Negative experiences during nursing may affect a student's response to her midwifery course. As a result, despite a career commitment to midwifery, the student may enter her programme with unresolved conflict. If such conflict is not resolved it may affect her future commitment to midwifery. Prior experience of this kind may also be a reason for the difficulty I had in identifying some student midwives' learning styles. Thus some may have felt the need during their nursing course to adapt their learning style to whatever learning opportunities were available, to the way in which teaching was provided and to the requirements of staff in the clinical areas. These strategies may then have been continued into life as a midwifery student.

Kolb (1984) defined learning style as the way in which individuals organize information and experience and believed that learning styles are acquired, consistent patterns of learner-environment interaction. Kolb also suggests, however, that people accommodate their styles to the learning opportunities presented. Active learners in this study were defined as using an accommodative style. This style entailed the acquisition of learning through concrete experience and active experimentation, with an approach to task accomplishment of risk-taking, trial and error and adaptation to changing situations. This appeared to be the style adopted by many students in this study.

Some students stated that they felt it necessary to behave in a compliant fashion in order to acquire learning opportunities. This accommodative behaviour, together with the fact that it emerged quite late in data analysis, meant I was able to identify only two styles of learning; these I described as active and passive. The active student learns best from new experiences, change, excitement and involvement in the experience. One student clearly identified herself with this style of learning:

I'm one you can sit and lecture me for days and it goes in one ear and out the other. I need to practise. Constructive teaching and practice are the methods by which I learn best.

(Merril, Set A, 16 months into course)

The passive learner is best illustrated by Linda, who described herself as being compliant, endeavouring to carry out, without question, tasks given to her by the midwife. Linda stated that at the beginning of her course she used to ask a lot of questions but was turned off by midwives who told her that she did not need to know the information at that time. Over a period of weeks she changed her style to one of compliance because she felt she would gain more knowledge and learning opportunities in this way.

Most nursing education research has identified student nurses as having active learning styles (Christensen, Lee and Bugg, 1979; Laschinger and Boss, 1984; O'Kell, 1988). One American study, however, has noted a passive learning style in a majority of university nursing students (Highfield, 1988). Kolb (1984) suggests that people enter disciplines which offer learning opportunities that are congruent with their learning styles. There has been little research, however, on what effects there are on learning styles when educators in the learning environment do not support a style of active learning. Laschinger and Boss (1984) suggest that nursing education can affect learning styles, while Highfield (1988) found it to have no effect whatever. Both studies had methodological problems which make it difficult to conclude whether the findings of one are more likely to be valid than those of the other. It would, however, be difficult to believe that teaching style would have no effect on students.

Evaluation and feedback Often it is not until a performance of a skill is complete that the student becomes aware that the outcome is other than the one she expected. She must then go back over the steps to identify what went wrong, and even the more experienced student may require help with this process.

Immediate feedback to help the student correct her performance of a skill can be provided by the midwife if she is present at the time. Providing the missing information is not easy, however, if she has not been present. Offering assistance through evaluation and feedback of a student's performance was not provided nearly as often as students required or wanted. Some students actively sought such information from their midwives, only to be rebuffed. Those midwives who did provide such insights were perceived in a very positive light by students who felt they were 'natural' teachers.

The majority of midwives appeared to believe they were providing sufficient feedback when they told the student they had 'got it wrong'. They would console students by saying that they would get it right with practice, but seemed unable or unaware of the need to obtain specific information on why or how the students had gone astray.

Factors interfering with learning

Communication was observed both to assist and to interfere with all types of learning throughout the study. Those midwives who knew how to communicate effectively with women and with their students were sought out by the latter. Unfortunately, many midwives did not have this facility, with the result that students were left to decode information or make up their own. As can be imagined this was not too successful, especially with the junior students. Poor communication enhanced the effect of many of the themes mentioned below; other findings on communication are available in Chamberlain (1992).

Anxiety The move from staff nurse to midwifery student created a great deal of anxiety in neophyte students because they lost not only status but also the security of the knowledge base of their previous profession. While most students expected to obtain some recognition for their previous nursing education, this rarely happened in the clinical environment. Indeed many midwives disabused students of the notion that such education was helpful in midwifery. Quite a few students had entered the programme knowing they would be treated as students but expecting to retain some of their previous status as staff nurses or sisters. More than one student complained of the lack of respect shown to her, given her previous professional experience:

> They forget that you're a qualified member of staff and they just see you as a student again, especially the more senior ones, and I feel it's a bit patronizing.
>
> (Myrtle, Set B, 9 months into course)

In addition, there was a difference in the way the students were treated by the educational staff and the service staff. Educators treated the students as professionals in the making and gave them some recognition for their previous career in nursing. This treatment created anxiety for students when the service staff then tended to dismiss previous professional experiences and yet treat them as staff able to provide a service. Post-registration student midwives will have had a period of experience of maternity care during their nursing course and it was surprising therefore that they experienced such an identity crisis. Midwifery teachers, when interviewing prospective students, usually emphasized role transition as a problem. The majority of students in this study claimed to be aware of this problem and to have prepared themselves for this eventuality. From the anxiety displayed, however, it was clear that such preparations were insufficient for this purpose. Other studies have similarly shown that student midwives receive little recognition of knowledge and experience gained during nursing, and that this is a source of discontent (Davies, 1988 and Chapter 5 in this volume; Robinson, 1991).

Anxiety was also engendered by the fact that the role and functions of the midwife, as taught by the staff in the school, bore little relationship to the realities of the clinical environment. Students, having been taught holistic midwifery and continuity of care, would find themselves expected to complete fragmented tasks in short periods of time in order to maintain efficiency and keep medical staff happy. How well the students 'fit in' in the clinical area at the beginning of their placements set the scene for their future placements and therefore was a source of great anxiety. One coping strategy used by some students to reduce anxiety was the threat to leave. Such threats were not carried out during the course of my study, but appeared to provide students with reassurance and with feelings of having some control over their programme.

Anxiety was also caused by placement in areas such as the labour ward or the special care baby unit, where the technology was complex and potential for problems enhanced. Few students felt adequately prepared for these areas, especially when staff shortages meant that they were often left to care for women on their own. Many midwives failed to recognize that students required a reorientation to clinical areas upon their return. Sometimes there had been a gap of six months from the time the student had last worked in the ward or clinic but midwives expected them to be able to carry on where they had left off many months previously. They failed to recognize that the students had had many different experiences during the interval and were unable to retain more than a minimal amount of information for that setting. The amount of information provided on their return was usually insufficient to enable the student to function competently. Few students felt able to identify this problem to a midwife and if they were asked often denied that such a problem existed in case they were thought of as stupid.

Conflict A major interference with student learning was caused by the presence of conflict in the workplace. Several conditions were identified as creating conflict, the first being the incongruence between students' and midwives' expectations as to what the student should accomplish in the clinical setting. The student had developed a set of expectations from the midwifery teachers concerning the clinical role of the midwife and this bore little relationship to the realities of practice in the clinical environment.

A second cause of conflict was that the student expected to be provided with clinical learning opportunities and then found these often did not provide effective learning or supervised practice. One reason for this was that the students and midwives held different goals concerning learning needs of the student. For the student the goal was competency in clinical skills. For the midwife the goal was to ensure that the student had sufficient skills to provide safe care for the women. Although the two goals need not be dichotomous they often were. In achieving her goal of competence the student would be complying with the goals of the midwife in providing safe care. Some midwives, however, stopped short of providing the student with the opportunity to obtain competence by teaching only the skill with no supervision, reflective time, rationale or feedback.

Conflict was also created when students' learning styles did not match the expectations of the midwives. Some midwives expected students to be passive recipients of teaching and rewarded students who behaved in this fashion. Midwives who expected students to be more active in learning would perceive students who had a passive style as not being interested in midwifery and in learning opportunities. In contrast, the active learning style of other students was threatening to some midwives and they would react by ignoring them or providing them with minimal information.

A previous career in nursing appeared to create its own drawbacks since many students felt demoralized by their change in status from managing care on a busy ward to being a student with little status or responsibility. Some students brought stereotypical nursing behaviours with them into midwifery which they were reluctant to dismiss and which were utilized in times of stress to reduce personal conflict. This tactic appeared to block the uptake of new midwifery knowledge and behaviour. One such example included a student who persisted in taking a woman's temperature despite the fact that she was having a very strong contraction at the time.

Many of the students received the same amount of close supervision regardless of the length of time they had been on the course and their level of expertise. This created conflict and frustration in the senior students and anxiety because of insufficient supervision in those who were more junior. Ogier (1989) similarly noted that senior student nurses became frustrated by not being provided with the freedom to plan their work and make their own decisions. Senior students in this study expressed the same frustration, complaining that one day they were students with no responsibility and the next they were midwives expected to make decisions and take full responsibility for a woman's care. For some the change was too drastic and resulted in newly-qualified midwives repeatedly requesting medical assistance for what should have been a midwifery decision.

Ward climate The ward climate has been identified clearly in studies of nursing education as a factor which could facilitate or inhibit learning (Howe, 1981; Jacka and Lewin, 1987; Ogier, 1989). The motivation of midwives to teach and the priority the institution placed on education were reflected in the climate of most wards. The ward climate was not a single entity but a composite of a variety of factors, such as the administrative structure, the aims of student learning, the methods of instruction and discipline and the teacher and the student. The ward teacher in this context was whichever midwife was working on the same shift as the student.

Students were able to identify fairly consistently those areas that provided them with the most effective teaching and learning opportunities. Wherever they worked within the institution their perception was that overall they had to initiate interactions to obtain learning opportunities. Community experience, however, was not perceived in the same manner. In only one ward in the institution was teaching time structured into the ward routine. Elsewhere it was rarely undertaken unless the ward happened to have a 'quiet period', Students felt that teaching was not a priority in the institution and they were looked upon as service staff rather than as students to be educated:

> I find you have to learn yourself – there's not much teaching and it's not up to much on labour ward. Considering it's a teaching hospital the teaching is poor. It's more trial and error.
>
> (Linda, Set A, 16 months into the course)

Senior students were very concerned that they had received training which prepared them only for work in the teaching institution. Many felt reluctant to consider a move elsewhere since the emphasis on technology had left them feeling too vulnerable for employment in hospitals which might place a heavier emphasis on midwifery skills. Hence those who wanted to practise 'midwifery' perceived a need to move to hospitals which supported such practices in order to learn how to be 'midwives'. In such cases, even though expecting to be qualified as midwives, the students said that they would not perceive themselves to be functioning as midwives, but to be still in a 'student' role.

The acceptance of inadequate learning conditions was fairly general and represented a widespread feeling of helplessness to effect change. All students were asked to evaluate their programme at the end of their course but each set recognized that their complaints were little different from those that had gone before. The complaints were made to both educational and service staff, but without follow-up from the educators changes rarely took place in the clinical area.

Reflection In the context of learning, 'reflection' is a generic term for intellectual and affective activities in which individuals engage to explore their experiences and to gain understanding. Boud, Keogh and Walker (1985) suggest that reflective time is needed in order to extract specific learning from an experience. It also enables the learner to identify other learning required in order to cope with additional experiences. The adoption of a reflective approach to learning has been associated with a deeper understanding of the knowledge inherent in learning experiences and with an individual having a more comprehensive approach to life.

My observations and the students' complaints clearly identified that little time was provided for reflective activity. When there is an absence of reflective time it is possible that students obtain only a superficial understanding of the knowledge that they should obtain from their clinical experiences. Students demonstrated a superficial approach in their attempts to 'copy' midwives' activities which they were not always able to integrate with the theory learned in the education department.

Some students performed tasks for which they were unable to provide a rationale. One teacher complained that when a student was asked why she was taking a blood pressure in the antenatal clinic she was unable to provide an answer. While a response of this nature was rare, it does serve to demonstrate that many students were unable to integrate theoretical knowledge provided in the classroom with the clinical skills utilized in the institution. It is to be expected that students in any profession will require expert help with this process of integration.

A method of reflective activity that students did find helpful was one identified as 'debriefing'. This entailed the educator, whether teacher or midwife, going over activities with the student in which they had both participated earlier. The educator would guide the student's understanding of the events that had occurred and the steps in the process in an objective fashion, attempting to remove any emotions that may have clouded the experience for the student. In this way the student was able to maximize the learning from her clinical experiences. In the event of a negative experience this strategy helped the student to come to terms with emotions engendered that might interfere with future learning. Unfortunately, as mentioned earlier, time was rarely made available for this exercise and this was to the detriment of student learning.

Organizational factors

Various organizational factors also inhibited student learning.

Staff shortages The amount of documentation required for admission, discharges and problems, combined with a shortage of staff, resulted in few midwives being available to students for teaching purposes. The rapid turnover of women as a result of 24- and 48-hour discharges also created a heavy workload for staff. The consequent lack of midwifery supervision meant that students continued with their 'trial and error' approach to learning.

Policies An added restriction in many areas, especially that of the labour ward, was the existence of hospital policies to determine practice. Simpson (1979) suggests that one of the reasons occupations such as nursing are only semi-professions is that the work is done largely in organizations in which tasks are defined and rules set out as to how they should be performed. In this respect midwifery is not unlike nursing. It is governed by policies often formulated by medical staff with varying amounts of input from midwives. Such policies, if adhered to by the midwife, provide little scope for independent professional judgement and for taking professional responsibility for care of women. The effect of policies on the role of the midwife has been explored in a number of studies (e.g. Robinson, 1989; Garcia and Garforth, 1991; Green *et al.*, 1994; Askham and Barbour, Chapter 3 in this volume). The fact that some policies were in fact only guidelines, and not to be treated as law, appeared to escape some midwives. They were too constrained by policies to demonstrate the art of decision-making and instead focused on a series of practical aspects of care. What was often role-modelled to the student was the request by the midwife for a medical consultation in situations that required a midwifery decision. As a result, some students were never exposed to learning opportunities which would have provided them with information on midwifery management of women in pregnancy, labour and the puerperium. Students were often more aware than staff of the appropriate use of such policies and the restrictive effect their use had on midwifery practice.

Medical interventions Few midwives or students appeared to be aware of the extent to which medical intervention interfered with student learning opportunities. This interference could be seen in medical interventions that interrupted midwifery care of a woman with a 'low-risk' pregnancy and in whose care a student might have been involved. In the antenatal clinic some women could not be discharged until seen by a doctor even though they had been thoroughly checked by a midwife. In one clinic very few women were discharged without being seen by doctors and in most cases the doctors were very junior, with far less experience than many of the midwives. Such policies meant that midwives often did not assess the women because they did not wish to subject them to two assessments: one by themselves and one by the doctor. All of these behaviours had an impact on students, who became very frustrated by the inability of the midwife to practise midwifery without medical supervision. It seems that in the study hospital circumstances in this respect have been very slow to change despite being a demonstrable source of concern nationally as far back as the late 1970s (Walker, 1976; Barnet, 1979; Robinson, Golden and Bradley, 1983).

Technology It was difficult to ascertain the extent to which midwives and students were aware of the inhibiting effects of technology on midwifery skills. Some midwives, trained in its use, were not conscious of how it had eroded their skills in midwifery. As a result, many students were taught the use of technology for monitoring women in labour and in antenatal care without being taught the appropriateness or otherwise of such use. Some midwives appeared to subscribe to the medical view that pregnancy and childbirth are normal only in retrospect. Monitoring, for example, was often taught in isolation and in a way that excluded an overall assessment of the woman and the course of her pregnancy.

Student as 'gofer' It was surprising that so few students complained of being treated as a 'gofer' (go for this and go for that). It was not uncommon for students to be interrupted in their care of a woman and be asked to fetch something from another ward, from medical records, or from haematology etc. While such treatment by midwifery staff was fairly common it was an expectation by the medical staff. Whatever the student was doing it was never considered important enough that it could not be interrupted for her to go on an errand. In the antenatal clinic one student I observed spent a great deal of her time running around getting equipment for doctors who would stand and wait for her return. Students were even expected to fill out laboratory forms which required medical signatures. If the student complained to a midwife she was rarely supported in her rebellion and actively encouraged to continue in order to 'keep the clinic moving'. For many students this activity reduced their sense of worth and left them questioning the independence of their new profession.

DISCUSSION

As noted at the beginning of the chapter this study took place at the end of the 1980s. Although a number of substantial changes in both practice and education have been instigated since that time, the importance of learning opportunities in the clinical environment remains unchanged. Hence, in this final section the implications of the findings for the education of student midwives are considered. The majority of midwives do remarkably well as teachers, considering the constraints under which they work. Teaching students to be competent midwives requires commitment and collaboration from both the education and the service staff. The education staff, however, cannot expect midwives providing services to teach students to function independently without providing more clinical assistance, support and physical presence in the wards than appeared to be the case in the research site.

An additional responsibility for educators is the appropriate selection of midwifery role models to act as mentors. Too often, midwives only recently qualified and feeling insecure in their own skills are expected to provide mentorship for students in the clinical area. Such midwives not only feel threatened by this responsibility but may react in a defensive fashion, which does not provide a positive or efficient learning experience for the student. Educators can help service staff recognize the needs of students and assist them to structure ward work in such a way that teaching is integrated into the routine. In addition, midwives need to be helped to understand what students need from them in order to learn skills. Better supervision is required in the early stages, with increasing independence as the student progresses through her course. Midwives have to ensure that students know where they went wrong and how it can be rectified. To be efficient in this area many midwives will need a course in communication skills.

The methods which midwives used to teach students clinical skills appear to have changed little over the years. However, the advent of technology has created a more anxiety-filled environment for the student. The way in which students learn skills is extremely important in how competent and self-directed they became subsequently. Students have to practise their skills to learn how 'to do' but such learning has to be focused. Students have to be helped to learn, just as most midwives have to learn how to teach and communicate not only with students but with their clients as well.

Midwives should be aware of how much anxiety students experience when exposed to new situations and skills. This type of anxiety, unless treated in a sympathetic way, can be disabling for the student and subsequently can interfere with her learning. It is also necessary to understand the anxiety and conflict experienced by those students who take up midwifery having first qualified as nurses. In the past the payment of salaries to student midwives may well have encouraged hospital administrators to regard students as staff and hence have insufficient numbers of qualified staff in post and expect students to make good the deficit. This type of situation results in insufficient teaching to meet the clinical needs of students. The move to making students supernumerary, and supporting them with education grants, can therefore only be viewed as a positive step for midwives as well as students.

Midwifery requires competent practitioners who can function independently if it is to move forward on the road to full professionalism. The creation of such practitioners requires motivation and the collaborative efforts of all midwives, whether educators, clinical staff or managers. It also means that midwives must continue to use and maintain their midwifery skills and decrease their dependence on technology. If midwives wish to regain and maintain their independence then they cannot be complacent about the education of those who follow. Not only do they owe it to themselves and the profession but also to the women and babies for whom they care.

REFERENCES

Barnett, Z. (1979) The changing pattern of maternity care and the future role of the midwife. *Midwives Chronicle and Nursing Notes*, **92**(1102), 381–4.

Bent, E.A. (1982) The growth and development of midwifery. In Allan, P. and Jolly, M. (eds), *Nursing, Midwifery and Health Visiting since 1900*. Faber & Faber, London.

Boud, D. Keogh, R. and Walker, W. (eds) (1985) *Reflection: Turning Experience into Learning*. Kegan Paul, London.

Chamberlain, M. (1992) Factors affecting students becoming competent in midwifery skills. In Robinson, S., Thomson, A.M. and Tickner, V. (eds), *Research and the Midwife: Conference Proceedings for 1991*. Department of Nursing, University of Manchester.

Chenitz, W.C. and Swanson, J.M.(1986) *From Practice to Grounded Theory? Qualitative Research in Nursing*. Addison-Wesley, Menlo Park. CA.

Christensen, M.G., Lee, C.A.B. and Bugg, B.W. (1979) Professional development of nurse practitioners as function of need motivation, learning style, and locus of control. *Nursing Research*, **23**, 51–6.

Cowell,B. and Wainwright, D. (1981) *Behind the Blue Door: The History of the Royal College of Midwives 1881–1981*. Ballière Tindall, London.

Davies, R.M. (1988) Midwifery: the happy end of nursing. An ethnographic study of initial encounters in a midwifery school. Unpublished Masters thesis, University of Wales.

Donnison, J. (1977) *Midwives and Medical Men: A History of Interprofessional Rivalries and Women's Rights*. Heinemann, London.

Donnison, J. (1988) *Midwives and Medical Men. A History of the Struggle for the Control of Childbirth*. Historical Publications, New Barnet, Herts.

Field, P.A. and Morse, J.M. (1985) *Nursing Research: The Application of Qualitative Approaches*. Croom Helm, London.

Garcia, J. and Garforth, S. (1991) Midwifery policies and policy-making. In Robinson, S. and Thomson, A.M. (eds), *Midwives, Research and Childbirth*, Vol. II. Chapman & Hall, London.

Glaser, B. and Strauss, A.L. (1967) *The Discovery of Grounded Theory*. Aldine, Chicago.

Green, J., Kitzinger, J. and Coupland, V. (1994) Midwives' responsibilities, medical staffing structures and women's choice in childbirth. In Robinson, S. and Thomson, A.M. (eds), *Midwives, Research and Childbirth*, Vol. III. Chapman & Hall, London.

Hammersley, M. and Atkinson, P. (1983) *Ethnography: Principles in Practice*. Tavistock, London.

Highfield, M. (1988) Learning styles. *Nurse Educator*, 13(6), 30–33.

House of Commons (1992) *Health Committee 2nd Report on Maternity Services*. HMSO, London.

Howe, C. (1981) *Acquiring Language in a Conversational Context*. Academic Press, London.

Jacka, K. and Lewin, D. (1987) *The Clinical Learning of Student Nurses* (NERU Report No. 6). King's College, University of London.

Kirkham, M. (1989) Midwives and information-giving during labour. In Robinson, S. and Thomson, A.M. (eds), *Midwives, Research and Childbirth*. Vol. I. Chapman & Hall, London.

Kolb, D.A (1984) *Experiential Learning: Experience as the Source of Learning and Development*. Prentice-Hall, Englewood Cliffs, NJ.

Lasching, H. and Boss, M. (1984) Learning styles of nursing students and career choices. *Journal of Advanced Nursing*, **9**, 375–8.

Lofland, L. and Lofland, J. (1984) *Analysing Social Settings: A guide to Qualitative Observation and Analysis* (2nd edn). Wadsworth, Belmont, CA.

Murphy-Black, T. (1991) Antenatal education: evaluation of a post-basic training course. In Robinson, S. and Thomson, A.M. (eds), *Midwives, Research and Childbirth*, Vol. II. Chapman & Hall, London.

Oakley, A. (1986) *The Captured Womb: A History of the Medical Care of Pregnant Women*. Basil Blackwell. Oxford.

Ogier, M. (1989) *Working and Learning: The Learning Environment in Clinical Nursing*. Scutari Press, London.

O'Kell, S.P. (1988) A study of the relationships between learning style, readiness for self-directed learning and teaching preference of learner nurses in one health district. *Nurse Education Today*, **8**, 197–204.

Orton, H.D. (1981) *Ward Learning Climate*. Royal College of Nursing. London.

Robinson, S. (1985) Responsibilities of midwives and medical staff: findings from a national survey. *Midwives Chronicle*, **98**(1116), 64–71.

Robinson, S. (1989) Caring for childbearing women: the inter-relationship between midwifery and medical responsibilities. In Robinson, S. and Thomson, A.M. (eds), *Midwives, Research and Childbirth*, Vol. I. Chapman & Hall, London, pp. 8–41.

Robinson, S. (1990) Maintaining the independence of the midwifery profession: a continuing struggle. In Garcia, J., Kilpatrick, R. and Richards, M. (eds), *The Politics of Maternity Care*. Clarendon Press, Oxford.

Robinson, S. (1991) Preparation for practice: the educational experiences and career intentions of newly qualified midwives. In Robinson, S. and Thomson, A.M. (eds), *Midwives, Research and Childbirth*, Vol. II. Chapman & Hall, London, pp. 302–345.

Robinson, S., Golden, J. and Bradley, S. (1983) *A Study of the Role and Responsibilities of the Midwife* (NERU Report No. 1). Nursing Education Research Unit, King's College, London.

Robinson, S., Thomson, A.M. and Tickner, V. (1989) Midwives' views and directions and developments in midwifery research. In Robinson, S. and Thomson, A.M. (eds), *Research and the Midwife: Conference Proceedings for 1988*. Nursing Research Unit, King's College, London University.

Rose, A.M. (1962) A systematic summary of symbolic interaction theory. In Rose, A.M. (ed.), *Human Behaviour and Social Processes: An Interactionist Approach*. Routledge & Kegan Paul, London.

Simpson, I. (1979) *From Student to Nurse: A Longitudinal Study of Socialisation*. Cambridge University Press, London.

Strauss, A. and Corbin, J. (1990) *Basics of Qualitative Research: Grounded Theory Procedures and Techniques*. Sage, Newbury Park.

Towler, J. and Bramall, J. (1986) *The Midwife in History and Society*. Croom Helm, London.

Vollman, A. (1989) The clinical instructor of nursing and the learning environment: a qualitative study. Unpublished doctoral dissertation, University of Ottawa. Canada.

Walker, J.F. (1976) Midwife or obstetric nurse? Some perceptions of midwives and obstetricians of the role of the midwife. *Journal of Advanced Nursing*, **1**(2), 129–38.

Wilson, H. (1985) *Research in Nursing*. Addison-Wesley, Don Mills, Ontario.

CHAPTER SEVEN

Progress and problems in midwifery education: some conclusions from published research

Sarah Robinson

Midwifery education is at a particularly challenging juncture in its history. Both the programmes leading to qualification as a midwife are now firmly linked to higher education, with courses offered at diploma and, increasingly, at degree level. Mergers with colleges of nursing and with institutions of higher education have presented opportunities for extending the knowledge base of midwifery and for increasing academic rigour (Roch, 1993). On the other hand difficulties have arisen over midwifery losing its unique identity in these larger institutions and in the often increased distance between educational facilities and the practice setting (Hall, 1994; Warwick, 1992). Those responsible for midwifery education are rising to the challenge of preparing students for the more independent role envisaged by the Expert Maternity Group (Department of Health, 1993). At the same time, midwife teachers are subject to an increasing range of pressures. They are required to attain graduate status, to maintain a credible clinical profile when often far removed from practice settings, and organize educational programmes within the complexities of the purchaser–provider system implemented by the NHS and Community Care Act of 1990.

Midwives in practice, like their colleagues in teaching, are also presented with various educational challenges. Continuing education opportunities have increased, and the range now includes post-graduate qualifications, post-basic teaching qualifications, National Board courses, a variety of diplomas in subjects such as counselling, study days and conferences on a diversity of topics, and updating for those who have been out of practice for a while. In addition to fulfilling statutory continuing education requirements, midwives may also find that demonstration of a high continuing education profile is increasingly important in relation to career prospects. At the same time, however, they may experience difficulties in obtaining funding and study leave to facilitate course attendance. Moreover, mentorship (or preceptorship) schemes have now been introduced in many maternity units, and midwives may find themselves asked to take greater responsibility for the guidance of students than hitherto (Kent, Mackeith and Maggs 1994a)

Although the present climate is very much one of change, nonetheless much in midwifery education remains constant. First-level preparation depends now, as it has always done, on the successful integration of clinical experience and theoretical knowledge. Continuing education, in the form of statutory refresher courses, has always been regarded as essential to the professional development of the midwife and to the delivery of high-quality care. In looking to the future, what evidence can midwives find from research upon which to base their educational strategies and policies? The purpose of this chapter is to try and answer that question by considering findings from published research on midwifery education in the United Kingdom.

At the outset criteria had to be determined as to what should be included in such a review. An initial problem was ascertaining whether or not a particular piece of research related to midwifery education. Research that at first appeared to relate only to nursing was found on further examination to have included midwifery respondents as well. In some instances data were provided separately for midwives, whereas in others this was not the case. Hence it was decided only to include work which focused on midwives and the processes involved in midwifery education. Research that focused primarily on midwifery practice, or an aspect of midwifery management, sometimes included an element concerned with midwifery education. Again a decision was made only to include studies with a primary focus on education.

The literature search indicated that a not inconsiderable volume of research into midwifery education is unpublished to date, mainly in the form of master's dissertations. Although a proportion of these dissertations are available centrally, for example in the Royal College of Midwives library, it is harder to ensure comprehensiveness than for published work, since many dissertations are available only from the institution in which the author was based. For the purpose of this chapter, a decision was made only to include published work.The following account therefore relates to published work which focused entirely or primarily on issues concerned with the education of midwives. Although an attempt has been made to be as comprehensive as possible, it is acknowledged that not all published work will have been included. It is also acknowledged that a more comprehensive review is required, that includes studies which focus on other health professionals as well as on midwives, together with unpublished work. Such a remit is in fact the first project to be undertaken at the recently established Midwifery Education Research and Development Unit at Surrey University (Pollock, 1992).

In looking at the volume of published midwifery research as a whole, it is striking that far fewer studies have focused on midwifery education than on either midwifery practice or on the role of the midwife in the maternity services. Attention was drawn to the paucity of research on midwifery education by those taking part in a 1989 survey of views about research developments in the profession (Robinson, Thomson and Tickner, 1989). Although a number of small- and large-scale projects have been completed since that time, recent reviews of midwifery research indicate that education still represents a small fraction of the total research output (e.g. Sims *et al.*, 1994). This is perhaps surprising, given that education is the basis upon which the provision of competent and knowledgeable practitioners depends. It is a matter of regret that the recent Delphi study of midwives' views of research priorities did not ask midwives for their views on priorities for midwifery education as well as for midwifery practice (Sleep and Clarke, 1993). A study by Hicks (1993) has shown that midwives who carry out research have often lacked the time or confidence to publish; it is possible that this may have had a greater impact on educational studies than on those other aspects of the profession.

The research reviewed in this chapter is divided into five main categories:

1. The kind of first-level courses that are required
2. Processes of recruitment and selection for first-level courses
3. Aspects of first-level courses – from curriculum design through to reasons why students leave
4. Opportunities for continuing education
5. Evaluation of particular continuing education courses.

In the following five sections, each of these categories is considered in turn. As well as a discussion of the findings, the aims and methods of the various studies are also presented in some detail, in order to provide the reader with an overview of the diversity of methods adopted and an indication of the confidence with which findings can be regarded. The format adopted for each of the above categories depends on the nature of the research studies which it comprises. In those categories consisting of several disparate studies, the methods and findings of each are considered in turn. In those in which several studies have addressed a similar range of topics, the methods of all the studies are considered together, followed by a discussion of the findings. Several studies addressed topics in more than one of the five categories of research. In these instances, the methods of the study are presented in the first category to which the study relates. The final section of the chapter considers those aspects of midwifery education to which the attention of researchers might now most usefully be directed.

Terminology in midwifery education has changed over the years; teacher is now used instead of tutor and education instead of training. Pre-registration midwifery programme has replaced direct entry course, and more recently the post-registration course has been renamed pre-registration midwifery programme (shortened) (UKCC 1994). For each of the studies reviewed in this chapter, the discussion uses the wording current at the time that the study was undertaken; to do otherwise might invite confusion when reference is made to the published work.

FIRST-LEVEL EDUCATION:
WHAT KIND OF COURSE IS NEEDED?

Two main questions have been asked about the kind of first-level education needed: the length of the post-registration course, and the rationale for introducing pre-registration courses for those without previous nursing qualifications. Decisions in these respects have not been based on research evidence, but studies have been undertaken to assess the extent to which the objectives of new courses have been met. Up until 1981, the main route to qualification as a midwife in the United Kingdom was a 12-month post-registration course and only a handful of courses were available for the direct entrant. Concern concentrated on the large numbers who took the post-registration course as a means of enhancing their nursing career and not because they wished to practise midwifery. Moreover, it was suggested that 12 months was too short a period to gain sufficient clinical confidence to wish to practise midwifery (Stewart, 1981). Consequently, the then Central Midwives Board decided to lengthen the course to 18 months, in the hope that this would increase confidence and deter those who took the course for collateral reasons.

A team at the Nursing Research Unit of King's College, London University, undertook a longitudinal comparative study of midwives qualifying from a 12-month course with midwives qualifying from an 18-month course, to determine whether the extended training did have the desired effect on midwives' confidence at the point of qualification, and on their career intentions and subsequent career paths (Golden, 1980; Robinson, 1986a, 1986b, 1991; Robinson, Owen and Jacka, 1992; Robinson, 1994; Robinson and Owen, 1994). A questionnaire was sent to a quarter of the midwives qualifying in England and Wales in 1979 after a 12-month course ($N = 932$), and the same questionnaire was then sent to a similar proportion of those qualifying in 1983 after an 18-month course ($N = 931$). Response rates of 84% and 89% were achieved for the two groups respectively. Topics investigated included the following: reasons for studying midwifery, intentions in relation to practising midwifery; aspects of clinical and classroom teaching; clinical experience; time for personal study; extent to which these newly qualified midwives felt adequately prepared for aspects of midwifery practice, and their enjoyment of the course. In 1986, a short questionnaire was sent to all members of the two cohorts who had returned the questionnaire sent to them at qualification. This second questionnaire sought the details of their career history in the intervening years. A subsequent questionnaire was then sent to those who had practised midwifery; response rates of 87% (319/394) and 82% (431/524) were obtained. In 1989 another questionnaire was sent to these respondents and response rates of 73% (288/394) and 78% (407/524) were achieved. The main findings in relation to course outcomes were small increases in the proportion who felt confident to practise, and in the proportion who intended to make a career in midwifery, but no difference in the proportion who subsequently remained in the profession. The King's College study provided information on many aspects of first-level and continuing education and these are discussed in subsequent sections.

Mander's Scottish study was similarly concerned with whether the longer course was associated with a greater likelihood of planning to practise midwifery and in subsequently doing so (Mander, 1989a, 1993). A questionnaire was sent to all those beginning the 12-month course in Scotland in December 1980 ($N = 303$) and all those beginning the 18-month course in December 1982 and March 1983 ($N = 397$). Seventy-two percent of these students returned the questionnaire sent to them at the start of their course; however, the response rate for those who completed the course ($N = 646$) was lower at 58%. The question focused on reasons for training as midwives, employment intentions and perceptions of various aspects of the course. Information from notification to practise records indicated whether respondents subsequently practised midwifery. Findings corroborated those of the King's College study; namely that the extended training made little difference to the proportion planning to practise midwifery and the proportion to do so.

The view that a new type of course should be introduced for those who did not wish to first train as nurses steadily gained ground during the 1980s. As Radford and Thompson (1988) observe, this view was driven by a number of imperatives: the projected decline in the number of school leavers from whom nursing and thus midwifery could draw and the need to recruit mature candidates who would not want first to qualify as a nurse; the continued waste of resources entailed in providing a course which many regarded as a stepping-stone in a nursing career; opposition to the inclusion of midwifery in the Project 2000 proposals for nurse education, and the view that desired changes in the role of the midwife in the maternity services required a different kind of educational preparation to the post-registration route. Taking up this latter point in more detail, then, the erosion of the midwife's role had been one of the profession's main concerns from the mid-1970s onwards. A number of studies had documented the disparity between the role for which the statutory body intended that the midwife be prepared and the one which she was able to fulfil in practice (Walker, 1976; Robinson *et al.*, 1983; Robinson, 1989; Green *et al.*, 1986; Garcia and Garforth, 1991). The main findings focused on the extent to which medical staff had eroded the midwife's responsibility for decision-making concerning the management of care of women who experience a normal pregnancy, labour and puerperium. The argument was advanced that direct entry would result in a more confident and independent practitioner and in one who was less 'doctor oriented', having not first been socialized to that effect in the course of nurse education (e.g. Association of Radical Midwives, 1986).

Despite commitment to the increased provision of direct entry courses by the English National Board (ENB), the Department of Health and Social Security and the Royal College of Midwives, little progress was made in this respect. Consequently, the ENB commissioned a research project to 'investigate what was inhibiting the implementation of direct entry courses and to recommend how development in this area could be fostered' (Radford and Thompson, 1988, 1994). The two researchers, Radford and Thompson, undertook their investigation by means of a three-phase study. The first phase comprised surveys by questionnaire of all regional and district health authorities and all schools of midwifery, in order to obtain information about current policy on course provision and factors that had encouraged or inhibited development. Response rates of 100%, 91% and 99% were obtained for regions, districts and schools respectively. In the second phase, questionnaires sent to a convenience sample of potential applicants for direct entry courses provided information about their background and reasons for wanting to train as a midwife. Interviews with key personnel in the profession and in a sample of schools comprised the third phase and provided information on a range of organizational issues concerning course provision.

Findings showed that overall there was a positive response to developing the new programmes, although only 13 were underway at the time of the research. Factors cited as sources of encouragement included assurance of financial support, evidence of demand for the course and a present and/or predicted shortage of midwives. Sources of constraint included uncertainty about funding, lack of information about demand, a shortage of tutors, and concerns about aspects of the organization and demands of the course. The last mentioned included availability of clinical placements, the preparation of education and service staff for the new course, and the need of students for supervision and support.

One of the main conclusions reached by Radford and Thompson was that the profession should clarify the kind of midwife that should be produced, since only then could appropriate target groups for recruitment be identified and appropriate courses designed. A diversity of view was indicated, in that some respondents felt nurse education was essential if the midwife was to cope with the full range of medical problems with which childbearing women might present, whereas others did not think this necessary. Moreover, if a more independent stance was to be assumed by the midwife, then greater educational investment in terms of quality and quantity was needed than if the midwife was to continue in the more restricted role identified by earlier studies.

In the period since the study was completed, the issue as to the role that midwives should fulfil has been resolved, following the publication of the Winterton Report (House of Commons Health Committee, 1992). This recommended that midwives should have greater professional independence – recommendations endorsed by the government with the publication of *Changing Childbirth* (Department of Health, 1993).

Radford and Thompson recommended that a programme of ongoing research was required to monitor the development of pre-registration midwifery education (Radford and Thompson, 1988) – a recommendation that has been heeded. A large-scale evaluation of many aspects of the implementation of pre-registration programmes was commissioned by the Department of Health in 1990, and reported in Kent, MacKeith and Maggs (1994a, 1994b), and the ENB commissioned a project in 1993 on the effectiveness of these programmes in terms of intended and actual outcomes (English National Board, 1993). Methods for the former study are discussed in the section on first-level education; the latter study has not yet been completed.

The study by Kent, MacKeith and Maggs (1994a, 1994b) showed nationwide provision of pre-registration courses, and a widespread commitment to their success, despite various problems that are described in subsequent sections of this chapter. This study also indicated a decrease in some areas in the number of post-registration courses offered. Research is now required to assess whether there is a demand for these courses from people qualifying as nurses via the Project 2000 route, but who decide subsequently to qualify as midwives.

FIRST-LEVEL EDUCATION: RECRUITMENT AND SELECTION OF STUDENTS

One of the main findings from the Radford and Thompson study (1988) was concern about recruitment and selection for pre-registration programmes. At many schools it was difficult to obtain information on how many people had enquired about the new courses, and the need for detailed records of enquiries to monitor demand was highlighted. Recommendations were made that resources of time and personnel were needed to deal with the process of advertising the course and handling enquiries and applications. Concerns were raised by respondents about the process of selection, since the diversity of applicant was likely to make this a more complex task than selection for the post-registration courses. Recommendations were made that staff should receive training in this respect.

Given the importance of the process of selection in determining the future composition of the profession, then those charged with responsibility for selecting students for pre-registration courses might perhaps have expected that they could turn to research for guidance on selection for post-registration courses. It is, however, a subject on which little research exists. The only major investigation on selection for post-registration courses is that undertaken by Phillips and reported in this volume (Chapter 4) and in Phillips (1993).

Phillips' study was undertaken by means of a survey by postal questionnaire sent to all Senior Midwife Teachers in England and Wales in 1988; a response rate of 95% was achieved. The study focused on the criteria which teachers believed to be important in applicants for midwifery and on the methods for selection. Findings demonstrated that selection of students entailed a vast information-gathering exercise that was not necessarily cost effective and that the decision to select was often based on relatively subjective criteria and processes. Phillips concluded that student selection merited further investigation.

Little subsequent research, however, has focused on the subject, with the exception of Kent, MacKeith and Maggs' study of pre-registration midwifery (1994a, 1994b). Investigation of recruitment and selection took place in five of the 16 sites offering pre-registration courses at that time. Methods included analysis of documentation pertaining to recruitment and selection processes, interviews with the key selector at each site and observation of interviews at four sites. A questionnaire on the topic was sent to key personnel at each of the 16 sites involved in the overall evaluation. Published findings to date do not include the observational data.

The findings demonstrated that centres offering the programme continued to receive large numbers of enquiries and that the potential source of applicants was not drying up, as some had originally feared. Midwifery teachers said that dealing with these enquiries, and arranging informal visits, were extremely time-consuming activities. The courses were advertised in a diversity of ways, but those which midwife teachers felt would be most valuable, such as presentations at careers fairs and visiting local secondary schools, were too time consuming to consider. As Radford and Thompson (1988) had suggested, this was an aspect of the new courses that would require resources, but Kent, MacKeith and Maggs (1994a) indicated that these were not always available. The latter study revealed that those involved in the process of selection were sometimes uncertain as to the qualities being sought. There was agreement, however, that evidence of motivation to become a midwife, and some awareness of what being a midwife would involve, were the most important criteria. Phillips' study, however, showed that ability to express an opinion verbally, an interest in current affairs and assertiveness were the three criteria cited most often as being important in the prospective student midwife (Chapter 4 in this volume).

Some findings do exist on the characteristics of those who are selected for midwifery courses. Information on those taking post-registration courses is provided in Robinson (1986b) and Mander (1989b), and those taking pre-registration courses in Kent, MacKeith and Maggs (1994a, 1994b). Direct comparisons are not always feasible, since question formats differed, but some general conclusions can be drawn on age structure and ethnic group. Findings show that pre-registration courses are, as anticipated, attracting a higher proportion of older entrants than did the post-registration courses. Moreover, half of the entrants to pre-registration courses had children under 16. Findings on ethnic group in the King's College study (Robinson, Owen and Jacka, 1992) showed that the proportion describing themselves as West

Indian, African, Indian, Pakistani or other Asian decreased from 28% of the 1979 cohort to 16% of the 1983 cohort. The question on ethnic group put to the pre-registration group differed in format from that used in the King's College study; findings showed that 97% gave 'white' as their ethnic origin (Kent, MacKeith and Maggs, 1994a). Findings on the representation of ethnic minorities in the student midwife population are open to a variety of interpretations. The pre-registration study, for example, indicated that midwife teachers felt that they had been unsuccessful in making information about the course accessible to potential recruits from these groups. Moreover, the development of equal opportunities policies in the selection process were at a fairly early stage in most sites (Kent, MacKeith and Maggs, 1994a). Recruitment and selection to midwifery courses is a subject which has been little researched, and completed studies indicate a range of issues, concerning diversity and subjectivity of criteria, that merit further investigation.

FIRST-LEVEL EDUCATION: ASPECTS OF THE COURSES

Most of the research on first-level education has focused on the post-registration route. This reflects the fact that by the time research in midwifery started to gather momentum, the pre-registration route had all but disappeared. By the mid-1980s only one school of midwifery offered courses for those without nursing qualifications (Radford and Thompson, 1988). By the late 1980s, the decision had been made to introduce pre-registration midwifery programmes which differed substantially from the earlier 'direct entrant' courses. As already observed, the factors inhibiting or encouraging the development of these courses were researched by Radford and Thompson (1988, 1994). The development of pre-registration programmes in fact rapidly gathered pace and by 1994 more than 30 courses were in progress. Consequently, the research focus is shifting towards the pre-registration route. As noted, a major evaluation of the implementation of these courses has recently been published (Kent, MacKeith and Maggs, 1994a, 1994b), and at least one other major study has been commissioned (English National Board, 1993). The next two sections of the chapter focus respectively on the aims and methods of this group of studies of post-registration and pre-registration courses, and on the main findings that have emerged.

Aims and methods of research on aspects of first-level courses

The studies concerned primarily with the effects of lengthening the post-registration course all drew samples on a national basis. The King's College study of midwives in England and Wales (Golden, 1980; Robinson, 1986a,

1986b, 1991) and Mander's study of midwives in Scotland (Mander, 1989a, 1993) both entailed comparisons of 18-month cohorts with 12-month cohorts. The methods for both of these studies have already been described, since findings related to other categories of research reviewed as well as to first-level education.

A second Scottish study (Pope, 1986) differed in design from the other two concerned with lengthening midwifery training, in that the perspectives of qualified midwives on the new training were sought as well as those of students, and only the 18-month course was investigated. Questionnaires were sent to the 1128 midwives working in institutions in Scotland, asking for their views on the style and content of the course and on the ability of newly registered midwives to function as competent team members. Only 53% responded which, as Pope comments, was disappointingly low from a group who might have been expected to have a particular interest in the subject. A second questionnaire, sent to all the 209 students who completed the course in January 1985, achieved a response rate of 64%. This focused on perceptions of course content, types of teaching, sequence and quantity of clinical experience, and how well prepared students felt to function as a midwife.

When the other post-registration studies were undertaken, comparison with the 12-month course was no longer an issue, and each was concerned with particular aspects of the 18-month course alone. Opoku and Davis (1988) reported on a study of the processes involved in designing a new 18-month course curriculum; as midwife teachers they undertook the research as participant observers. Leong (1989) focused on the introduction of computer-assisted learning into the midwifery curriculum in one college. The study entailed a small-scale qualitative evaluation of the usefulness of a computerized care plan programme to assist students in learning about the management of pre-term labour; eight students were observed using the programme and then interviewed about their perceptions of its usefulness. Mitchell (1994) similarly undertook a small-scale study in one college to explore students' and teachers' perceptions and experiences of portfolios as a means of student assessment. Questionnaires were sent to 24 post-registration students and interviews held with the eight teachers who worked with them.

Three studies (Chamberlain, 1992, and Chapter 6 in this volume; McCrea *et al.*, 1994; West and Thomson, 1995) focused on student experiences in the clinical settings. Chamberlain's study adopted a qualitative approach and entailed both observation and interviewing. Twenty-five students from six stages of a post-registration course at one college were observed while practising midwifery skills during an eight-month period, and interviewed at regular intervals throughout this time about their perceptions of learning experiences. Interviews were also held with qualified staff and with midwife teachers and managers. Findings took the form of themes that emerged from a process of analytic induction. Similarly, studies undertaken by McCrea *et al.* (1994) and West and Thomson (1995) were based in one unit. McCrea *et al.* (1994) sent questionnaires to 66 student midwives at varying points of a course, 64% of whom responded. West and Thomson (1995) sent question-naires to 10 student midwives, their 9 labour ward mentors and 2 midwife teachers; all respondents were subsequently interviewed.

The research by Davies (1991 and Chapter 5 in this volume) and Raymond and Ananda-Rajan (1993) focused on both the clinical and the academic aspects of the post-registration course. Davies undertook a small-scale qualitative study of nine student midwives during the first 18 weeks of their course. By means of observation, interview and respondents' diaries she explored their perceptions of the world of midwifery. Raymond and Ananda-Rajan (1993) sent questionnaires to 85 student midwives in one college at different stages of the course. The questionnaire focused on stu-dents' needs and views in the light of developments in midwifery education at that time; an 80% response rate was achieved.

As observed earlier, research interest is now focusing on the pre-registration programmes, and the first major evaluation of this important development in midwifery education has recently been published (Kent, MacKeith and Maggs, 1994a, 1994b). This evaluation was commissioned and funded by the Department of Health for England and Wales, undertaken by an independ-ent research organization, and sought to answer two questions:

1. What are the workforce implications of the introduction of pre-registration midwifery education?
2. What are the views of those involved in pre-registration midwifery?

The project team adopted an ambitious multi-method design, comprising six main elements. The first was a survey of all midwifery units and regional health authorities to explore the workforce implications of the new programme. This part of the research had to be abandoned, since many respondents were either unwilling or unable to provide the information requested (Kent, MacKeith and Maggs, 1994a). The second element was a sur-vey undertaken in 1991 in the 16 sites in which courses were then established; this entailed sending questionnaires to midwifery students, teachers and man-agers, together with analysis of course documentation. Seventy-seven per cent (557) of students returned a questionnaire; the number of respondents are given for the other groups, but not the proportion this represented of those eligible to participate. The third element was an in-depth case study of six of the 16 sites; this comprised the substantive part of the study and adopted what the authors described as a democratic, responsive and reflexive approach to evaluation (Kent, MacKeith and Maggs, 1994a). Data collec-tion at the six sites was by means of semi-structured interviews with mid-wifery students, mentors, teachers, service and clinical managers and with non-midwife teachers and obstetricians. Group enquiry with students in two of the six sites formed the fourth element of the study; these groups met every three to four months over a two-year period to discuss what they perceived as important issues in their course. Recruitment and selection formed the subject of the fifth part of the study; this was undertaken in five of the sites that had not been included in the in-depth phase. Finally a survey of students who had left the course sought to determine the reasons for making this decision. Most of the reported data from this study are presented in the form of themes that emerged from the case study interviews, supplemented by the questionnaire survey, and provided information on many aspects of pre-registration courses.

In 1993 the ENB commissioned a three-year study to examine the effectiveness of pre-registration midwifery programmes with a focus on actual and intended outcomes. The project is a collaboration between a University Faculty of Education and a College of Nursing and Midwifery, and comprises two phases. The first seeks to establish whether the programmes are effective in producing midwives who are confident and competent to practise at the point of registration, and the second focuses on evaluating progress in the first year after registration (Fraser, Murphy and Worth-Butler 1994). At the time of writing the project is at the mid-point; publications to date have focused on the concept of competence (Worth-Butler, Murphy and Fraser, 1994, 1995) and an analysis of curriculum documents from 23 institutions (Mountford *et al.*, 1995).

The foregoing has shown that published research into aspects of first-level courses encompasses studies of varying size and scope, which have employed a diversity of methods: questionnaire surveys, document analysis, interviewing and observation. Most of the research has taken the form of survey by questionnaire and, in the main, high response rates have been achieved. This, combined with the fact that much of the questionnaire data have been corroborated by interview material, means that findings overall can be regarded with confidence. These are discussed in the next section, grouped into the following six themes: the midwifery curriculum; the clinical learning environment; college experience; integration of theory and practice; adequacy of preparation for midwifery practice, and students who leave before course completion.

Findings from research on aspects of first-level courses

The midwifery curriculum Research has focused on both the process of designing curricula for midwifery programmes and on cross-centre analysis of curriculum documents in order to identify commonalities and differences. Opoku and Davis's study (1988) shows that if a new curriculum is to be successfully implemented, then its underlying philosophy has to be negotiated with all those who will be involved – service staff, midwife teachers and students. The study also demonstrated, however, that this is a time-consuming process if ongoing commitment to curriculum development is to be maintained.

The process of negotiation in curriculum design is explored in detail in the case study phase of Kent, MacKeith and Maggs' (1994b) evaluation of pre-registration midwifery programmes and two main findings emerge. First, midwife teachers were likely to have to negotiate curriculum design not only with service colleagues, but also with staff of the colleges and institutions of higher education with which midwifery schools have been amalgamated. Secondly, the process of negotiation was likely to centre on concerns about midwifery control of the curriculum, in particular that the needs of student midwives might not always be the prime focus of those who have an input into teaching.

Both of the large-scale evaluations of pre-registration programmes (Kent, MacKeith and Maggs, 1994a, 1994b; Mountford *et al.*, 1995) have involved analysis of curriculum documents at an early stage of the project. Following the identification of a framework of categories, each document was then considered within this context. Mountford *et al.*'s first category focused on the purpose and presentation of the document; each represented a very substantial amount of work, yet in the main appeared to have been written primarily for the validating body, rather than in a format and style which could be used effectively by staff and students of the institution. Both studies demonstrated that all curricula emphasized childbirth as a natural process, and the role of the midwife as a reflective practitioner able to provide total woman-centred care on her/his own responsibility. Another category in both analyses focused on the relationship between theory and practice and on curriculum structure. The main distinction between courses related to whether there was an initial period for 'foundation' knowledge upon which midwifery knowledge was then developed, or whether pure subjects and 'application to midwifery' were taught in parallel from the outset of the course (Kent, MacKeith and Maggs, 1994b; Mountford *et al.*, 1995). Finally, Mountford *et al.*'s analysis focused in particular on information provided about methods of assessing competence, since this was the main focus of the larger project (Fraser, Murphy and Worth-Butler, 1994). All documents described a progression of intellectual, practical and professional competencies to be achieved, although there were differences in the way the levels of progression were defined. The analysis similarly indicated that student profiles had been designed by all institutions to assess competence in practice, but that the details varied.

The clinical learning environment The majority of published research findings on post-registration courses focus on students' experiences in clinical settings. This is not surprising, since it is primarily in this environment that students develop clinical skills and gain the confidence that may well lead to a decision to practise after qualification. As observed earlier, it was concern that the 12-month course afforded insufficient time to gain clinical confidence that lay behind the decision to extend the length of the course

(Stewart, 1981). The King's College study (Robinson, 1986a, 1991) showed that the majority (73%) of those qualifying after an 18-month course still felt that they had not had enough time in clinical areas, although the proportion was smaller than that for the 12-month qualifiers (85%). Areas in which 18-month respondents were most likely to want more time were obstetric theatre (50%), special care baby unit (37%) and the labour ward (28%). The comments made most frequently in relation to labour ward experience were an over-emphasis on obtaining the required number of deliveries and insufficient time in caring for the baby after delivery. Both these comments were echoed by the 34% of respondents in Pope's study who felt that they needed more time in the labour ward (Pope, 1986). West and Thomson (1995) found that students had insufficient experience of antenatal wards and of the special care baby unit. Findings for labour ward experience showed concerns about an over-emphasis on deliveries at the expense of care during labour, and insufficient experience of performing episiotomies, perineal suturing and caring for women with a breech presentation. The study by Raymond and Ananda-Rajan (1993), showed that most respondents wanted a flexible course design, that allowed them to identify and return to those areas in which they felt they needed more time to consolidate clinical skills.

Turning to teaching in clinical areas, the research studies reviewed have varied in the amount of detail in which this topic has been addressed. One of the most detailed accounts of teaching strategies employed by staff is provided by Chamberlain (Chapter 6 in this volume). The main finding to emerge from all studies is that the majority of student midwives feel they do not have enough clinical teaching. The study by Robinson (1986a, 1991) looked separately at helpfulness and amount of clinical teaching. The majority of those who took an 18-month course found clinical teaching helpful; figures were 61% for teaching from paediatric medical staff, 66% for obstetric medical staff, 83% for midwifery tutors, 91% for hospital midwives and 93% for community midwives. Respondents were, however, much less likely to say that they had had enough clinical teaching; the proportion who said they had too little was 58% for teaching from paediatric medical staff, 56% for obstetric medical staff, 54% for hospital midwives, and 42% for midwifery tutors. Only 16% said they had insufficient teaching from community midwives, no doubt reflecting the fact that there is usually a one-to-one relationship between midwife and student during community experience.

The participants in Pope's study were asked a generic question about clinical teaching; 66% of respondents said that they did not have enough (Pope, 1986). When asked from whom they would have liked more clinical teaching, then clinical teachers, midwives, doctors and midwife teachers were cited in that order. All the respondents in Raymond and Ananda-Rajan's study (1993) expressed a desire for more teaching in clinical areas, and they all wanted more contact with, and support from, midwifery teachers, especially in clinical areas. McCrea *et al.,* (1994) asked only about teaching from qualified staff in the wards; 67% of their respondents felt that they had not had enough. Similar findings emerge from interviews held with students participating in Chamberlain's study (Chapter 6 in this volume).

Several of the studies discussed above offered reasons why qualified staff and midwifery tutors might not be able to provide the amount of clinical teaching that students desired; these were based on respondents' comments and on researchers' observations. Turning first to midwifery tutors, comments made by 18-month qualifiers in Robinson's study suggested that there were not enough tutors for them to spend sufficient time teaching in clinical settings (Robinson, 1986a, 1991). This perception was corroborated by other research undertaken at the time the courses were in progress (Standon-Batt, 1979; Robinson, 1980). The view that there are not enough midwife teachers in post to meet the many demands on their time has persisted throughout the 1980s and early 1990s, and has been highlighted recently by those concerned about current developments in midwifery education (Hall, 1994; Warwick, 1992). Findings from the Kent, MacKeith and Maggs (1994a, 1994b) evaluation suggest that this situation is likely to get worse; midwifery teachers were finding it much more difficult to spend time in clinical settings, due to the increased distance between these and the educational institutions in which teachers were based.

Short-staffing on wards has similarly been cited as a reason why qualified staff are unable to meet students' needs for teaching. Respondents in the studies by Robinson (1986a, 1991), Raymond and Ananda-Rajan (1993) and Chamberlain (Chapter 6 in the volume) drew attention to the problem. McCrea *et al.* (1994) asked participants in their study to rate the level of staffing in the clinical areas in which they had been placed: 67% said day duty shifts were understaffed or very understaffed; the corresponding figure for night duty was 78%. From an analysis of the ratio of qualified to unqualified staff in the wards, the authors concluded that the problem was one of qualified staff having to spend so much time on administration that they were not available for clinical teaching, rather than one of short staffing (McCrea *et al.*, 1994). The other reason suggested for lack of teaching by qualified staff is that they feel ill prepared to do so. Walker (1990) comments that little research has focuses on the extent to which staff are prepared for their teaching role. Her own study focused on two aspects of this preparation: attendance at specific courses and keeping up to date.

Recent years have seen the introduction of a mentoring system in many midwifery units, in which each student is paired with a qualified midwife who acts as a personal teacher and, in some instances, also as an assessor of progress. Chamberlain (Chapter 6 in this volume) highlights the problem of recently qualified midwives acting as mentors. Raymond and Ananda-Rajan (1993) comment from their own experience, that newly qualified midwives do not feel adequately prepared to take on the role of effective mentor to students, and that time is needed to consolidate their own knowledge and experience before doing so. Problems with mentorship is one of the main themes to emerge from the Kent, MacKeith and Maggs (1994a, 1994b) evaluation of pre-registration midwifery programmes. Difficulties identified included the following: widespread confusion about objectives of the scheme; lack of understanding about the process of assessment; students feeling that mentors had no overview of the course; mentors struggling with heavy workloads and staffing shortages, and lack of access to midwife teachers. Mentorship is clearly an area which requires further and ongoing research; a useful review of the methodological problems confronting researchers in this field is provided by Maggs (1994).

College experience The earlier studies on post-registration courses showed that classroom teaching was much less likely than clinical teaching to be problematic. Eighty-four per cent of the 18-month qualifiers who took part in Robinson's study said the amount of classroom teaching by midwifery tutors was about right and that it was helpful or very helpful (Robinson, 1986a, 1991). Pope (1986) found that students expressed satisfaction with the content and composition of study blocks, although some would have liked more teaching in college from midwife teachers and from midwives working in specialist fields.

Leong's study of computer-assisted learning showed that following an introductory session, students found a computer-assisted learning programme to be both user friendly and an aid to learning (Leong, 1989). The introduction of computer-assisted learning is in keeping with the general trend towards a more student-centred, self-directed approach (e.g. Royal College of Midwives, 1987). However, Raymond and Ananda-Rajan's study (1993) showed that in the early weeks of the course the majority of respondents would have preferred more formal teaching and less self-directed learning. As some of their respondents observed, self-directed learning is a skill that needs to be taught if it is to be an effective approach. The majority of respondents in this study felt that courses could be more academically challenging, with many commenting that they would have welcomed the opportunity to make a more thorough review of research-based practices (Raymond and Ananda-Rajan, 1993).

Students participating in the evaluation of pre-registration midwifery programmes generally regarded the content of classroom teaching as helpful and appropriate (Kent, MacKeith and Maggs, 1994a, 1994b). One of the main concerns raised in this study, by both midwifery students and teachers, was shared learning with non-midwifery students. While recognizing the benefits of shared learning in promoting good inter-professional relationships, concerns were expressed that the needs and interests of midwifery students would be neglected, particularly since they were usually in a minority in the class.

Integration of theory and practice Another theme addressed in studies of post-and pre-registration courses is the integration between the theoretical and practical components of the course. This has had two aspects: the sequencing of teaching in relation to corresponding clinical experience, and the extent to which the content of classroom teaching matches the reality experienced in the clinical situation. Programme sequencing was explored by Pope (1986) and by Kent, MacKeith and Maggs (1994a, 1994b). The majority of students and qualified staff participating in the former study expressed themselves as satisfied with the sequence (Pope, 1986). The Kent, MacKeith and Maggs (1994a, 1994b) study explored the pattern of placements in detail in the six case study sites; the main findings were that the sequence of placements was sometimes out of step with planned teaching of theory in the classroom; there was uncertainty about what was most beneficial to students keen to gain practical experience, and placement patterns were influenced by managerial needs to move students and by staffing levels.

A key finding from studies of both post-and pre-registration courses has been the disparity between the role of midwife as promulgated in classroom teaching and the role actually fulfilled in clinical practice. The former has tended to portray the midwife as a 'practitioner in her own right', whereas the latter, as discussed earlier in this chapter, has been characterized by an erosion of that level of responsibility by the involvement of medical staff in normal maternity care. The two qualitative studies included in this volume (Davies in Chapter 5 and Chamberlain in Chapter 6) demonstrate the way in which this is made manifest to student midwives as their course progresses, and it was a key theme to emerge from the group discussions held with students on pre-registration courses (Kent, MacKeith and Maggs, 1994a, 1994b). For a few students this disparity has been cited as a reason for deciding not to practise midwifery after qualification (Robinson, Owen and Jacka, 1992; McCrea *et al.*, 1994).

Adequacy of preparation for midwifery practice Earlier studies (Pope, 1986; Robinson, 1986a, 1991; Mander, 1989b) focused on the extent to which students themselves felt that their course had prepared them for practice. The main conclusion was that student midwives did feel well prepared by their course, although they identified some aspects of care for which they did not feel confident. Pope (1986) reports that 71% of students considered that they were able to 'function as full members of the midwifery team' and that 99% thought they had learned 'how to provide an acceptable standard of care for mothers and babies'. Eighty-one per cent of qualified midwives participating in the study concurred with the students' assessment of their capabilities. Robinson (1986a, 1991) asked students how well prepared they felt for 15 aspects of responsibility for practice and Mander (1989b) asked students how confident they felt in relation to 12 essential midwifery tasks.

The findings from the first study, reported in full in Robinson (1986a, 1991 and Robinson, Owen and Jacka 1992) showed that the majority of the 12-month and 18-month qualifiers felt that their course had prepared them adequately or more than adequately for the various aspects of care listed, with the exception of home confinements and special care baby units. For most items, the 18-month qualifiers were significantly more likely to feel adequately prepared than the 12-month qualifiers. This difference between the two cohorts, however, appeared to be a transient phenomenon. As already described, the 1979 and 1983 cohorts also took part in a longitudinal study which followed their careers after qualification for 10 and six years respectively (Robinson, Owen and Jacka, 1992; Robinson and Owen, 1994). Respondents were asked how well their course had prepared them for the responsibilities of their first midwifery post. For each clinical setting the majority of respondents said that their course had prepared them adequately, but the difference between the two cohorts observed at qualification had disappeared or decreased to a level that was not statistically significant. This finding emphasizes the importance of assessing whether differences observed at course completion persist over time; this point is returned to in the section on continuing education.

There was some indication from the study by Robinson *et al.* that adequacy of preparation was associated with intentions to practise midwifery (reported in Robinson, 1991; Robinson, Owen and Jacka, 1992), but this association was not found for the respondents in Mander's study (1989b). The relationship between perceptions of adequacy of a course and intentions about post-qualification employment is complex and requires more detailed investigation than has been carried out hitherto.

In studies of course outcomes the focus is now moving to methods of assessment of competence, rather than students' reports of their feelings of adequacy. A number of studies have been undertaken to assess the competencies of student nurses (While, 1994; Bedford *et al.* 1993); the latter study also involved midwives, although the findings were not presented separately. Reviews of the extensive literature on competence have attempted to define how the construct differs from those of performance and capability, and have considered the difficulties in assessing competence (While, 1994; Worth-Butler, Murphy and Fraser, 1994; 1995). Consequently findings from studies of competencies of student midwives are awaited with interest.

Systems of continuous assessment have been incorporated into the midwifery curriculum in recent years; one aspect of this development has been the introduction of student portfolios. Mitchell's study (1994) of perceptions of portfolios indicates the importance of evaluating innovations in education. Findings from her study showed that students were more likely to hold negative than positive perceptions of portfolios: in particular that they were time consuming to complete, students were anxious and uncertain about what was required and use of portfolios identified weaknesses in performance without indicating strategies for improvement. On the other hand students found that the use of portfolios encouraged further reading and led to increased communication with teachers. The teachers themselves had a much more positive assessment of portfolios than students. Mitchell recommended that students should be given adequate guidance and support in using their portfolios (Mitchell, 1994).

Students who leave Reasons for leaving a midwifery course before completion have been investigated in two studies (Mander, 1984; Kent, MacKeith and Maggs 1994a, 1994b). Mander's study of employment intentions of student midwives had, as noted earlier, involved sending questionnaires to some 700 students at the start of their course. A comparison of questionnaires returned at this time by those who went on to complete the course, with questionnaires returned by those who subsequently left, revealed differences between the two groups (Mander, 1984). Those who left were more likely than those who stayed to have made the decision to train as a midwife within the year prior to course commencement. Moreover, the leavers were more likely than the stayers to perceive childbirth as a natural, home-based event. Mander suggests that these students left because they may have entered midwifery with what, at that time, were unrealistic expectations about the profession. Leavers from the pre-registration courses studied by Kent, MacKeith and Maggs (1994a, 1994b) were interviewed about their reasons for doing so; reasons cited included unmet expectations about the course, failing an assessment, or personal reasons such as a partner having to move. Interviews with leavers led the authors of the report to conclude that these problems might have been overcome with support and counselling.

In retrospect: research on aspects of first-level courses

Looking back at the findings discussed in this section on first-level courses, then, lack of satisfaction with the amount of teaching in clinical settings has been a recurring theme. Findings from recent studies indicate that control over midwifery education may now be the main area of concern. However, it is important not to lose sight of the fact that the majority of respondents had reached the end of their course feeling confident to practise midwifery. Moreover, the majority of those completing post-registration courses did so with the intention of practising midwifery, even if not to make a career in the profession (Robinson, 1986b; Mander, 1989a). Those taking pre-registration courses are even more likely to want to practise midwifery upon qualification, since most entered with the specific intention of wanting to become a midwife (Kent, MacKeith and Maggs, 1994a).

CONTINUING EDUCATION: VIEWS AND EXPERIENCES
OF OPPORTUNITIES

Research projects that focus on continuing education are considered here as comprising two main categories: first, those that have studied views and experiences of opportunities for continuing education generally; second, projects that have investigated particular courses. This section concerns the former; taken together these studies address the following issues:

1. Availability and uptake of courses
2. Views on the importance of continuing education
3. Views on course content and format
4. Keeping in touch with professional developments while having a break for child care

Aims and methods of research on opportunities
for continuing education

Concern about the paucity of post-basic midwifery courses available in Wales led Maclean (1980) to undertake a survey of midwives' views as to the importance of continuing education and their experiences of the availability and uptake of both post-basic and in-service courses. Information was obtained from a questionnaire sent to a 10% random sample of midwives in practice in Wales, plus all the midwifery tutors working there; an 88% response rate overall was achieved ($N = 147$). Opportunities for continuing education was one of the main aspects of post-qualification experience explored in the King's College longitudinal study of midwives' careers, in particular its possible relationship to retention (Robinson and Owen, 1994; Robinson, 1994).

A study by Parnaby (1987) centred on midwives' views of the content of refresher courses and was undertaken in response to concerns identified by Mander (1986) about the usefulness of these courses. Questionnaires were sent to all senior midwife teachers in England of whom 95% responded (141/149) and to all midwives attending one refresher course, 98% of whom responded (117/119). Both groups of midwives were presented with a total of 45 topics and asked to rate their importance for inclusion in the refresher course curriculum.

A number of smaller-scale studies have also been undertaken; each used questionnaires and focused on continuing education opportunities for midwives in one health district/area (Sugarman, 1988; McCrea, 1989; Clarke and Rees, 1989). Sugarman's study was prompted by concerns about decreasing levels of attendance at a series of study days provided specifically for staff midwives. Questionnaires were sent to the 59 staff midwives employed in one health district; 71% (42) replied. In a study to redress the lack of information about continuing education for midwives in Northern Ireland, McCrea (1989) investigated the participation of midwifery sisters and staff midwives in formal continuing education opportunities, such as courses and study days, as well as time spent reading journals and using libraries. Responses were obtained from 43 midwives, representing a 72% return from a sample in one area health board in Northern Ireland. A subsample of respondents was also interviewed in both the Sugarman and McCrea studies. In order that a proposed programme of continuing education for midwives in South Glamorgan should meet staff needs, Clarke and Rees (1989) sought information from the district's 178 midwives on their experiences of continuing education to date and views about which topics would be of most use in future courses. The overall response rate was low at 56% and this was primarily attributable to a very low response rate from night staff (21% compared with 74% of day staff). As the authors comment, the low response for night staff might well reflect a lack of access to courses for this group.

Findings from these six studies considered as a whole can be viewed with confidence since all, with the exception of the latter, achieved high response rates. A seventh study focused specifically on the continuing education needs of practitioners who were not working (Midgley, 1993). This was a small-scale exploratory study in which 10 non-working midwives were interviewed.

Findings from research on opportunities for continuing education

Availability and uptake of courses The studies by Maclean (1980) and Robinson (1994) investigated the uptake of in-service courses and obtaining post-basic qualifications; the other studies focused only on in-service courses. Maclean's survey of midwives in Wales demonstrated a lack of available courses in some areas, but also inaccurate knowledge as to what was available. The published findings do not provide an overall figure for the number of midwives in practice who had attended an in-service and/or post-basic course since qualifying, but do show that the number who had attended each kind of course was small, ranging from 37% for Family Planning Appreciation courses to 2% for the Advanced Diploma in Midwifery (Maclean, 1980).

Midwives who took part in the 1986 phase of the King's College study (Robinson, 1994) were asked whether they had attended any in-service courses relevant to midwifery, apart from statutory refresher courses, since qualifying as midwives; these courses were defined as those organized by the respondent's hospital or employing authority but which received no nationally recognized certificate. Less than half had in fact done so: 41% of both cohorts. All respondents were asked if they had successfully completed any National Board courses since qualifying. A quarter (79) of the 1979 respondents had done so in the seven years since they qualified and 13% (57)

of the 1983 respondents had done so in the three years since they qualified. The two courses most likely to have been taken were Special and Intensive Care of the Newborn (44) and Family Planning (47).

The other three studies found varying proportions who had attended courses. McCrea (1989) reported that 30% (13/43) of respondents had attended a course, other than a refresher course. Fifty-seven per cent of those participating in Sugarman's (1988) study had attended at least one of the staff midwife study group sessions. Clarke and Rees' (1989) findings on previous attendance showed that 63% of respondents overall had attended a course within the health authority in the last year, but that this varied by grade; hospital sisters were most likely to have done so, community midwives and newly qualified staff the least likely.

Barriers to attending continuation education events were identified in some of these studies. Sugarman (1988) found that respondents were often precluded from attending by family responsibilities and, to a lesser extent, by short staffing on their wards. McCrea, like Sugarman (1988), found that family responsibilities and staff levels militated against course attendance; but many respondents also said that encouragement from managers to attend courses was not always forthcoming. Moreover, the latter study also showed that although 51% of respondents said courses were available, only 30% said that they were accessible, mainly because of the 'take your turn' system. This meant that a midwife might not be allowed to attend a course of particular relevance to her educational needs, because she attended the last course that had been available. Clarke and Rees' (1989) study highlighted the particular difficulties encountered by night staff and community staff in making arrangements to attend courses.

Views on the importance of continuing education Although the above studies show that midwives may experience difficulties in attending courses, it was a consistent finding that midwives perceive continuing education to be of value. The view that their own professional education was not complete, and that continued study was of benefit to career development and to the quality of care delivered, were expressed by over 80% of respondents who took part in Maclean's (1980) survey of midwives in Wales. The importance attached to continuing education by midwives was indicated in Robinson's study (1994) in that 70% of respondents who had attended in-service courses and over 70% of those who had not done so perceived a need for greater provision of courses.

Midwives taking part in Robinson's study (1994) were provided with a list of factors identified as relevant to retention and asked to ring those that they felt were important. Although pay, staffing levels and the availability of creche facilities and flexible hours featured most prominently, nonetheless the increased provision of in-service education was indicated as important to retention by 51% of the 1979 cohort and 58% of the 1983 cohort. More refresher courses for updating of skills were similarly indicated as of importance by 49% and 45% of the two cohorts respectively (Robinson, 1994). The majority of respondents in Sugarman's (1988) study said that study days were beneficial, whether or not they themselves had been able to attend. Nearly all respondents in Clarke and Rees' study (1989) felt there was a need for a set programme of continuing education, and were more likely to support compulsory rather than voluntary attendance.

Views on course content and format Questions of varying degrees of depth were asked in these studies about the kind of courses respondents would like to see provided. The most consistent finding was an emphasis on clinical subjects. Respondents in Maclean's (1980) study were asked to specify the kinds of course for which they felt the need was most urgent, and short courses on keeping up to date were cited most frequently (52%). All respondents in Clarke and Rees' study (1989) were given a list of five broad topic areas and asked to rate them from 'of a great deal of interest' to 'no interest' in relation to forming the content of future continuing education courses. Clinical practice was the topic most likely to be cited as 'of great interest' to respondents (84%). The percentage of respondents rating other topics as 'of great interest' were 62% for teaching and assessment, 54% for communication skills, 37% for management and 36% for personal development (Clarke and Rees, 1989).

Parnaby's research focused specifically on midwives' views on the content of refresher courses, and entailed asking respondents to rate 45 items in terms of being essential to inclusion in the refresher course curriculum. Findings from respondents (141 midwifery teachers and 117 refresher course members) showed that 14 topics were rated by 50% or more as being essential for curriculum content. The most highly rated topic of the 14 was 'recent changes in midwifery practice' (90%), and this was followed by new policies/rules of statutory bodies (83%) and new government legislation on reports related to midwifery practice (83%). The majority (88%) of both groups said that refresher courses should offer participants a choice of sessions. Parnaby proposed three solutions as to how this could be achieved: by parallel sessions on existing courses; by offering specialist courses; or by allowing midwives to choose a number of separate courses that they perceived as relevant to their continuing education needs (Parnaby, 1987). The last option has now been introduced as an alternative for those who do not wish to attend a course of five consecutive days.

Respondents in the King's College study (Robinson, 1994) who had attended in-service courses were asked to specify the main topics of each; these were then grouped into broad categories and indicated that management courses were the most likely to have been attended (36% and 38% for the two cohorts) followed by parentcraft (27% and 19%). All respondents were asked to specify the topics that they would like to see addressed at future courses. As in Maclean's (1980) study, this was an open-ended question; respondents were not provided with a list of possible topics and to rate importance for inclusion, as were those who participated in the studies by Parnaby (1987) and Clarke and Rees (1989). Findings revealed some interesting differences between the frequency of topics of courses taken and those desired in future. Management courses had been taken by just over a third of each group but desired in future by less than 10%. Very few respondents had attended courses concerned with clinical updating (8% of the 1979 group and 1% of the 1983). This, however, was the topic listed by far the most frequently as desired in the future – by just over half (53%) of both groups of respondents. Given the rapid developments in the management of childbirth, and the new policies and procedures with which midwives need to become familiar, it is perhaps not surprising that clinical subjects are cited most often when midwives are asked for their preferences for the content of continuing education courses. Moreover the research literature on continuing education for nurses similarly reveals an emphasis on clinical practice topics when respondents are asked for their views about future course content (Bariball, While and Norman, 1991).

Keeping in touch with professional developments while having a break for child care Opportunities for midwives to keep in touch while having a break for a period of child care were explored by Robinson (1994). Respondents were asked whether they had left midwifery for family reasons and then subsequently returned. Further questions, relevant to professional development, included whether employers had kept in touch during breaks about developments in the field. By 1989, respondents from the cohort of midwives who had qualified in 1979 ($N = 288$) had taken a total of 129 completed periods of absence from midwifery, and the corresponding figure for the 1983 cohort ($N = 407$) was 157. Employers had provided opportunities and facilities for midwives to keep in touch about professional developments in less than 10% of these periods of absence: 6% of those taken by the 1979 cohort and 9% of those taken by the 1983. Of those periods of absence in which opportunities had not been available, for 52% of those taken by the 1979 cohort, respondents said that they would have liked some form of contact; the corresponding figure for periods of absence taken by the 1983 cohort was 64%. It appears therefore that during the majority of breaks for child care midwives did want to keep in touch with professional developments, but certainly up until 1989 little provision in this respect had been made.

Midgley's study similarly showed that midwives do want opportunities to keep in touch while taking a break. Nine of the 10 members of her group of interviewees said that they would be interested in a 'keep in touch' programme and that it would be important for such a programme to attract credit accumulation (Midgley, 1993). Learning methods favoured were learning packages (8), attending midwives' study days (8), loan of videos (7) and tutorial groups with clinical and teaching staff (6).

EVALUATION OF SPECIFIC CONTINUING EDUCATION COURSES

Published research includes at least four studies that have focused on particular courses. Kilty and Potter (1975) and Balch (1982) both examined aspects of the then Midwife Teacher's Diploma (MTD); Murphy-Black (1991) studied courses on antenatal teaching and Hicks (1994) investigated a study day to increase research mindedness.

Kilty and Potter's study (1975) was commissioned in response to concerns about the examination failure rates of students in the early 1970s. Following discussions with an 'expert group', the authors identified several areas that might be relevant to the low pass rate, four of which were then investigated in the course of a multi-method project. Questionnaires completed by midwives attending a refresher course ($N = 33$), midwives attending a practical teachers course ($N = 22$) and interviews with groups of midwife teachers (number not stated) provided information on potential deterrents to course application. These included the high failure rate, difficulties in obtaining secondment, lack of guidance about teaching as a career, lack of information about the course and problems in combining course attendance with family commitments. Interviews with small groups (numbers not given) of senior midwife teachers, course tutors, MTD students and examiners, together with observation of the oral part of the final examination, showed that many of the changes occurring in the midwife's role in the 1960s and 1970s were reflected in course aims and objectives, but that the same was not true of the written and oral examinations. The content of both examinations was in some respects poorly matched to course objectives. Analysis of written material and observation at oral examinations demonstrated that the marking scheme was weighted towards failure and that lack of agreed criteria led to inconsistency of marking between examiners. Finally the possible relationship of student variables to pass rates was studied by means of examining records for 77 students from three colleges. These data revealed no significant association of pass rates with age or previous midwifery experience. Interviews with tutors, however, revealed concerns that some students embarked on the course with inadequate basic midwifery knowledge and that this contributed to the high failure rate.

As Sweet (1994) has commented, despite the fact that the Kilty and Potter research is now some 20 years old it is still of interest. This is not only because the project addressed many aspects of the MTD course that might have a bearing on the course pass rate, but also because, unlike many projects, most of the recommendations were implemented. Changes were made to the content and conduct of the examination system, the course length was extended, a greater emphasis was placed on educational as opposed to professional subjects, and more attention paid to pre-course preparation.

The second published research project on the Midwife Teachers' Diploma focused on views and experiences of those who had taken the course at the Royal College of Midwives during the period 1975–1979 (Balch, 1982). Questionnaires were sent to 60 midwives who had taken the course and subsequently worked as tutors, and 80% (48) were returned. Findings showed that enjoyment of teaching was specified most frequently (23) as the reason for taking the course. When asked about their expectations of the course, learning about teaching and increasing professional knowledge were each mentioned by the same number of respondents (29). The author commented in particular on the latter finding, given that the course emphasis was ostensibly educational. However, given the prominence of professional as opposed to educational topics in the course (Kilty and Potter, 1975), it is perhaps not surprising that a majority of Balch's respondents perceived that attendance would increase their professional knowledge. Moreover, until the Advanced Diploma in Midwifery was introduced, the MTD was the only course available to those who wished to increase their professional knowledge. When respondents were asked to recommend changes to the course, two of the five that came up most often corroborated Kilty and Potter's conclusions: namely the need for a period of pre-course preparation and for the course itself to be lengthened.

Bariball *et al.*'s review of research on continuing education for nurses showed that very few studies have attempted to assess whether course attendance has any impact on subsequent behaviour (Bariball, While and Norman, 1991). Two exceptions in the midwifery literature are studies of courses on antenatal teaching (Murphy-Black, 1991) and study days on research awareness (Hicks, 1994). Murphy-Black's study investigated the effect that a course on antenatal education had on participants' teaching styles (Murphy-Black, 1991). The course philosophy emphasized the value of group work and interactive teaching methods. The research sought to determine whether expectations of course members were met and to assess course outcome by means of an observation study of participants' pre- and post-course teaching styles.

Expectations were studied by means of questionnaires given to course members ($N = 65$) at two centres: responses from a 94% pre-course return and a 78% post-course return showed a high degree of satisfaction, with most participants saying they had learnt about teaching, leading a group and communicating with women. The observation study was carried out with a third of the course members and used Flanders Interaction Analysis Categories (Flanders, 1970). Findings showed a small post-course increase in interactive teaching and this difference reached a significant level for those members who had chosen to go on the course but not for those who had been sent. This finding may have important implications for selection of participants, if resources invested in course provision are to be cost-effective. Murphy-Black argues that evaluation studies comprising process measures only, are useful to identify strengths and weaknesses of a course, but satisfaction with a course does not necessarily mean there will be any subsequent change in practice. Outcome studies are needed to assess whether or not this is the case (Murphy-Black, 1991).

Hicks (1994) sought to assess the value of brief training days in developing midwives' competencies in reading research articles critically. The study was prompted by a concern that midwives did not integrate research findings into practice, because they lacked knowledge and confidence about how to interpret and use published research. The research had two aims: to establish whether following attendance at the study day midwives were better able to critically evaluate a research article; second, whether the study day had a longer-term impact on midwives' use of published findings. A before and after design was employed. Nineteen midwives in clinical practice were sent a questionnaire that asked about the frequency with which they read research articles, how confident they felt when doing so and the potential use their reading had for influencing their clinical practice (Hicks, 1994). The study group members were also sent a research article which they were asked to evaluate along various criteria; the article had previously been evaluated by expert raters. The midwives then attended a study day which provided a synopsis of key issues in research methodology, together with guidelines for evaluating research papers. At the end of the study day they were asked to evaluate the article again, and two months later were asked again about their use of research articles to inform practice. The findings indicated that the study day did have an impact. Evaluations of the article made at the end of the day were closer to those of the expert raters than those made earlier. Moreover, there was an increase in participants' reported frequency of reading research, their confidence in its evaluation and the influence it had when reviewing their current practice (Hicks, 1994). Although this was a small-scale study of one study day, it does, as Hicks concludes, demonstrate the value that such events can have in increasing research-mindedness.

DISCUSSION

This chapter has sought to provide a review of published research on midwifery education, with the aims of indicating the range of subjects studied, the diversity of methods used and the main conclusions that have emerged. Although the volume of published research on midwifery education is comparatively small, nonetheless a very wide range of issues have been investigated. This means, of course, that most issues are represented by one study only, and thus there is a need for replication. The research reviewed has used a variety of methods, although surveys by questionnaire are the most common. Recent studies are adopting more challenging methods, in particular to assess outcomes of both first-level and continuing education courses. A number of conclusions can be drawn from the published work and these, together with some of the major areas of omission, are discussed here.

Research on the kind of course needed demonstrated that lengthening the post-registration course had no impact on subsequent retention in the profession, and identified difficulties in setting up the new pre-registration programmes. Two questions about the courses as a whole can be posed for the future. Will there be a possibly unmet demand for post-registration courses (now known as pre-registration (shortened) courses), since some may qualify as Project 2000 diplomates and then decide to pursue midwifery? Second, how will the long-term careers of those qualifying from pre-registration courses compare with those who have qualified via the shortened route?

Research into recruitment and selection for both courses was notable by its absence. Studies that have been undertaken indicated concerns about time available for these two time-consuming activities, some uncertainty about qualities desired in student midwives, and differing criteria for selection across colleges. Given the importance of recruitment and selection for the composition of the midwifery workforce, these are clearly subjects which merit increased research attention.

Work on analysing curriculum documents indicated that further research might usefully focus on how the process of curriculum design could serve more purposes than satisfying the validating body, in particular the production of a 'working' document for use during the course by staff and students. A consistent finding, spanning research on student cohorts over a 15-year period, was that students perceive the amount of clinical teaching to be inadequate. Attention needs to focus on ways of overcoming the problem, rather than continuing to document its continued existence. Lack of preparation to teach and anxieties about mentoring were important and consistent findings; both require further research. Classroom teaching was less likely to be the subject of criticism, but the importance of evaluating new styles of teaching and learning strategies has been indicated. Research on assessment of competencies is still in relatively early stages and more work is likely to be needed when current studies are completed. At a broader level, the move to higher education has raised many questions about the control of midwifery education, and these too will need to be researched.

The years since many of the studies reviewed were undertaken have seen the publication of the *Changing Childbirth* Report (Department of Health, 1993), with its recommendations of a midwifery-led service for those women who experience a normal pregnancy, labour and puerperium. The extent to which these recommendations are implemented will determine the nature of the clinical environment in which students learn their midwifery skills; research will be required to assess the extent to which the disparity between classroom rhetoric and the reality of practice decreases in the future.

Commitment to continuing education is espoused from all quarters; studies reviewed, however, show that midwives may experience barriers to course attendance. Midwives' needs and preferences in relation to continuing education need to be researched, and more studies than have been undertaken hitherto are required to assess the effect of course attendance on subsequent behaviour. Midwife teachers feature prominently in research findings, but very little research has focused on them as a group. Thus little is known about their views on their own development needs and the extent to which they feel able to fulfil their demanding remit. Much emphasis has been placed in recent years on providing opportunities for midwives to keep up to date while taking a break for child care responsibilities. Research to date has indicated that such opportunities have often not been available. Research is needed to assess the kinds of courses that midwives would like while taking a break, and how these might best be provided.

In conclusion, research evidence exists on many aspects of midwifery education upon which strategies and policies can be formulated. However, given the many unanswered questions surrounding midwifery education and the challenges faced by those engaged in its various dimensions, it is essential that the research attention devoted to the subject begins to equal that devoted to other aspects of the profession. Moreover, those who do undertake research into midwifery education should be provided with the facilities and support to publish, in order that their findings can benefit the profession as a whole.

ACKNOWLEDGEMENTS

Some of the ideas that informed the content of this chapter were developed in the course of discussions with Judith Lathlean, Julia McGill-Cuerden, Lesley Page, Betty Sweet and Beryl Thomas. I should like to record my thanks to them and to Paul Robinson for typing the manuscript.

REFERENCES

Association of Radical Midwives (1986) *The Vision: Proposals for the Future of the Maternity Services*. Association of Radical Midwives, London.

Balch, B. (1982) Teacher training for midwives: an investigation of the midwife teacher's diploma course 1975–79 at the Royal College of Midwives, London, with special reference to teaching practice. In Thomson, A.M. (ed), *Research and the Midwife Conference Proceedings for 1981*. Department of Nursing, University of Manchester.

Barriball, K.L., While, A. and Norman, I. (1991) Continuing professional education for qualified nurses: a review of the literature. *Journal of Advanced Nursing*, **17**, 1129–40.

Bedford, H., Phillips, T., Robinson, J. and Schostak, J. (1993) *Assessing Competencies in Nursing and Midwifery Education*. English National Board, London.

Chamberlain, M. (1992) Factors affecting students becoming competent in midwifery skills. In Thomson, A., Robinson, S. and Tickner, V. (eds), *Research and the Midwife Conference Proceedings for 1991*. Department of Nursing, University of Manchester.

Clarke, J. and Rees, C. (1989) The midwife and continuing education. *Midwives Chronicle and Nursing Notes*, **102**(1220), 228–290.

Davies, R. (1991) Perspectives on midwifery: students' beginnings. In Robinson, S., Thomson, A. and Tickner, V. (eds), *Research and the Midwife Conference Proceedings for 1990*. Department of Nursing, University of Manchester.

Department of Health (1993) *Changing Childbirth: Report of the Expert Maternity Group Parts 1 and 2 (Cumberledge Report)*. HMSO, London.

English National Board (1993) *Project Specification: An Outcome Evaluation of the Effectiveness of Pre-registration Midwifery Programmes of Education*. English National Board, London.

Flanders, N. (1970) *Analysing Teaching Behaviour.* Addison Wesley, Massachusetts.

Fraser, D.M., Murphy, R.J.L., Worth-Butler, M. (1994) Evaluation of the effectiveness of pre-registration midwifery programmes of education. A joint project between the Faculty of midwifery, Mid Trent College of Nursing and Midwifery, and the school of Education, University of Nottingham. Interim report to the English National Board Research and Development Group. English National Board, London.

Garcia, J. and Garforth, S. (1991) Midwifery policies and policy-making. In Robinson, S. and Thomson, A.M. (eds), *Midwives, Research and Childbirth*, Vol. 2 Chapman & Hall, London.

Green, J., Kitzinger, J. and Coupland, V. (1986) *The Division of Labour: Implications of Medical Staffing Structures for Doctors and Midwives on the Labour Ward*. Child Care and Development Group, University of Cambridge.

Golden, J. (1980) Midwifery training: the views of newly qualified midwives. *Midwives Chronicle and Nursing Notes*, **93**(1109), 190–94.

Hall, J. (1994) Midwifery education: where is it going. *MIDIRS Midwifery Digest*, **4**(4), 384–6.

Hicks, C. (1993) A survey of midwives' attitudes to, and involvement in, research: the first stage in identifying needs for staff development programmes *Midwifery*, **9**(2), 51–62.

Hicks, C. (1994) Bridging the gap between research and practice: an assessment of the value of a study day in development of critical research reading skills in midwives. *Midwifery*, **10**(1). 18–25.

House of Commons Health Committee (1992) *Second Report, Session 1991–92. Maternity Services (Winterton Report)*. HMSO, London.

Kent, J., MacKeith, N. and Maggs, C. (1994a) *Direct but Different: Volume 1 – The Discussion*. Maggs Research Associates, Bath.

Kent, J., MacKeith, N. and Maggs, C. (1994b) *Direct but Different: Volume 2 – The Evidence*. Maggs Research Associates, Bath.

Kilty, J.M. and Potter, F.W. (1975) The midwife teacher's diploma project. University of Surrey, Guildford.

Leong, W. (1989) The introduction of computer-assisted learning in a school of midwifery using the Wessex Care Plan Program. *Nurse Education Today*, **9**, 114–123.

Maggs, C. (1994) Mentorship in nursing and midwifery education: issues for research. *Nurse Education Today*, **14**(1), 22–29.

Mander, R. (1984) Stop and consider: student midwife wastage in training. In Thomson, A. and Robinson, S. (eds), *Research and the Midwife Conference Proceedings for 1983*. Department of Nursing, University of Manchester.

Mander, R. (1986) Refresher course: unfulfilled potential. *Midwives Chronicle*, **99**(1176), 4–5.

Mander, R. (1989a) Who continues? A preliminary examination of data on continuation of employment in midwifery. *Midwifery*, **5**(1), 26–35.

Mander, R. (1989b) The best laid schemes: An evaluation of the extension of midwifery training in Scotland. *International Journal of Nursing Studies*, **26**(1), 27–41.

Mander, R. (1993) Midwifery training and employment decisions. In Robinson, S. and Thomson, A.M. (eds), *Midwives, Research and Childbirth*, Vol. 3, Chapman & Hall, London.

McCrea, H. (1989) Motivation for continuing education in midwifery. *Midwifery*, **5**(3), 134–5.

McCrea, H.,Thompson, K., Carswell, L. and Whittington, D. (1994) Student midwives' learning experiences on the wards. *Journal of Clinical Nursing*, **3**, 97–102.

Maclean, G. (1980) *A Study of the Educational Needs of Midwives in Wales and How They Might be Met*. West Glamorgan Health Authority.

Midgley, C. (1993) Continuing education for non-practising midwives. In Robinson, S., Thomson, A. and Tickner, V. (eds), *Research and the Midwife Conference Proceedings for 1992*. Department of Nursing, University of Manchester.

Mitchell, M. (1994) The views of students and teachers on the use of portfolios as a learning and assessment tool in midwifery education. *Nursing Education Today*, **14**(1), 38–43.

Mountford, B. in collaboration with Fraser, D.M., Murphy R.J.L. and Worth-Butler, M. (1995) *An Interpretative Comment on 23 Pre-registration Midwifery Education Curricula Documents*. EME project, English National Board, London.

Murphy-Black, T. (1991) *Antenatal Education: Evaluation of a Post-basic Training Course*. In Robinson, S. and Thomson, A.M. (eds), *Midwives, Research and Childbirth*, Vol. 2. Chapman & Hall, London.

Opoku, D. and Davis, K. (1988) Exploring other perspectives in the midwifery curriculum. In Robinson, S. and Thomson, A.M. (eds), *Research and the Midwife Conference Proceedings for 1987*. Department of Nursing, University of Manchester.

Parnaby, C. (1987) Surveying the opinions of midwives regarding the curriculum content of refresher courses. *Midwifery*, **3**(3), 133–42.

Phillips,. R. (1993) Choice or chance? An exploratory study describing the criteria and processes used to select midwifery students. In Robinson, S., Thomson, A.,and Tickner, V. (eds), *Research and the Midwife Conference Proceedings for 1992*. Department of Nursing, University of Manchester.

Pollock, M. (1992) *Establishment of a Midwifery Education Research and Development Unit*. Department of Education Studies, University of Surrey.

Pope, V. (1986) Midwifery training in Scotland: An opinion survey. *Midwives Chronicle*, **99**(1184), 198–200.

Radford, N. and Thompson, A. (1988) *Direct Entry: A Preparation for Midwifery Practice*. ENB, London.

Radford, N. and Thompson, A. (1994) A study of issues concerning the implementation of direct entry midwifery education. In Robinson, S. and Thomson, A.M. (eds), *Midwives, Research and Childbirth*, Vol. 3. Chapman & Hall, London.

Raymond, R. and Ananda-Rajan, K. (1993) Learning practice. *Nursing Times*, **89**(31), 36.–7.

Robinson, S. (1980) Are there enough midwives? *Nursing Times*, **76**(17), 726–30.

Robinson, S. (1986a) Midwifery training: the views of newly qualified midwives. *Nurse Education Today*, **6**(2), 49–59.

Robinson, S. (1986b) Career intentions of newly qualified midwives *Midwifery* **2**(1), 25–36.

Robinson, S. (1989) Caring for childbearing women: the inter-relationship between midwifery and medical responsibilities. In Robinson, S. and Thomson, A.M. (eds), *Midwives, Research and Childbirth*, Vol. 1. Chapman & Hall, London.

Robinson, S. (1991) Preparation for practice: the educational experiences and career intentions of newly qualified midwives. In Robinson, S. and Thomson, A.M. (eds), *Midwives, Research and Childbirth*, Vol. 2. Chapman & Hall, London.

Robinson, S. (1994) Professional development in midwifery: findings from a longitudinal study of midwives' careers. *Nurse Education Today*, **14**, 161–76.

Robinson, S., Golden, J. and Bradley, S. (1983) *A study of the Role and Responsibilities of the Midwife*. NERU Report No 1, Nursing Education Research Unit, King's College, London.

Robinson, S. and Owen, H. (1994) Retention in midwifery: findings from a longitudinal study of midwives' careers. In Robinson, S. and Thomson, A.M. (eds), *Midwives, Research and Childbirth*, Vol. 3. Chapman & Hall, London.

Robinson, S., Owen, H. and Jacka, K. (1992) *The Midwives' Career Patterns Project*. Report to Department of Health, Nursing Research Unit, London University.

Robinson, S., Thomson, A.M. and Tickner, V. (1989) Midwives' views on directions and developments in midwifery research. In Robinson S. and Thomson, A.M. (eds), *Research and the Midwife Conference Proceedings for 1988*. Nursing Research Unit, London University.

Roch, S. (1993) Excellence in midwifery education. *Modern Midwife*, March–April, 36–8.

Royal College of Midwives (1987) *The Role and Education of the Future Midwife in the United Kingdom*. Royal College of Midwives, London.

Sims, C., McHaffie, H., Renfrew, M. and Ashurst, H. (1994) *The Midwifery Research Database MIRIAD*. Books for midwives Press, Hale.

Sleep, J. and Clark, E. (1993) Major new survey to identify and prioritize research issues for midwifery practice. *Midwives Chronicle* **106**(1265) 217–218.

Standon-Batt, M. (1979) Where are the tutors? *Midwives Chronicle and Nursing Notes*, **92**(1,100), 304.

Stewart, A. (1981) The present state of midwifery training. *Midwife, Health Visitor and Community Nurse*, **17**(7), 270–72.

Sugarman, E. (1988) The case of the disappearing midwives. *Nursing Times*, **84**(8), 35–6.

Sweet, B. (1994) A critical review of research related to midwifery education. In Thomson, A., Robinson, S. and Tickner, V. (eds), *Research and the Midwife Conference Proceedings for 1993*. Department of Nursing, University of Manchester.

Walker, J. (1976) Midwife or obstetric nurse? Some perceptions of midwives and obstetricians of the role of the midwife. *Journal of Advanced Nursing*, **1**(2), 129–38.

Walker, P. (1990) How midwives prepare to teach. *Nursing*, **4**(14), 22–4.

Warwick, C. (1992) Reflections on the current management of midwifery education. *MIDIRS Midwifery Digest*, **2**(3), 251–4.

West, S., Thomson, A.M. (1995) Midwifery Competencies – Why 40 deliveries. In Robinson, S., Thomson, A.M., Silverton, L. (eds) Research and the Midwife Conference Proceedings for 1994. Department of Nursing Studies, University of Manchester.

While, A. (1994) Competence versus performance: which is more important? *Journal of Advanced Nursing*, **20**, 525–31.

Worth-Butler, M., Murphy, R.J.L. and Fraser, D.M. (1994) Towards an integrated model of competence in midwifery. *Midwifery*, **10**(4), 225–31.

Worth-Butler, M., Murphy, R.J.L., Fraser, D.M. (1995) The need to define competence in midwifery. *British Journal of Midwifery* **3**(5): 259–62.

UKCC (1994) Midwifery programmes of education: changes in terminology. Registrar's letter. UKCC, London.

CHAPTER EIGHT

The Southampton randomized controlled trial of breast shells and Hoffman's exercises for inverted and non-protractile nipples

Jo Alexander

I first became interested in the treatment for inverted and non-protractile nipples while working as a midwife teacher in the midwives' antenatal clinic of a large maternity hospital. I had been taught as a student midwife that women who intended to breast feed should have their nipples examined antenatally and that if they proved to be inverted or non-protractile they should be offered 'shells'. From their reactions it appeared that many of the women did not relish the idea of wearing these shells and some asked about their efficacy. As the standard textbooks indicated quite clearly that they worked, I had no hesitation in reassuring the women and it came as quite a shock when I investigated the literature!

PREVIOUS WORK ON NIPPLE INVERSION AND PROTRACTILITY

The importance of good nipple protractility

A full description of the breast-feeding 'suck' cycle has been given by Woolridge (1986), the precise role of the nipple first being illustrated by the cineradiographic work of Ardran, Kemp and Lind (1958). The latter stated that the baby forms a 'teat' from the nipple and much of the areola, and that it is only the very end of the 'teat' which is formed by the nipple. The attachments of the nipple to the breast are stretched to form the rest of the 'teat', as demonstrated by the observation that when the 'nipple' is withdrawn from the baby's mouth it is found to be very elongated. These observations were also confirmed ultrasonically (Weber *et al.*, 1984).

Further evidence of the importance of this protractility was provided by Hytten and Baird (1958), who used quarter-inch diameter ball-ended callipers to compress the areola just behind the nipple. This was done to a point just short of discomfort for the woman and the investigators considered that the measurement obtained (or 'bite' size) could be regarded as a quantitative assessment of nipple protractility. The smaller the 'bite' the greater the ability of the tissue to elongate. If the 'bite' was large it appeared to be related to difficulty with fixing the baby to the breast. Of 170 primiparous women who had this measurement made on their first postnatal day, 26 had a 'bite' size of 6 mm or above, and nine of these (35%) had fixing difficulties; of the 144 who had a 'bite' size of less than 6 mm, only four (3%) had fixing difficulties.

Waller (1939) was aware of the importance of protractility in preventing damage to the nipple and to illustrate this suggested that the reader should put his thumb (flexor surface upwards) into his mouth until his lips met round the base of the first phalanx. On sucking virtually no suction is felt on the tip of the thumb. This ceases to be the case when the thumb is pulled forwards.

Hytten (1954) studied 6456 women who were delivered in the Aberdeen Maternity Hospital of singleton babies who survived the lying-in period. These women received no systematic antenatal treatment of their breasts. He found 'poor nipples' to be an important cause of breast-feeding failure (Table 8.1) and the fourth commonest reason for not leaving hospital fully breast feeding (the first being 'poor lactation'). In a further study of 1075 primiparae carried out in Aberdeen between 1954 and 1955, Yorston (1956) found that 16% had discontinued breast feeding while in hospital, and that of those who had discontinued 19% were considered to have done so because of poor nipples. This was the second commonest cause of discontinuing, the first again being poor lactation. A survey of 7950 births in Great Britain in 1990 (White, Freeth and O'Brien, 1992) also found that 4% of women who

Table 8.1 'Poor nipples' as a cause of breast-feeding difficulty (Hytten, 1954)

	Feeding difficulties in hospital due to 'poor nipples'		Not leaving hospital fully breast feeding because of 'poor nipples'		'Poor nipples' as a percentage of all reasons given for not leaving hospital fully breast feeding (by parity)	'Poor nipples' as a percentage of all reasons given for not leaving hospital fully breast feeding
	No.	%	No.	%		
Primiparae (N=2461)	105	4	62	2	16	10
Multiparae (N=3995)	67	2	43	1	7	

Source: Compiled by the author.

discontinued breast feeding during the first week and 3% of women who discontinued in the second gave inverted nipples as at least one of their reasons for doing so. Jones (1989) reports that poor protractility has been recognized as a problem at the breast-feeding clinic set up by the Lactation Research Group of the Department of Child Health, University of Bristol.

Many authors (e.g. Waller, 1946; Blaikley *et al.*, 1953; Otte, 1975; Sweet, 1988) state that inverted or non-protractile nipples predispose to nipple soreness and damage on breast feeding; however, two reports call this supposed link into question. In the first, L'Esperance (1980) examined 102 women within 24 hours of delivery and found that 23 (22%) had flat or inverted nipples. At 48 hours postnatally, only 4 of these 23 women (17%) were complaining of moderate or extreme discomfort compared with 32 (40%) of the 79 women with protractile nipples ($\chi^2 = 4.17$, $p < 0.05$). At first glance it would appear from these figures that inversion or non-protractility had a protective effect against soreness, but two cautionary comments should be made. First L'Esperance herself suggests that the women with problematic nipples may have had more difficulty with fixing their babies and therefore have been breast feeding less frequently than those with protractile nipples. Second, her report does not specify whether the assessment of nipple protractility was made before the first breast feed. We are told that the assessment took place within 24 hours of delivery, and several authors suggest that a baby with a vigorous suck can improve anatomically poor nipples (Waller, 1946; Hytten and Baird, 1958; Gunther, 1973; Otte, 1975; Riordan, 1983; Helsing and Savage King, 1984). It is therefore possible that some women with nipples which were 'poor' at the time of delivery had protractile nipples by the time of the examination, as several feeds may have taken place, and Otte (1975) suggests that nipples which are 'corrected' by vigorous sucking are at especial risk of persistent soreness and cracking. For these reasons this aspect of the study by L'Esperance needs to be treated with caution.

The second report to call into question the supposed link between inverted and non-protractile nipples and nipple soreness caused by breast feeding is that by Hytten (1954). He states that the incidence of soreness was no higher in those with poor nipples than in the rest. He does not state whether examination of nipple protractility was conducted antenatally or postnatally, although from a subsequent study (Hytten and Baird, 1958) it appears to have been his practice to carry out an examination on the first postnatal day (precise time unspecified). One can therefore have reservations similar to those given in relation to the data presented by L'Esperance. The prevalence of poor nipple protractility in early pregnancy has been the subject of a number of studies (Waller, 1946; Blaikley *et al.*, 1953; Hytten, 1954; Hytten and Baird, 1958), the figures quoted for nulliparous women ranging from 14% to 35%.

Definitions of nipple inversion and non-protractility

Inverted nipples, which are situated on a plane below the areola (Hauden and Mahler, 1983), are thought to be a persistence of the original invagination of the mammary dimple (Waller, 1946; Lawrence, 1985; Williams *et al.*, 1989). Riordan (1983) describes basically two types of inversion: simple and complete. In simple inversion 'the nipple moves outward to protraction with manual pressure or when cold'. Complete inversion is where adhesions binding the nipple to the deeper structures of the breast prevent it from responding to manual pressure.

A non-protractile nipple is less easy to define. The most widely advocated test is that described by Waller (1946): 'in imitation of the action of the baby's jaws the areola is pinched (between the thumb and forefinger) just beyond the nipple's base'; if this causes the nipple to project it is considered as satisfactory and classed as being protractile. This 'pinch test' has been used by many investigators (Blaikley *et al.*, 1953; Gunther, 1973; Lawrence, 1985; Samuel, 1985; Walker, 1989; Larsen, 1990) to make their assessment of nipple protractility and most stress that simple inspection is not enough. Riordan (1983) describes two types of non-protractility, minimal being when 'instead of protracting the nipple moves inward' and moderate to severe, when the nipple 'retracts to a level even with or behind the surrounding areola'. There is considerable disagreement between the authors as to the gestation at which the test should be carried out. Many (e.g. Waller, 1946; Naish, 1948; Blaikley et al., 1953; Larsen, 1990) advocate that it should be done early in pregnancy, Otte (1975) the second trimester and Gunther (1973) at about 20 weeks.

The predictive value of antenatal nipple examination in relation to subsequent breast-feeding success

Hytten conducted two studies (Hytten 1954; Hytten and Baird, 1958) from which he concluded that antenatal examination of the nipples has some predictive value. He notes, however, that the majority of those who are considered to have 'poor' nipples in early pregnancy appear to have no subsequent difficulty in breast feeding, even if they have no antenatal treatment of their nipples.

An additional question mark over the need to treat inverted and non-protractile nipples antenatally was raised by Hytten and Baird (1958) who found that in a group of women who apparently carried out no antenatal treatment there was a marked trend towards spontaneous improvement in protractility (Table 8.2); interestingly, a few women had nipples which 'regressed'. Hytten (1990) has suggested that oestrogen is responsible for the connective tissue adhesions absorbing water and thus becoming softer and more mobile. The association with oestrogen is also supported by animal research (Burrows, 1949).

Table 8.2 Spontaneous changes in nipple protractility during pregnancy (Hytten and Baird, 1958)

	Poor protraction				Change in prevalence
	At 8–15 weeks gestation		On first postnatal day		
	No.	%	No.	%	
Primigravidae (N = 170)	50	35	13	8	–27%
Primiparae (N = 75)	8	11	3	4	–7%
>parity one (N= 29)	0		0		0

Source: Alexander (1991).

Treatment for poor protractility

Shells Breast shells (or Woolwich shells) are the most widely described method of antenatal treatment. Waller (1946) wrote about the use of Victorian glass shells: 'worn during pregnancy under a firm [bra] it serves our purpose by pressing the nipple through the opening and gradually stretching and loosening its attachment to the deep structures of the breast'. Gunther (1973) postulated that the edges of the aperture may induce hormonal changes by a mechanism similar to that triggered by the baby's mouth. She therefore suggested that the hole should be of such a size that the nipple and about a third of the areola are left free from pressure.

Advice about when women should begin to wear shells varies from the end of the first trimester (Dutton, 1979; Riordan, 1983), right through to the last weeks of pregnancy (Lawrence, 1985) but authors appear to agree that they should be used for gradually increasing periods until they are worn throughout the day (Gunther, 1973; Otte, 1975; Riordan, 1983; Lawrence, 1985; Larsen, 1990). Helsing and Savage King (1984) are so enthusiastic about the use of shells that they urge rural Indian heath workers to have them made locally out of wood, ceramics, plastic or glass.

I was surprised to find that there had been no controlled trials to investigate the effectiveness of breast shells. Waller (1946) had conducted a controlled trial to investigate the effect of antenatal expression of colostrum on postnatal engorgement. However, women from both the control and the experimental groups were also given shells if they 'were thought likely to benefit'. He states that 'in all but the worst kinds of deformity the results are good', but gives no supporting evidence for this claim.

Blaikley *et al.* (1953) conducted a controlled trial to investigate the effects of the 'Woolwich methods' on the success of breast feeding. Unfortunately, as with Waller's study (1946), all those with inverted or non-protractile nipples were given shells regardless of whether they were in the control or experimental group.

Antenatal manipulation This is another method used to treat inverted or non-protractile nipples (DeLee and Greenhill, 1947; Eastman, 1950; Applebaum, 1969; Dutton, 1979; Cadwell, 1981; Riordan, 1983; Helsing and Savage King, 1984; Lawrence, 1985; Sweet, 1988; Larsen, 1990). Hoffman (1953) gives the most detailed description of nipple-stretching exercises and describes thus: 'The procedure is one of placing the thumbs, or the forefingers, close to the inverted nipple, then pressing into the breast tissue quite firmly and gradually pushing the fingers away from the areola' and thus from each other. This is done five times in succession with the fingers first in a horizontal and then in a vertical position (Figure 8.1). He recommends that the woman should then grasp the nipple at its base and ease it out a bit further.

Figure 8.1 Hoffman's exercises.

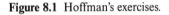

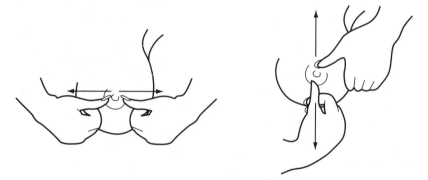

Source: Reproduced from Alexander (1990). By permission of the Macmillan Press.

Opinion as to the time during gestation at which manipulation should begin varies from 'as early in pregnancy as possible' (Larsen, 1990) through to 34 weeks gestation (Lawrence, 1985). Hoffman (1953) reports that during the previous two years in which he had taught the exercises, no woman had had to stop breast feeding because of inversion. Unfortunately neither his research, nor any other that I could find, involved a control group. Riordan (1983) and Lawrence (1985) caution that nipple stimulation may cause uterine contractions and this is borne out by the work of Jhirad and Vago (1973), Viegas *et al.* (1984) and Frager and Miyazaki (1987).

Other methods of treatment These include the antenatal wearing of nipple-shaped shields (Naish, 1948; Lawrence, 1985) the use of mechanical suction (Cotterman, 1976; Gangal and Gangal, 1978; Poole, 1987), the use of oral suction (Gaskin, 1980; Riordan, 1983; Lawrence, 1985) and surgical elevation (Hauden and Mahler, 1983). These methods do not appear to have been as widely advocated as the use of breast shells or Hoffman's exercises.

The psychology of antenatal examination for and treatment of non-protractility

The view has been expressed that too much emphasis on preparation of the breasts might actually discourage women from breast feeding (Cunnane, 1938; Ministry of Health, 1944; Stone, 1946), and that if a woman is led to believe that she may have difficulty this could damage her confidence and become a self-fulfilling prophecy (Royal College of Midwives, 1988).

In view of this and the assertion by Hytten and Baird (1985) that 'the effectiveness of treatment [of inverted and non-protractile nipples] could be assessed only by a closely controlled trial on a sufficient scale'. I decided to embark on the randomized controlled trial described below.

METHODS

Hypotheses

The management trial was to test the hypotheses that women with inverted or non-protractile nipples, when treated with breast shells and/or Hoffman's exercises begun between 25 and 35 completed weeks of pregnancy, would be: (a) more likely to have nipples which had ceased to be inverted or non-protractile by the time of delivery than if no such intervention had taken place; and (b) more likely to succeed with breast feeding until at least six weeks postnatally than if no such intervention had taken place.

Shells and Hoffman's exercises were chosen for study as they were considered the most commonly used and acceptable forms of treatment.

Study design

The study had a two-treatment by two-level factorial design with four basic management groups, as shown in Figure 8.2. This allowed all those who were advised to use exercises to be compared with all those who were not advised to use them, and all those who were advised to use shells to be compared with all those who were not advised to use them. Such a design allows several therapies to be compared simultaneously without increasing the required number of participants and has a greater chance than a non-factorial design of demonstrating a statistically significant difference if it exists (it has greater 'power') (Cochran and Cox, 1957; Pocock, 1983). With such a design one can estimate the separate effects of the different factors (i.e. shells or exercises) – the main effects – and find out whether combining the factors has an effect beyond that of the individual factors alone (an interaction effect) (Cochran and Cox, 1957).

Figure 8.2 Design of the management trial.

	No shells	Breast shells
No exercises	1	2
Hoffman's exercises	3	4

Source: Compiled by the author.

Setting

Pregnant women were examined by myself, midwives and student midwives in the antenatal clinic of the Princess Anne Hospital, Southampton and three outlying antenatal clinics. Recruitment took place over 23 months between 1987 and 1989. Five community midwives also collected data. The delivery rate in the Southampton district remained fairly constant at about 6000 babies a year throughout the period of recruitment; the population was primarily Caucasian. The health authority encompassed both areas of considerable affluence and of considerable social deprivation, high unemployment and poor housing. The predominant areas of employment were manufacturing, distributive trades and catering (Southampton and South West Hampshire Health Authority, 1990).

Nipple examination

Women who were intending to breast feed and who gave consent had their nipples observed for inversion. If inversion was not found, a version of the 'pinch test' was carried out. This test was based on the instructions given by Waller (1946) and described above, but added the detail that if when the compression was completed the nipple was sticking out half a centimetre or more above the areola then it was to be considered protractile; if it was not then it was non-protractile. It was also felt important that the woman should carry out the compression herself. This test was chosen as it had already been used by midwives for many years and it involved no apparatus which might reduce its acceptability, or hamper the subsequent further spread of its clinical use should this prove desirable.

Ideally all the assessments of nipple protractility would have been made by the same observer, but as I was in full-time employment this was not possible. However, the other recommendations made by Gore (1982) to limit inter-observer variation were followed: the test technique and the criteria for interpreting the test were standardized, the observers were trained by the researcher and each observer was given a typed copy of the test instructions. In addition the observers assisted in the formulation of the instructions and experimented with them for a period before data collection began. The reliability of the 'pinch test' was not, however, investigated as the literature review had demonstrated that it was already in widespread use and the main purpose of the study was to investigate the value of the treatments advised as a result of the test currently used.

In all, 3006 women were examined but only 96 of them finally participated in the management trial; the reasons for this are discussed below. This could have been very dispiriting but data were also recorded about each woman examined (whether each nipple was inverted, non-protractile or protractile; age; parity; gestation; any previous experience of breast feeding). The prevalence study (Alexander, 1991) is beyond the scope of this chapter but the fact that there was a record made each time an examination was carried out (whether or not the woman was suitable for recruitment to the management trial), and thus there was visible evidence available demonstrating the effort expended by the observer, was probably a very important factor in maintaining momentum. A regularly updated chart illustrating the number of women examined was displayed in the main antenatal clinic and a celebration held each time another thousand was added to the total! Twenty-three months is a very long time over which to maintain data collection and the dedication of the midwives was greatly to be praised; the fact that they were involved with the planning of the study from the very beginning and seemed to feel 'ownership' of it was probably important.

Trial eligibility

Only nulliparous women were recruited to the trial because the work of Hytten and Baird (1985) had shown that the prevalence of poor protractility diminished with increasing parity and this suggested that recruitment from higher-parity groups might be poor. The prevalence study showed that increasing parity does not of itself result in a reduction in prevalence but rather the reduction is associated with previous breast feeding (Alexander, 1991). It was decided not to instigate treatment earlier than 25 completed weeks of gestation in view of Hytten and Baird's (1985) work which suggested that there might be spontaneous improvement in nipple protractility during pregnancy. Women were not recruited after 35 completed weeks of gestation as the time available for treatment would have been short. Women with multiple pregnancies were not recruited as it was considered that the increased hormone levels present might cause a greater increase in protractility than those of a singleton and that, as anatomical change was to be used as one of the measures of the success of treatment, there would be difficulty in interpreting the findings. The subsequent success of feeding (the other outcome measure) was also likely to be influenced, this time adversely

(Grant B., 1989). Women who had surgery involving the nipple or areola were not recruited as it was felt such surgery might adversely affect both the outcome measures.

Thus women were considered eligible for recruitment provided they met the following inclusion criteria:

1. had at least one inverted or non-protractile nipple
2. were nulliparous
3. were intending to breast feed
4. were not intending to have their baby adopted
5. were not already using shells or any kind of nipple exercises during the current pregnancy
6. were between 25 and 35 completed weeks of gestation
7. had a singleton pregnancy
8. had not had surgery involving the nipple or areola

Consent and random allocation

While an eligible woman was being invited to take part in the trial, special emphasis was laid on the need for random allocation (words such as 'taking pot luck' were occasionally used to describe this). It was also emphasized to the woman that if she decided not to participate her general care would not suffer as a result.

If the woman gave consent, her name was recorded in the trial log along with the number on the outside of the next available trial envelope; this was the only place where the woman was identified by name and I removed the sheets of the log at regular intervals. After this had been done, thus committing the woman to the allocation contained within the envelope, the latter was opened. The envelopes were opaque and sealed, all were of the same thickness and there were no other external features which made it possible to determine which trial allocation was contained within. In order to allow interim analysis of data the allocations were randomized (using a table of random numbers) in blocks of 16, but the midwives were not aware of this blocking. In fact no interim analysis was carried out as the number of women recruited was much smaller than anticipated.

Trial documentation

Each envelope contained an antenatal data sheet, a postnatal data sheet to be attached to the notes, a letter giving the woman details of the allocation which she had drawn and a letter giving details of the trial for her to give to her GP at her next visit. If the trial allocation included the use of shells, these were given to the woman (they were kindly provided free of charge by the manufacturer, Eschmann Brothers & Walsh Limited). Women prone to eczema were advised to stop wearing them should an eruption occur; the letter also explained that the shells were not suitable for postnatal use.

Outcome measures

After delivery the labour ward reassessed the woman's nipples using instructions identical to those used antenatally. The same measures were taken to limit inter-observer variation except that the observers were not involved in the formulation of the instructions. Both the midwives and the women were requested not to discuss the trial allocation prior to the reassessment in order to minimize bias. The examination was to be conducted prior to the first feed so that the protractility would not have been affected by suckling.

During the sixth week after delivery I sent the woman a questionnaire requesting details of her baby feeding. Assessing the success of breast feeding is difficult but national studies have shown that the sharp decline in the prevalence of breast feeding which occurs over the first few weeks becomes somewhat less acute six weeks after delivery (Martin, 1978; Martin and Monk, 1982; Martin and White, 1988; White, Freeth and O'Brien, 1992).

The envelope containing the questionnaire and that for its return were handwritten with ordinary postage stamps attached, as it has been found that typewritten 'Freepost' envelopes have a less satisfactory response rate (Sleep, personal communication). The covering letter was hand signed and thanked the woman for her assistance. The visit which I made to each woman and baby before they left hospital was referred to and their first names were used, which helped to personalize the letter further.

The questionnaire, like all the data sheets, was pilot tested and modified before the trial began. Its design was based on that used in the national survey by Martin and White (1988). To avoid the questionnaire being sent to the parents of a baby who had subsequently died, the local Department of Immunization and Vaccination informed me of all baby deaths occurring within the District.

The eventual 'response' rate was 100% but five of the questionnaires were in fact completed by telephone interview. The original mailing had failed to achieve a response from these participants and it became evident that this other method of 'completion' was much more acceptable to these five women.

Sample size

Before the study no data were available about success rates for breast feeding at six weeks after delivery among women with antenatal nipple inversion or non-protractility. Because of time constraints, recruitment ceased when 96 women had joined the trial. A trial of this size had 50%

power to identify an increase in successful breast feeding of 20% ($p<0.05$) due to one or other of the policies (Polit and Hungler, 1991).

Data-processing and statistical analysis

This was performed at the Department of Medical Statistics and Computing of Southampton General Hospital. The data were entered onto a DBase II spreadsheet on an IBC PC AT. Statistical tests were two sided and 95% confidence intervals were calculated (Gardner and Altman, 1986). Continuous variables were analysed by Student's t test when a parametric test was appropriate or by the Mann–Whitney U or Kruskal–Wallis non-parametric tests. Categorical variables were analysed by the χ^2 test with Yates' correction two × two tables.

In the postnatal questionnaire women were asked to what extent they had complied with their treatment allocation but for the main outcome measures they were analysed as belonging to the group to which they had been originally assigned; that is, the study was analysed by 'intention to treat' (Peto *et al.*, 1976). Withdrawals after trial entry for reasons related to a specific treatment may introduce selection bias (Gail, 1985) and analysis of this trial based on 'treatment received' would almost certainly have been biased in this way.

Ethical aspects

There had been no ill effects reported concerning the 'pinch test' and it was already widely used. It was judged ethical to investigate the treatment methods as there is evidence (see literature review) that poor nipple anatomy hampers breast feeding. It was not thought unethical to withhold one or both of the treatments according to trial allocation as the benefit of neither had yet been proven. In fact it could be argued that, in view of the lack of evidence supporting the use of shells or exercises, it would have been unethical not to have undertaken the trial.

Participants were identified by trial number only on their data sheets. The data on computer were subject to the Data Protection Act 1984. The research was approved by the Local Research Ethics Committee.

Derivation and description of the trial groups

During the 23 months of recruitment, 3006 women had the protractility of their nipples recorded. Of these women 1926 were nulliparous and thus potentially eligible for recruitment to the management trial. One hundred and thirty women fulfilled the inclusion criteria (Figure 8.3). Two of the eligible women were never invited to participate because of a misunderstanding concerning the eligibility criteria. Thirty of the 128 women approached to participate declined to do so, the majority of those who declined being unwilling to accept random allocation to a treatment group (Table 8.3). Only women who were intending to breast feed were examined and it is noteworthy that 11 women immediately changed their mind and decided to artificially feed on being told the result of their examination.

Figure 8.3 Source of participants.

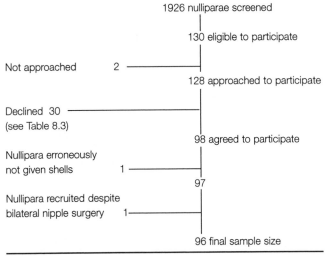

Source: Compiled by the author.

Table 8.3 Principal reason for declining invitation to participate in management trial

Reason	($N = 30$)	
	No.	*%*
Unwilling to wear shells	9	30
Unwilling to use shells or exercises	4	13
Requested both shells and exercises	5	17
Requested shells alone	1	3
Decided to bottle feed	11	37

Source: Alexander (1991).

Of the 98 women who agreed to participate in the trial, one (allocated shells with exercises) was almost certainly never given her shells and thus not formally enrolled, and another (allocated exercises) was found to be ineligible having had bilateral nipple surgery. Full data were collected about both these women but they were excluded from the analysis and thus 96 nulliparae constituted the final study sample.

The characteristics of the final study sample are shown in Table 8.4. Overall, 27 women had at least one inverted nipple and 80 at least one non-protractile nipple. There were no statistically significant differences between the groups.

Table 8.4 Characteristics of pregnant women with inverted or non-protractile nipples allocated to four treatment groups. Values are medians (ranges) unless stated otherwise

Characteristics	Shells (N=24)	Exercises (N=24)	Shells plus exercises (N=24)	Control (N=24)
Maternal age (years)	24(16–32)	25(17–33)	24(18–38)	25.5(17–37)
Anatomical state of nipples*:				
No. (%) inverted	8(33)	8(33)	7(29)	4(17)
No. (%) non-protractile	21(88)	19(79)	19(79)	21(88)
Interval between recruitment and delivery (days)	59.5(32–107)	60.5(14–112)	65.5(3–102)	52.5(31–103)
Gestational age at delivery (weeks)	40(37–42)	40(33–42)	39.5(34–42)	40(34–42)
Mean (SD) birth weight (g)	3299(535)	3415(461)	3262(593)	3228(532)
Type of delivery (no.(%) of women):				
Normal vaginal	18(75)	18(75)	12(50)	15(63)
Instrumental vaginal	4(17)	4(17)	7(29)	3(13)
Caesarean	2(8)	2(8)	5(21)	6(25)

*Some women were in both categories.
Source: Reproduced from Alexander, Grant and Campbell (1992). By courtesy of the British Medical Journal.

FINDINGS

Compliance

Sixty-three per cent (30/48) of the women allocated shells reported using them as instructed all or most of the time, whereas 75% (36/48) allocated exercises reported doing so. The reasons given by those who failed to carry out their trial instructions all of the time are shown in Table 8.5. It can be seen that only one woman (2%) forgot her shells, as compared with 42% (20) of women who forgot to use the exercises on occasions. Conversely 44% of women did not use their shells 'all of the time' because they found them painful or uncomfortable, as opposed to 4% (2) who gave this reason in relation to exercises. Considerable numbers of women failed to use their shells 'all of the time' because of embarrassment, their prominence beneath clothing or because they caused sweating, rash, eczema or soreness.

No woman in the control group ever used shells or exercises.

Table 8.5 Reasons for failing to carry out trial instructions 'all of the time'

Reason	All women commenting on exercises (N=48)		All women commenting on shells (N=48)	
	No.	%	No.	%
Maternal illness (did not include preterm labour)	2	4	0	0
Forgot	20	42	1	2
Too tired	4	8	0	0
Did not have time	3	6	0	0
Treatment made no difference	3	6	0	0
Treatment already worked	1	2	0	0
Treatment painful/uncomfortable	2	4	21	44
Other	2	4	0	0
Embarrassment			13	27
Evident under clothing			19	40
Slipped out of place			1	2
Caused sweating, rash, eczema or soreness beneath them			11	23
Promoted or allowed milk leakage			5	10
Total No. of reasons	37		71	

Some women gave more than one reason.
Source: Alexander (1991).

Changes in nipple anatomy

Ninety-five per cent confidence intervals (Gardner and Altman, 1986) were calculated in order to give a more accurate indication of where the true difference between the groups is likely to lie. In essence they indicate that there is a 95% chance that the value which would result, if the total population of women with inverted or non-protractile nipples was to be studied, would lie between these values. The larger the sample size the narrower the confidence interval becomes.

The effects of treatment allocation on nipple anatomy are shown in Table 8.6. It can be seen that sustained improvement in nipple anatomy was more common in the untreated groups (8% fewer (–8%) of those recommended to use shells having a sustained improvement than those not recommended to use them; 4% fewer (–4%) of those recommended exercises than those not recommended them). However, in both cases the 95% confidence intervals span zero, thus indicating that the possibility of a lack of effect or even of a positive effect from recommending the treatments cannot be ruled out. For example, in the case of recommending shells the 95% confidence intervals indicate that the true result might lie anywhere between 28% fewer (–28%) of those recommended shells having a sustained improvement than those not recommended them, through to 11% more of them having an improvement.

Table 8.6 Effects on nipple anatomy of recommending breast preparation with shells and Hoffman's exercises

| | *Shells* | | | |
| | *Recommended shells (N=48)* | | *Not recommended shells (N=48)* | | *% Difference (95% confidence interval)* |
	No.	*%*	*No.*	*%*	
Sustained improvement in nipple anatomy after delivery*	25	52	29	60	–8(–28 to 11)

| | *Exercises* | | | |
| | *Recommended shells (N=48)* | | *Not recommended shells (N=48)* | | *% Difference (95% confidence interval)* |
	No.	*%*	*No.*	*%*	
Sustained improvement in nipple anatomy after delivery*	26	54	28	58	–4(–24 to 16)

*Not known for one woman in the control group. Sustained improvement defined as at least a unilateral improvement without a balancing regression on the other side.
Source: Compiled by the author.

Breast feeding six weeks after delivery

The effects of treatment allocation on the success of breast feeding six weeks after delivery are summarized in Table 8.7. It can be seen that recommending exercises seemed to have no effect on the success of breast feeding. However, the estimate is imprecise and compatible with both a 20% decrease and a 20% increase in breast feeding success.

Table 8.7 Effects on breast feeding of recommending breast preparation with shells and Hoffman's exercises

Breast feeding six weeks after delivery	*Shells*		*% Difference (95% confidence interval)*
	Recommended shells (N=48)	*Not recommended shells (N=48)*	
	No. *%*	*No.* *%*	
Successful*	14 29	24 50	−21(−40 to −2)
Discontinued	29 60	23 48	
Never started	5 10	1 2	

Breast feeding six weeks after delivery	*Exercises*		*% Difference (95% confidence interval)*
	Recommended shells (N=48)	*Not recommended shells (N=48)*	
	No. *%*	*No.* *%*	
Successful*	19 40	19 40	0(−20 to 20)
Discontinued	27 56	25 52	
Never started	2 4	4 8	

*Includes women giving supplementary or complementary bottle feeds.
Source: Compiled by the author.

Ten (21%) fewer of the women recommended shells were breast-feeding six weeks after delivery than the women not recommended shells ($p=0.05$). The 95% confidence intervals (−40% to −2%) did not encompass the possibility that recommending shells would have a positive effect on breast feeding rates. The poor outcome for those recommended shells reflected both more women discontinuing breast feeding and more women who had changed their mind before delivery and decided not to attempt to breast feed. Four of the five women recommended shells who had decided by the time of delivery to feed artificially mentioned the problems which they had had with shells as one of the reasons for their decision. For three of these women their inability to tolerate wearing shells was the major reason for their decision not to attempt to breast feed. No women reported that exercises had been a factor in their decision not to breast feed.

There was some evidence that exercises, when recommended in combination with shells, mitigated the adverse effect of shells when recommended alone (see Table 8.8). It is interesting to note that the breast feeding rate was highest amongst the control group. In all, 40% (38) of the women were breast feeding at six weeks postnatally.

Table 8.8 Breast feeding in the four groups at six weeks after delivery

	Control (N=24)		Exercises (N=24)		Shells (N=24)		Shells and exercises (N=24)	
	No.	%	No.	%	No.	%	No.	%
Breast feeding*	15	63	9	38	4	17	10	42
Discontinued	8	33	15	63	17	71	12	50
Never started	1	4	0	0	3	13	2	8

*The term 'breast feeding' includes those giving supplementary bottles.
Source: Alexander (1991)

The women were also asked in the questionnaire if they had experienced nipple bleeding, latching difficulties or 'breast infection needing antibiotics'. There were no significant differences between the groups in relation to these; however, slightly more women recommended breast shells had breast infections postnatally than other women (14% (6/43) of women who had attempted breast feeding in the 'shell groups' compared with 6% (3/47) in the 'no shell' groups).

Data were also collected concerning any complementary or supplementary feeds which had been given and, if breast feeding had been discontinued, the reasons for this and the age of the baby at which the last breast feed had been given. No important differences were found between the groups.

DISCUSSION

Generalizability

Of the 3006 women screened in the Southampton area, 130 were eligible to participate in the management trial and all but two of these were approached. It therefore seems likely that the findings of the trial are generalizable at least to the population of Southampton. In generalizing to any other group of women it is possible that the findings might differ quantitatively but there is no reason to think that they would differ qualitatively.

Randomization

This study was the first randomized controlled trial of either shells or Hoffman's exercises (see review of previous work). It was conducted in this way with the aim of avoiding systematic differences between the two groups and it would appear from the data in Table 8.4 that this was successful. It is particularly noteworthy that the gestational age at delivery of the women in the groups recommended exercises was not statistically lower than that of the groups not recommended to use them. Previous authors (Riordan, 1983; Lawrence , 1985) had cautioned that the nipple stimulation caused by exercises could result in uterine contractions.

Avoiding bias in the measurement of outcome

The measurement of outcome constitutes another potential source of bias. Instructions were given both to the women recruited to the trial and to the midwives that the assessment of the anatomical state of the nipples after delivery should be conducted blind to allocated group. There is no reason to believe that this was not done. If there had been any element of bias one might have expected the midwives to be less likely to find inverted or non-protractile nipples still present in women who had been allocated to an active treatment group; this did not prove to be so. The details collected by questionnaire concerning feeding are also unlikely to have been biased; if they had been, one might have expected women from the groups who received active treatment to be more likely to have reported continuing breast feeding as they may have considered this the outcome desired by the researcher; again this was not the case.

Compliance with trial allocation

The control group All reported complying with their trial allocation 'all of the time'. This is perhaps surprising as, although a full discussion concerning the lack of evidence to support the use of the treatments under investigation took place before trial entry, one might have expected some recruits to assume that shells or exercises were effective and to use them regardless of their allocation.

The acceptability of exercises Seventy-one per cent (17) of women in the exercise (alone) group reported carrying them out on all or most occasions. The instructions were that the exercises should be done twice a day. There was evidence that some participants did the exercises only once daily and hence, despite being very conscientious, could not claim to have done them as instructed 'all of the time'. The acceptability of exercises appeared to be good, and out of the nine women who declined to participate in the management trial for fear of being allocated shells, eight recorded unprompted that they would be happy to use exercises. It is perhaps not surprising that (as shown in Table 8.5) exercises were more likely to be forgotten than shells.

The acceptability of shells Shells proved to be less acceptable than exercises, but 14 (58%) women in the shell (alone) group reported wearing them all or most of the time. Nine (30%) of the 30 women who declined to enter the management trial did so because of their unwillingness to risk allocation to a shell group, and four (13%) because they were unwilling to use either shells or exercises. Thirty-eight per cent of those assigned to a policy involving shells reported wearing them only occasionally or not at all. It must be stated, however, that five of those who declined the trial (17%) did so because they wished to use both shells and exercises, and one woman because she wished to use shells alone.

Of the 48 women allocated to a treatment group involving shells, 21 (44%) said that they had failed to wear them 'all of the time' because they caused pain or discomfort (only two women (4%) failing to follow the instructions regarding exercises 'all of the time' for this reason (Table 8.5)). This is in contrast to the claims of Waller (1946) and Blaikley *et al.* (1953) that shells are painless. Contrary to Blaikley *et al.* (1953), Gunther (1973), Poole (1987) and Larsen (1990), who assured readers that shells are surprisingly inconspicuous, 19 of the women (40%) stated that they failed to wear them 'all of the time' because they were evident beneath clothing, and 13 (27%) because of embarrassment. Eleven women (23%) did not wear their shells 'all of the time' because sweating, soreness, a rash or eczema occurred beneath them, similar problems being mentioned by Gunther (1973), Otte (1975), Lawrence (1985), Levi (1988) and the manufacturer's own product literature. Five women (10%) did not wear their shells 'all of the time' because they found that they caused colostrum leakage; this is a problem that the researcher has not found in the literature. The above casts some doubt on Waller's (1946) observation that 'in many years experience no ill effects whatever from [the use of(glass) shells] have been seen', although he did caution about the occurrence of eczema in 1957 (Waller, 1957).

The decision not to breast feed

Six of the women recruited to the trial had decided not to breast feed by the time they delivered. Whereas exercises did not play a major part in the decision of any of these women, five were allocated shells and three of these stated that their inability to tolerate shells was of major importance.

The opinion of some authors (Hytten, 1954; L'Esperance, 1980) that there may be doubt about the link between inverted and non-protractile nipples and nipple soreness caused by breast feeding has already been discussed. In the light of this it seems tragic that 11 (37%) of the 30 women who declined to enter the trial told the midwife at the time of their examination that they had decided to feed artificially on the basis of having been found to have inverted or non-protractile nipples (Table 8.3). A further six women who were recruited to the trial had also decided not to breast feed by the time they delivered, three of them stating that this was due, at least in part, to their nipple anatomy continuing to be poor. Thus 17 (13%) of the 128 women approached to participate in the trial decided to feed artificially. Unless the treatments can be shown to result in a significant improvement in the outcome variables, it would seem that the practice of examining the protractility of nipples during the antenatal period should be seriously questioned, as an adverse examination can result in a number of women not even attempting to breast feed.

The size of the trial and the trial results

The numbers of women recruited to the trial were smaller than planned due to time constraints and, because of the small numbers involved, the risk of being misled by random errors increased. The factorial design of the study proved especially important as it increased its statistical power. The 95% confidence intervals indicate the range in which the true differences are likely to lie. Sizes of effect outside the confidence intervals are therefore very unlikely. Because the trial results tend to suggest no benefit (or even an adverse effect) it would appear that quite moderate positive effects from treatment can, in fact, be ruled out (Detsky and Sackett, 1985).

Change in nipple anatomy between recruitment and delivery

The policy of recommending Hoffman's exercises, that of recommending shells and that of recommending a combined allocation, all failed to result in any statistically significant difference in anatomical change when compared with that occurring following a policy of not recommending these treatments. When examining the 95% confidence interval (exercises versus no exercises −24% to +16%, shells versus no shells −28% to +11%) it can be seen, however, that the upper end is compatible with some moderate improvement (Table 8.6).

Nipple anatomy at outset of breast feeding

When assessed after delivery there was no significant difference in nipple anatomy between the allocation groups (Table 8.6). Thus, at least in this respect, no group was advantaged in comparison with the others at the outset of breast feeding.

Type of feeding at questionnaire completion (six weeks after delivery)

There was no significant difference between the policies of recommending and not recommending Hoffman's exercises when the type of feeding at questionnaire completion was examined (Table 8.7). The 95% confidence intervals (–20% to +20%) were just as likely to include a negative as they were to include a positive effect on breast feeding rates. However, when the policy of recommending shells was compared with the policy of not recommending them, the former group was significantly less likely (p=0.05) to be breast feeding at questionnaire completion than the latter (Table 8.7). The 95% confidence intervals (–40% to –2%) exclude 'no difference' and indicate that there is at least a 95% chance that the policy of recommending shells is associated with an adverse effect on breast feeding rates at six weeks postpartum.

The lower rate of breast feeding amongst those allocated shells was both because more women had discontinued breast feeding by the time of questionnaire completion and because more had decided to feed artificially by the time they delivered. From the comments made by the women who had decided to feed artificially by the time they delivered, poor acceptability of shells appears to have been an important issue. The statement made by the Ministry of Health in 1944 – 'We think it possible that with an anxious type of woman too much stress on [antenatal] preparation of the breasts may alarm and discourage her to such an extent that she will refuse even to initiate breast feeding' – seems to be vindicated at least in respect of shells. It appears that women who cannot tolerate shells presume that any attempt they make to breast feed will be doomed and therefore have a tendency not even to start, or to give up should they run into any problems. The adverse effect of shells on breast feeding appears to be partially mitigated when women use both shells and exercises (Table 8.8). It is difficult to explain this and it may reflect a chance difference. Alternatively, women who cannot tolerate shells have a second method of treatment to use, and, having expended this effort in the treatment of their 'problem', may feel more positive about their likelihood of success.

Latching difficulty, nipple bleeding and 'breast infection needing antibiotics'

No statistically significant differences were found between the main effect groups in relation to these, nor when the combination of these three problems was considered.The effect of the combined allocation was as expected from studying the effect of each treatment separately. The confidence intervals were wide, however, and quite large effects in either direction cannot be ruled out.

IMPLICATIONS FOR FURTHER RESEARCH

There are two major problems with relatively small trials such as the one described above (Grant, A., 1989). First, they may over-estimate the true effect of an intervention when the difference observed in the trial is statistically significant. For example, the apparent adverse effect of shells identified in this trial may be exaggerated. Second, they tend falsely to ascribe real differences between treatments to chance. This trial cannot, for example, rule out up to a 20% improvement in breast-feeding rates being associated with exercises. For these reasons it was important that the experiment should be replicated on a larger scale.

Therefore, when it became evident that the target of 400 recruits could not be achieved, I approached the National Perinatal Epidemiology Unit (Oxford) concerning the possibility of extending the trial to other centres. A core group consisting of Mary Renfrew (midwife researcher), Adrian Grant (epidemiologist) and myself was set up; we were soon joined by Rona McCandlish (research midwife). The development which resulted at the time of writing had two components: one involving a multi-centre and international hospital-based study, the other involving women contacted through the National Childbirth Trust. The findings from this longer trial have now been published, and support those of the research reported here. The longer trial showed that neither Hoffman's exercises nor shells is 'certain to improve the chances that a woman will be breast feeding at six weeks after birth' (MAIN Trial Collaborative Group, 1994).

IMPLICATIONS FOR CLINICAL PRACTICE

It is ironic that in 1947, Waller, who popularized breast shells, stated that 'if anything unfavourable to success should gain entry, however unwittingly, into the management of breast feeding ... and especially should it become incorporated in the teaching of training schools for nurses and midwives, its effects may become disastrously widespread' (Waller, 1947). In relation to the antenatal examination of nipple protractility and the treatment of inversion and non-protractility this appears to have happened, particularly in the case of shells.

This trial provides no good evidence that either the policy of recommending shells or the policy of recommending exercises conveys any benefit in terms of anatomical change occurring between recruitment and delivery. In terms of the success of breast feeding as assessed at six weeks postnatally, those who were recommended to wear shells were significantly (p=0.05) less likely to be breast feeding at this time than those who were not recommended to wear them (see Table 8.7). On the basis of this, the use of shells should be abandoned, other than in the context of further well-controlled trials. The trial also failed to identify any benefit from the policy of recommending exercises but a moderate and clinically useful effect of up to a 20% improvement in breast feeding success rates cannot be ruled out. As 13% of those approached to participate in the trial decided not even to attempt to breast feed, antenatal examination of nipples for protractility (regardless of subsequent management) may actually have a negative effect on breast feeding rates. For this reason the present findings suggest that an antenatal examination of the nipples in women who intend to breast feed is not only unnecessary but may in fact be counter-productive and should be discontinued. There would appear to be no need even to raise the topic for discussion unless the woman does so herself.

ACKNOWLEDGEMENTS

I owe a tremendous debt of gratitude to the women and midwives who took part in this study and particularly for the advice and support given to me by Adrian Grant and Michael Campbell. I am also most grateful for advice and support from Fred Anthony, Iain Chalmers, Diana Elbourne, Chloe Fisher, Frank Hytten, Sally Inch, Chris James, Rona McCandlish, Mary Renfrew, Jennifer Sleep, Timothy Wheeler, Sarah Roch and the late John Dennis; and colleagues in the Department of Midwifery Education, Southampton.

This study was supported by a Royal College of Midwives/Maws Research Scholarship and the Iolanthe Trust. Eschmann Brothers & Walsh provided the breast shells.

REFERENCES

Alexander, J. (1990) Antenatal preparation of the breasts for breastfeeding. In Alexander, J., Levy, V. and Roch, S. (eds), *Antenatal Care: A Research-Based Approach*. Macmillan, Basingstoke, p. 68.

Alexander, J. (1991) The prevalence and management of inverted and non-protractile nipples in antenatal women who intend to breastfeed. Unpublished PhD thesis, University of Southampton, Faculty of Medicine.

Alexander, J.M., Grant, A.M. and Campbell, M.J. (1992) Randomised controlled trial of breast shells and Hoffman's exercises for inverted and non-protractile nipples. *British Medical Journal*, **304**(6833), 1031.

Applebaum, R.M. (1969) *Abreast of the Times*. Applebaum, R.M. (private publication), Miami.

Ardran, G.M., Kemp, F.H. and Lind, J. (1958) A cineradiographic study of breast feeding. *British Journal of Radiology*, **31**(363), 156–62.

Blaikley, J., Clarke, S., MacKeith, R. and Ogden, K.M. (1953) Breast feeding: factors affecting success – a report of a trial of the Woolwich Methods in a group of primiparae. *Journal of Obstetrics and Gynaecology of the British Empire*, **60**, 657–69.

Burrows, H. (1949) Biological Action of Sex Hormones, 2nd edn. Cambridge University Press, London.

Cadwell,K. (1981) Improving nipple graspability for success at breastfeeding. *Journal of Obstetric, Gynecologic and Neonatal Nursing*, **10**(4), 277–79.

Cochran, W.G. and Cox, G.M. (1957) *Experimental Designs*, 2nd edn. Wiley, New York.

Cotterman, J. (1976) Intensive preparation for inverted or retracting nipples. *Keeping*

Abreast Journal, **I**, 330–2.

Cunnane, M. (1938) Letter. *British Medical Journal*, **ii**, 1112.

DeLee, J.B. and Greenhill J.P. (1947) *Principles and Practice of Obstetrics*, 9th edn. Saunders, Philadelphia.

Detsky, A.S. and Sackett, D.L. (1985) When was a 'negative' clinical trial big enough? How many patients you needed depended on what you found. *Archives of Internal Medicine*, **145**, 709–12.

Dutton, M.A. (1979) A breastfeeding protocol. *Journal of Obstetric, Gynecologic and Neonatal Nursing*, **8**(3), 151–5.

Eastman, N.J. (1950) *Williams Obstetrics*, 10th edn. Appleton-Century-Crofts, New York.

Frager, N.B. and Miyazaki, F.S. (1987) Intrauterine monitoring of contractions during breast stimulation. *Obstetrics and Gynecology*, **69**(5), 767–769.

Gail, M.H. (1985) Eligibility exclusions, losses to follow-up, removal of randomized patients, and uncounted events in cancer clinical trials. *Cancer Treatment Report*, **69**, 1107–13.

Gangal, H.T. and Gangal, M.H. (1978) Suction method for correcting flat nipples or inverted nipples. *Plastic and Reconstructive Surgery*, **61**(2), 294–96.

Gardner, M.J. and Altman, D.G. (1986) Confidence intervals rather than P values: estimation rather than hypothesis testing. *British Medical Journal*, **292**, 746–50.

Gaskin, I.M. (1980) *Spiritual Midwifery*, revised edn. The Book Publishing Company, Summertown.

Gore, S.M. (1982) Assessing clinical trials – between observer variation. In Gore, S.M. and Altman, D.G. (eds), *Statistics in Practice: Articles Published in the British Medical Journal*. British Medical Association. London.

Grant, A. (1989) Reporting controlled trials. *British Journal of Obstetrics and Gynaecology*, **96**, 397–400.

Grant, B. (1989) Multiple pregnancy. In Bennett V.R. and Brown L.K. (eds), *Myles Textbook for Midwives*, 11th edn. Churchill Livingstone, Edinburgh.

Gunther, M. (1973) *Infant Feeding*. Penguin Books, Harmondsworth.

Hauden, D.J. and Mahler, D. (1983) A simple method for the correction of the inverted nipple. *Plastic and Reconstructive surgery*, **71**(4), 556–9.

Helsing, E. and Savage King, F. (1984) Preparing mothers for breastfeeding. *Nursing Journal of India*, **75**(7), 155–6.

Hoffman, J.B. (1953) A suggested treatment for inverted nipples. *American Journal of Obstetrics and Gynecology*, **66**(2), 346–8.

Hytten, F.E. (1954) Clinical and chemical studies in human lactation; IX Breast feeding in hospital. *British Medical Journal*, **ii**(4902), 1447–52.

Hytten, F.E. (1990) Is it important or even useful to measure weight gain in pregnancy? *Midwifery*, **6**, 28–32.

Hytten, F.E. and Bird, D. (1958) The development of the nipple in pregnancy. *Lancet*, **i**, (7032), 1201–4.

Jhirad, A. and Vago, T. (1973) Induction of labour by breast stimulation. *Obstetrics and Gynecology*, **41**(3), 347–50.

Jones, W.E. (1989) Setting up a breastfeeding clinic. *Midwives Chronicle and Nursing Notes*, **102**(1216), 138–41.

Larsen, L.L.V. (1990) Prenatal breastfeeding counselling: nipple inversion. *International Journal of Childbirth Education*, February, 33–4.

Lawrence, R.A. (1985) *Breast-feeding: A guide for the medical profession*, 2nd edn.

Mosby, St Louis.

L'Esperance, C.M. (1980) Pain or pleasure: the dilemma of early breastfeeding. *Birth and the Family Journal,* **7**(1), 21–6.

Levi, J. (1988) Establishing breast feeding in hospital. *Archives of Disease in Childhood,* **63**, 1281–5.

MAIN Trial Collaborative Group (1994) Preparing for breast feeding: treatment of inverted and non-protractile nipples. *Midwifery,* **10**(4), 200–14.

Martin, J. (1978) *Infant feeding 1975: attitudes and practice in England and Wales.* Office of Population Censuses and Surveys, HMSO, London.

Martin, J. and Monk, J. (1982) *Infant feeding 1980.* Office of Population Censuses and Surveys, London.

Martin, J. and White, A. (1988) *Infant feeding 1985.* HMSO, London.

Ministry of Health, January (1944) *The Breast Feeding of Infants: Report of the Advisory Committee on Mothers and Children.* Public Health Medical Subjects, Report 91. HMSO, London

Naish, F.C. (1948) *Breast Feeding: A Guide to the Natural Feeding of Infants.* Oxford University Press, London.

Otte, M.J. (1975) Correcting inverted nipples: an aid to breast feeding. *American Journal of Nursing,* **75**(3), 454–6.

Peto, R., Pike, M.C., Armitage, P., Breslow, N.E., Cox, D.R., Howard, S.V., Mantel, N., McPherson, K., Peto, J. and Smith, P.G. (1976) Design and analysis of randomized clinical trials requiring prolonged observation of each patient: I. Introduction and design. *British Journal of Cancer,* **4**, 585–614.

Pocock, S.J. (1983) *Clinical trials: A Practical Approach.* Wiley, Chichester.

Polit, D.F. and Hungler, B.P. (1991) *Nursing Research: Principles and Methods,* 4th edn. Lippincott, Philadelphia.

Poole, K. (1987) A matter of confidence. *New Generation,* **6**(1), 33–4.

Riordan, J. (ed.) (1983) *A Practical Guide to Breastfeeding.* Mosby, St Louis.

Royal College of Midwives (1988) *Successful Breastfeeding: A Practical Guide for Midwives (and Others Supporting Breastfeeding Mothers).* Holywell Press, Oxford.

Samuel, P. (1985) *Thinking About Breastfeeding?* National Childbirth Trust, London.

Southampton and South West Hampshire Health Authority (1990) *Annual Report of the Director of Public Health.*

Stone, E.L.(1946) *The New-born Infant.* Lea & Febiger, Philadelphia.

Sweet, B.R. (1988) *Mayes' Midwifery: A Textbook for Midwives.* Baillière Tindall, London.

Viegas, O.A.C., Arulkumaran, S., Gibb, D.M.E. and Ratnam, S.S. (1984) Nipple stimulation in late pregnancy causing uterine hyperstimulation and profound fetal bradycardia. *British Journal of Obstetrics and Gynaecology,* 91, 364–6.

Walker, M. (1989) Management of selected early breastfeeding problems seen in clinical practice. *Birth* **16**(3), 148–58.

Waller, H. (1939) Clinical Studies in Lactation. Heinemann, London.

Waller, H. (1946) The early failure of breast feeding: a clinical study of its causes and their prevention. *Archives of Disease in Childhood,* **21**, 1–12.

Waller, H. (1947) Incidence, causes and prevention of failure of breast feeding. *British Medical Bulletin,* **5**, 181–5.

Waller, H. (1957) *The Breasts and Breast Feeding.* Heinemann, Medical Books, London.

Weber, F.,Woolridge, M.W., McLeod, C.N., Rochefort, M.J. and Baum, J.D. (1984) An ultrasonographic study of the organisation of sucking and swallowing in newborn infants (an abstract). *Pediatric Research*, **18**(8), 806.

White, A., Freeth, S. and O'Brien, M. (1992) *Infant Feeding 1990*. HMSO, London.

Williams, P.L., Warwick, R., Dyson, M. and Bannister, L.H. (eds) (1989) *Gray's Anatomy*, 37th edn. Churchill Livingstone, Edinburgh.

Woolridge, M.W. (1986) The 'anatomy' of infant sucking. *Midwifery*, 2, 164–71.

Yorston, J. (1956) A study of breast feeding. Unpublished MD thesis, University of Aberdeen.

CHAPTER NINE

Care in the third stage of labour*

Diana Elbourne

This chapter discusses my involvement in research concerning care in the third stage of labour, leading up to the Bristol third-stage trial (Prendiville *et al.*, 1988), and its aftermath. Although the perspective is personal, I hope my experience of how decisions about research priorities were arrived at, about which research methods were used, and about the interface between research and policy and practice, has wider relevance for researchers with different backgrounds, and for areas other than the third stage of labour.

BEFORE THE BRISTOL THIRD-STAGE TRIAL

For the mother, [delivery of the placenta] is the most dangerous stage of labour when the skill and expertise of the midwife will be crucial factors in ensuring her safety.

(Sleep, 1989)

As the above quotation makes clear, the third stage of labour is a crucial period as seen from a midwifery perspective, as postpartum haemorrhage (PPH) can lead to death or serious morbidity in many countries in the world. For most mothers giving birth today in the UK and similar countries, however, delivery of the placenta is not a cause of either great joy or of great interest – unless something goes wrong. Certainly, my own involvement in this area was not sparked off by being the mother of two children. Nor, as a social statistician working on perinatal trials at a Department of Health funded research unit in Oxford (the National Perinatal Epidemiology Unit (NPEU)) in 1984, had any of my previous research suggested that the third stage would take up a considerable proportion of my time over the next decade.

I did have a long-term interest in the Third World, and was aware that PPH was one of the major reasons for women dying in their childbearing years (see Kwast, 1991a, 1991b). The trigger for my research interest, however, was the request of an obstetrician (Walter Prendiville), then working in the Bristol Maternity Hospital (BMH), for help from the NPEU with the design of a trial concerning the use of Syntometrine (0.5 mg ergometrine with 5 IU oxytocin) in the third stage of labour. His interest had, in turn, arisen from the request by a woman for whom he was caring in labour to withhold the routine administration of Syntometrine with delivery of the anterior shoulder.

Initially my role was, with the help of Iain Chalmers (then director of the NPEU), to persuade Walter Prendiville first to conduct a formal review of the research evidence. For all three of us, this was our first major experience in developing the methods for what was then called an overview or a meta-analysis (and is now more often called a structured or systematic review). Within the review, we decided to broaden the question to include all oxytocics used in the third stage of labour, rather than just Syntometrine.

A key component of this review was a wish to reduce the risk of being misled by selection biases. This involved, first, ensuring that the individual studies included were methodologically rigorous. This necessitated the use of a contemporaneous control group chosen by random or quasi-random allocation. Secondly, we wanted to aim for comprehensiveness in the review, because of the recognition that many reviews selectively include some studies but not others. We were lucky that, at just about the same time, the Oxford Register of Perinatal Trials (Chalmers, 1989) was becoming established. From this, we were able to identify all controlled trials comparing the use of prophylactic oxytocics to no prophylactic oxytocics.

We then worked to produce three sets of tables. The first table included a description of the individual studies in terms of the population, the interventions (and any associated or co-interventions) and the outcomes considered. The second table showed an assessment of the methodological quality of the studies. Although there are many ways to describe the quality, we chose to concentrate on three issues: first, the avoidance of selection bias at allocation to treatment, preferably by using secure random allocation secondly, the avoidance of selection bias in the analysis, preferably b including virtually all the women randomized; and thirdly, the avoidance of assessment bias, either by using such unambiguous endpoints (for instanc maternal death) that there was almost no danger of biased assessment, ensuring that the assessment was made without knowledge of which tre ment had been allocated or received. The final set of tables presented data in terms of the incidence of the outcomes of interest in the two gro being compared in each study. In situations in which data were missing unclear in the report of the trial, we wrote to the authors for information

clarification. Even though some of the studies had been conducted several years ago, many authors replied helpfully.

On the basis of this work, we published two overviews in the *British Journal of Obstetrics and Gynaecology* (BJOG) early in 1988. The first (Prendiville, Elbourne and Chalmers, 1988) concentrated on the evidence from all the trials comparing the use of prophylactic oxytocics to no prophylactic oxytocics; it was found that their use reduced the risk of PPH by about 40% and reduced the need for therapeutic oxytocics. There were also suggestions that oxytocics led to more hypertension, nausea and vomiting but there were insufficient data to be definitive.

The second paper (Elbourne, Prendiville and Chalmers, 1988) compared different oxytocics in four broad categories: ergot alkaloids, oxytocin, Syntometrine and prostaglandins, to explore which were the most effective and had fewest side-effects. The overview provided no evidence of any benefit of ergot alkaloids over Syntometrine or oxytocin alone, but more side-effects of ergot alkaloids, and therefore did not recommend their use. There was almost no evidence comparing prostaglandins with alternatives. The evidence comparing Syntometrine with oxytocin was based on trials of questionable methodological quality, and suggested that Syntometrine had a small advantage over oxytocin alone, in terms of a reduction in the risk of PPH, but Syntometrine had more side-effects.

Conducting research nearly always leads to a demonstration of the need for further research, and these overviews were no exception. This later research went in two directions. One was an extension of the reviewing work into other aspects of third-stage management. The other was primary research which involved conducting new randomized controlled trials (RCTs) to address questions for which reliable answers were not forthcoming from overviews of existing evidence. These two branches proceeded in parallel.

PRIMARY RESEARCH

The Bristol third-stage trial

Many of the reports of the trials included in the overview of oxytocics (Elbourne, Prendiville and Chalmers, 1988) did not provide full details of the context in which the oxytocics were administered. As oxytocics are only one part of a total package of active third-stage management, and there was no research evidence at that time about the effectiveness of that package, we began to design a trial to take place in Bristol to compare the then current policy of active management with expectant (physiological) management. Active management was the norm in England and Wales at the time (Garcia, Garforth and Ayers, 1987) and involved the use of a prophylactic oxytocic

(usually Syntometrine), early cord clamping and controlled cord traction. In contrast, expectant management used none of these interventions routinely, but encouraged maternal effort with an upright posture to allow the aid of gravity, followed by early breast feeding.

The protocol development took place over several months, with considerable input not merely from colleagues in the NPEU and the BMH, but also from representatives of consumer groups, and a number of midwives (usually 'independent' midwives) who were then practising expectant management (although not necessarily exactly the same versions). As the prime rationale for using active management was its presumed effect on the rate of PPH, we used PPH as the outcome measure on which to calculate the sample size required. We hypothesized that active management might reduce the incidence of PPH from 7.5% to 5%. A sample size of 3900 would then give an 80% chance of detecting this difference at the 5% level of statistical significance. This meant that it was feasible to carry out the trial in a single centre – the BMH. We secured project funding from the Regional Health Authority, and appointed Jo Harding as the research midwife.

Her role was crucial in the success of the trial (Harding, 1988). In addition to becoming involved in the later stages of protocol development, she was responsible for the day-to-day management of the trial in Bristol. This particularly included involving the midwives, primarily in the labour ward. Midwives were also involved in the antenatal clinic as women were initially recruited into the trial at this point, and in the postnatal wards and the community as some data collection related to the period after leaving the labour ward. There was a period of 'training' before the trial began (with updating during the trial) for those midwives who were not completely confident with both of the third-stage policies being compared. Jo Harding was also responsible for ensuring that the recruitment and data collection systems ran smoothly.

At the outset, an independent data-monitoring committee (DMC) was appointed. This consisted of a midwife, an obstetrician and an epidemiologist. This committee planned to meet to review the data about halfway through the recruitment period.

The first woman was randomized on 1 January 1986, and because of concerns about a high incidence of PPH in the expectant group the DMC had an early meeting in April 1986. They met on three subsequent occasions and in January 1987 recommended that the trial should cease recruitment as there was already an answer to the main trial question. The trial organizers, once shown the statistical data, accepted this recommendation, and the trial ended on 31 January 1987.

The principal report of the trial was published very speedily in the *British Medical Journal* (BMJ) late in 1988 (Prendiville *et al.*, 1988). In summary, it showed that the active management policy greatly reduced the rate of PPH, but increased the rate of nausea, vomiting and hypertension caused by the ergometrine component of Syntometrine.

To say there was considerable interest in the trial is rather a British understatement. Walter Prendiville left Bristol to take up an appointment on the other side of the world (Perth, Western Australia), but continued to work with us long distance on further publications arising from the trial over the next few years. In the UK, however, Jo Harding and I was in constant demand to talk about the trial. Some of these talks were to obstetricians, but the 'liveliest' ones were to midwives and consumer groups, often addressing issues which, although pre-specified and mentioned in the BMJ report, were not discussed in detail in that paper.

One question which was raised by several audiences concerned the actual managements used. This was less of an issue with active management than with expectant management. The controversy was both in terms of the management as stated in the protocol, and also its implementation in practice.

The definitions in the protocol were based on extensive and helpful discussions with many proponents of expectant management, particularly independent midwives. No one definition could reflect the variety of individual variations, but one was finally agreed for the protocol. Although not unfamiliar with the disappointment obstetricians sometimes faced when a trial report did not support a cherished belief, this was the first occasion in which I had met the same phenomenon among midwives. The reaction of a few, admittedly small in number but certainly vociferous, was to say that the reason the Bristol trial had not found in favour of expectant management was that the sort of expectant management in the trial protocol was not the sort of management that they would consider to be expectant management. This criticism, based on 'moving the goalposts after the match was over' is, in some senses, unanswerable, as the managements were very carefully defined and agreed beforehand as described above. For those proponents of a different form of expectant management who felt that it was different enough from those stated in the Bristol trial to invalidate the results, the only solution would be for them to try to put their preferred alternatives to the test in another well-designed trial. To the best of my knowledge, the only place where this has happened is in Hinchingbrooke, where a trial is in progress (see below).

The other criticism about the managements was less that they were 'wrongly' defined in the protocol but, instead, that they were not correctly implemented in practice. Again, this related almost entirely to the expectant management arm. Before the trial started recruitment, we had asked a number of midwives practising this management either to come to Bristol or to meet Jo Harding to discuss and demonstrate their skills. This was the basis for a training period of several weeks in the BMH. This training was continuously updated as new staff came into the labour ward. A survey of the views of the BMH labour ward midwives (Harding, Elbourne and Prendiville, 1989) showed that, by the time the trial began, they felt confident about their competence with both managements. In addition, it was clear from this survey that the prior assumption that they would all already be skilled in active management as this was the current policy, but not in expectant management was not entirely correct. Many of the midwives were very familiar with expectant management either because they had trained at a time when active management was not quite so all-pervasive, or they had trained abroad and had to learn about active management when they started to work in Britain, or they had practised as independent midwives using expectant management, or they would occasionally use it at the request of a labouring women, or ... In other words, there were many reasons for believing that familiarity with and competence in the two managements was not biased against expectant management. The only really valid part of these criticisms was in terms of the current policy of the BMH which was certainly, in common with virtually all UK hospitals, active management. We ended the BMJ report by suggesting that the Bristol trial needed to be repeated in a setting in which expectant management was the norm, as in most Third World countries. New research is now proceeding in this area (see below).

Another comment often made was that whereas virtually all of the women allocated to active management received this management, a much smaller proportion of the other trial arm successfully received expectant management in the sense of delivering the placenta without needing an oxytocic, without controlled cord traction and without the cord being clamped before placental delivery. Whereas this was undoubtedly true, the contrast was hardly surprising as, if active management was not working, it was not possible to go back to expectant management, whereas if expectant management was not successful in delivering the placenta, the protocol set out guidelines for the use of oxytocics, controlled cord traction and cord clamped. It was extremely important to draw attention to this phenomenon as a result of the two policies being compared, but some of the commentators clearly expected that the primary analysis of the trial should have been in terms of the actual management received, rather than that as randomly allocated (Gyte, 1989; Inch, 1989; Isherwood, 1989a, 1989b). Whereas the former was clearly stated in the protocol as a secondary analysis, it is difficult to interpret (Elbourne and Harding, 1990). What it shows is that those allocated to active management and for whom this management led to a successful placental delivery had a   successful placental delivery; and those allocated to expectant management and for whom this management led to a successful placental delivery had a successful placental delivery; and those allocated to expectant management and for whom this management did not lead to a successful placental delivery had more problems and therefore needed more interventions – a rather circular analysis which is not helpful as a guide to future policy! The scientifically correct analysis based on the randomly allocated groups not only avoids the problems of selection bias after randomization but, by demonstrating that the effects of a policy of expectant management leads to more problems which need more interventions to deal with them, does provide a basis for decisions about policy.

Other comments related to the population of women eligible for trial entry. Whereas there was some literature about which women are most likely to have complications such as PPH in the third stage (Hall, Halliwell and Carr-Hill, 1985), this research was mainly based on women receiving an active third-stage management, and hence it is possible that their problems were as much as result of that management as due to their demographic or obstetric characteristics. We could not, therefore, be confident about which women might be at increased risk of complications in the context of the trial. Hence, we only considered women ineligible for entry if they were likely to have risk factors which led to one or other management being either indicated or contraindicated, or if the clinician responsible for the woman in labour felt that there was a good reason why trial entry was not appropriate for this woman. However, we also predefined a secondary analysis based on the previous work about the risk status of the woman in terms of third-stage complications. In this analysis we showed that, although women deemed to be a lower risk did, in fact, have fewer third-stage complications, the benefits of active over expectant management were just as marked within both the low- and the high-risk strata (Elbourne and Harding, 1991). This was also the case in the Dublin third-stage trial (Begley, 1990a, 1990b), although there were differences between the two trials in other respects (see 'Systematic reviews', below).

The other major concern expressed by those commenting on the Bristol trial was in terms of the principal outcome – PPH. We chose this because it was the basis upon which an active management policy had been justified, albeit without good research evidence. However, there are good reasons to question exclusive concentration on this outcome. One argument is that clinical estimations of blood loss are unreliable (Newton, *et al.*, 1961; Brant, 1966, 1967; Quinlivan, Brock and Sullivan, 1970; Moore and Levy, 1983). This is doubtless true, but the (usually) more accurate estimations based on elution techniques are expensive, time-consuming and not feasible in normal clinical practice. Moreover, clinical estimation, however imperfect, is usually the basis on which clinical decisions are made, and is likely to be as imperfect in one arm of the trial as in the other. A serious concern arises, however, if this assumption is not correct because the person (usually the midwife) making the estimations knows the trial managements and so may, potentially, be biased. As it was not possible to blind the midwives, we also arranged that a more objective measure of blood loss, the woman's postpartum haemoglobin level, was also considered. This objective measure was completely in line with the trial result based on the subjective assessment, i.e. active management reduces maternal blood loss.

Perhaps even more important is the question of whether or not maternal blood loss of 500 ml is of clinical relevance. First, the advantage of active management was not just linked to this cut-off point, but true at 1000 ml and above also. In addition, such loss may lead to interventions such as blood transfusions which, while potentially life saving, have hazards and are therefore not given lightly. But in addition to reducing serious maternal morbidity (and even mortality), active management may also reduce longer-term consequences of postpartum blood loss in terms of fatigue and depression. We were not able to secure the resources necessary to investigate this in Bristol, but it is a major part of the Hinchingbrooke trial (see below).

The Perth third-stage trial

While I was involved in the Bristol trial aftermath in the UK, Walter Prendiville was setting up a trial in his new home in Western Australia. This trial was to compare two oxytocics used in the active management of the third stage of labour. In the BJOG review (Elbourne, Prendiville and Chalmers, 1988) we had shown that evidence comparing Syntometrine with oxytocin was not based on trials of good quality. Hence, Walter Prendiville set up a double-blind randomized controlled trial in Perth with Sue McDonald, a local midwife. My role in this was merely advisory at the early and later stages, although I helped to service the Data-Monitoring Committee when I was in Perth in the middle of the trial. The trial showed that Syntometrine greatly increased the rate of maternal nausea and vomiting, at the cost of a slight (and not statistically significant) increase in the risk of PPH (McDonald, Prendiville and Blair, 1993). On the basis of these results, the policy of active third-stage management in the participating hospitals was changed from Syntometrine to oxytocin.

The Salford third-stage trial

As part of my role as reviewer for the Oxford Database of Perinatal Trials (ODPT), later called the Cochrane Collaboration Pregnancy and Childbirth (CCPC) Database (see below), I came across details of an unpublished trial also comparing Syntometrine with oxytocin in the third stage. I made contact with the principal investigator, an obstetrician called Grant Mitchell in Salford. He explained that this trial had begun some years ago and the field-work had been completed, but local circumstances had not allowed the resources to analyse the data, write it up and publish it. I offered to help with this process, little realizing that the next post would bring the data, in the form of what looked to all intents and purposes like several supermarket till rolls, except that in place of prices the figures were trial numbers and blood loss (and a few other relevant variables). Over the next few months, the Introduction, Materials and Methods were drafted in Salford, and the Results and Discussion drafted in Oxford. Unlike the Perth trial, the Salford trial data found a statistically significant reduction in the rate of PPH for the women allocated to Syntometrine compared to oxytocin alone (but administering half the dose of oxytocin used in the Perth trial). The paper was published in a new electronic journal: the *Online Journal of Current Clinical Trials* (Mitchell and Elbourne, 1993).

The Hinchingbrooke third-stage trial

The most recent primary research in the third stage of labour with which I have been involved is the Hinchingbrooke third-stage trial (Simms *et al.*, 1994). This arises from the interest and enthusiasm of two midwives, Jane Rodgers and Juliet Wilson, working in an unusual hospital in the UK, the Hinchingbrooke Health Care Trust – unusual in that this is a hospital in which midwives use both active and expectant third-stage management routinely for women for whom either is relevant or requested. This trial is basically a replication of the Bristol trial in this different setting, and addressing some of the additional questions which remained after the Bristol trial – in particular the longer-term effects (there is a six-week follow-up questionnaire to mothers). As there have been suggestions that the additional blood loss associated with expectant management may be related to an upright posture, the Hinchingbrooke trial also incorporates a comparison between upright and supine postures. This trial began recruiting in June 1993, and is expected to continue until June 1995. No results are therefore available as yet.

SYSTEMATIC REVIEWS

As indicated above, my work within the field of the third stage of labour includes not just primary research but also systematic reviewing, following on the BJOG reviews. Of course, these two branches are not separate, as the reviews feed and inform into primary research and vice versa. The context of these reviews varies, some appearing in paper publications such as journals (Elbourne, Prendiville and Chalmers, 1988; Prendiville, Elbourne and Chalmers, 1988; Elbourne and Harding, 1991), but more recently the reviews appear in electronic publications in ODPT, (Chalmers, 1989) and now CCPC (Enkin *et al.*, 1993), so that they may be continuously updated.

The reviews consider a range of interventions aimed at preventing or treating PPH and retained placenta.

Active versus expectant management

Following the Bristol trial, a further trial was set up in Dublin (Begley, 1990a, 1990b). This used an almost identical protocol to the Bristol trial, with two points of difference. First, the entry criteria specified women deemed to be a low risk of third-stage problems. Second, and perhaps most importantly, the oxytocic of choice was not intramuscular Syntometrine but intravenous ergometrine. This trial also showed conclusively that active management greatly reduced the rate of PPH and increased the rate of nausea, vomiting and hypertension. In addition however, it suggested that active management increased the likelihood of retained placenta. This is almost certainly a result of the particular oxytocic and route of administration (Elbourne and Harding, 1991). The systematic reviews incorporating both these trials and a later smaller one (Thiliganathan *et al.*, 1993) came to much the same conclusions as the Bristol trial alone, both for all women in the trials (Elbourne, 1993a) and specifically for those considered at reduced risk (Elbourne, 1993b).

Choice of oxytocics

These reviews build on the second BJOG paper (Elbourne, Prendiville and Chalmers, 1988). There has been little more information for many of the possible comparisons. In particular, there has been very little research about the role of prostaglandins. However, even if they are shown to have advantages over other oxytocics (and there is certainly no evidence to suggest this so far), the high costs of prostaglandins mean they are never likely to be generally available worldwide.

As indicated above, there has been a recent increase in good-quality evidence comparing Syntometrine with oxytocin (Elbourne, 1993e). A further trial (similar to the Perth trial) has been conducted by Khan and colleagues in Abu Dhabi and will also be reported shortly. Taking all the available evidence together, the picture is now much clearer. Syntometrine has a small (but definite) advantage over oxytocin alone, in terms of a reduction in the risk of PPH. However, Syntometrine also has a large and definite disadvantage in comparison with oxytocin alone: namely an increase in nausea and vomiting, and a strong suggestion of an increase in hypertension. These competing advantages and disadvantages need to be balanced in different settings and for different individuals. It is likely that the differences between the two policies in terms of PPH would be diluted if a higher dose of oxytocin is used. This may be the subject of future trials.

Route and timing of oxytocic administration

The most common route of administration in the UK is intramuscular, although intravenous is sometimes preferred if there is already an intravenous line in place. There is interest in administration via the umbilical vein (Elbourne, 1994), mainly in the context of the treatment for retained placenta (see below). Other possible routes being explored are oral and rectal. While these might be particularly useful in non-hospital settings, they are still at the research stage. Hence, as yet, there is no good information about the relative value of the different alternatives.

Another as yet unanswered question in this field concerns the timing of prophylactic oxytocics: whether they should be given before placental delivery, as is common in the UK, or immediately after placental delivery (the so-called fourth stage of labour), as in common in Canada. A trial to assess different timings has started in Perth (McDonald, personal communication).

Timing of cord clamping

Although there have been well over 20 trials looking at the timing of cord clamping, many are of poor methodological quality, and most have concentrated on neonatal effects; therefore there is insufficient evidence to draw conclusions about its effects on PPH (Elbourne, 1993c). A trial to assess different timings has started in Perth (see above).

Controlled cord traction

A small number of trials have compared controlled cord traction to a less active approach (albeit one which sometimes entailed the use of fundal pressure), but again these provide insufficient evidence from which to draw conclusions about practice (Elbourne, 1993d).

Early suckling and/or nipple stimulation

In principle, the idea that early suckling and/or nipple stimulation might release natural oxytocics, which might in turn reduce the risk of PPH, seems a very attractive, non-invasive proposition. However, there are a number of cultures in which this practice is unacceptable. Also, a recent trial by Bullough and his colleagues using a 'cluster' randomization based on traditional birth attendants in Malawi was unable to demonstrate any beneficial effect (Bullough, Msuku and Karonde, 1989).

Maternal posture

Most of the work concerning the value of an upright posture using gravity to help delivery relates to the first and second stages of labour, when upright posture is associated with more PPH (Nikoden, 1993, 1994). In the third stage of labour, the value of upright postures (on its own) has not been examined, so again there is insufficient evidence on which to base clinical practice. The Hinchingbrooke trial (see above) should help clarify this issue.

Treatment for retained placenta

Up to now, I have concentrated on aspects of the prevention of problems in the third stage. But as prevention does not always work, there has been some recent work about the treatment of these problems.

Once the decision that the placenta is retained has been reached, the usual procedure in UK hospitals is to give further oxytocics, encourage maternal effort and gentle controlled cord traction. If these are unsuccessful, the placenta is manually removed, usually under general anaesthetic. Manual removal is not without risks, and the chances of an unsuccessful outcome are vastly increased if the woman is labouring some distance from operative facilities and personnel.

Previous trials have suggested that an intra-umbilical vein injection containing oxytocin may help to deliver the placenta without resort to operative procedures. It is unclear, however, whether it is the oxytocic or just the volume of fluid which is effective. Hence, a WHO-funded RCT is currently recruiting in Latin America to compare different managements for retained placenta. The trial has three arms comparing umbilical vein oxytocin with umbilical vein saline with expectant management. My role was advisory, particularly at the stage of designing the protocol, and I chair the Data-Monitoring Committee. (Results were not available at the time this volume was in press.)

CONCLUSIONS

This description of my research work in the third stage of labour has been from a personal viewpoint. Taking a slightly wider perspective by looking at the UK first, the vast majority of women cared for by midwives are at low risk of complications of the third stage of labour, and at infinitesimally small risk of maternal death. So it is essential that they should not be unnecessarily exposed to risks of the side-effects of treatments for conditions to which they are extremely unlikely to succumb. Such iatrogenic risks might include the effects of the ergometrine component of Syntometrine: nausea, vomiting, hypertension or even life-threatening situations such as the need for manual removal of the placenta. The decision about the balance of risks and benefits needs to be taken by the woman in conjunction with the clinicians caring for her.

The main burden arising from the complications of the third stage of labour falls on women in developing countries, where the risks of serious consequences, such as maternal death, are much greater (see Kwast, 1991a, 1991b). The stark facts are that more than half a million women die from complications of pregnancy and childbirth each year, mostly in developing countries. Complications of the third stage of labour are a major cause, and PPH is responsible for about 50% of maternal deaths in some places such as rural China.

It is not clear, however, whether the research findings concerning effective prophylaxis and treatment in the UK are directly transferable to the very countries in which they could potentially have the greatest benefit. For instance, oxytocics are not commonly available to rural health workers, and there is the possibility that they could do harm if used incorrectly. The best time of administration is also not certain in this context.

However, it must always be remembered that women and their families do not exist just in a clinical context. Many women who die following PPH or retained placenta do so for reasons outside the arena of clinical interventions. For instance, they succumb because they are malnourished, or because there is a poor transport system to take them to a place with medical help, or because they could not afford such help even if they could reach a hospital (Kwast 1991a). This makes it even more imperative that the appropriateness of clinical interventions in the third stage of labour are thoroughly tested in the settings in which they might be applied. Plans for research to compare active with expectant management of the third stage in settings in which the latter is the norm are currently under discussion with the WHO.

ACKNOWLEDGEMENTS

I would like to thank many colleagues who have contributed to my work on the third stage of labour, particularly Iain Chalmers, Murray Enkin, Jo Garcia, Adrian Grant, Jo Harding, Sue McDonald, Walter Prendiville, Mary Renfrew, Jane Rogers, Jennifer Sleep and Juliet Wilson. I am especially grateful to Sarah Robinson and Ann Thomson for their help with this chapter. The Perinatal Trials Service is funded by the Department of Health.

REFERENCES

Begley, C.M. (1990a) A comparison of 'active' and 'physiological management of third stage of labour. *Midwifery*, **6**, 3–17.
Begley, C.M. (1990b) The effect of ergometrine on breast feeding. *Midwifery*, **6**(2), 60–72.
Brant, H.A. (1966) Blood loss at caesarean section. *Journal of Obstetrics and Gynaecology of the British Commonwealth*, **73**, 456–7.

Brant. H.A. (1967) Precise stimulation of post-partum haemorrhage difficulties and importance. *British Medical Journal*, **i**, 398–400.

Bullough, C., Msuku R.S. and Karonde, L. (1989) Early suckling and postpartum haemorrhage: controlled trial in deliveries by traditional birth attendants. *Lancet*, **ii**, 522–5.

Chalmers, I. (ed.) (1989) *Oxford Database of Perinatal Trials*. Oxford Electronic Publishing, Oxford.

Elbourne, D.R. (1993a) Active vs conservative 3rd stage management. In Enkin, M., Keirse, M.J.N.C., Renfrew, M. and Neilson, J.P. (eds), *Cochrane Database of Systematic Reviews*. Review No. 5352. Cochrane Updates on Disc. Oxford.

Elbourne, D.R. (1993b) Active vs conservative 3rd stage management: low risk women. In Enkin, M., Keirse, M.J.N.C., Renfrew, M. and Neilson, J.P. (eds), *Cochrane Database of Systematic Reviews*. Review No. 5353. Cochrane Updates on Disc. Oxford.

Elbourne, D.R. (1993c) Early umbilical cord clamping in third stage of labour. In Enkin, M., Keirse, M.J.N.C., Renfrew, M. and Neilson, J.P (eds), *Cochrane Database of Systematic Reviews*. Review No. 3818. Cochrane Updates on Disc, Oxford.

Elbourne, D.R. (1993d) Cord traction vs fundal pressure in third stage labour. In Enkin, M., Keirse, M.J.N.C., Renfrew, M. and Neilson, J.P. (eds), *Cochrane Database of Systematic Reviews*. Review No. 3004. Cochrane Updates on Disc, Oxford.

Elbourne, D.R. (1993e) Prophylactic syntometrine vs oxytocin in third stage of labour. In Enkin, M., Keirse, M.J.N.C., Renfrew, M. and Neilson, J.P. (eds), *Cochrane Database of Systematic Reviews*. Review No. 2999. Cochrane Updates on Disc, Oxford.

Elbourne, D.R. (1994) Umbilical vein oxytocin for retained placenta. In Enkin, M.W., Keirse, M.J.N.C., Renfrew, M.J. and Neilson, J.P. (eds), *Pregnancy and Childbirth Module, Cochrane Database of Systematic Reviews*. Review No. 05831, 3 April 1992. Published through 'Cochrane Updates on Disk', Update Software, Oxford. Disk Issue 1.

Elbourne, D. and Harding, J. (1990) The Bristol third stage study. In Thomson, A.M., Robinson, S. and Tickner, V. (eds), *Proceedings of the 1989 Research and the Midwife Conference*. Department of Nursing, University of Manchester.

Elbourne, D. and Harding, J. (1991) Routine management for the third stage of labour: evidence from two randomised controlled trials. *Journal of Obstetrics and Gynaecology*, **11**(Suppl. 1), S23–7.

Elbourne, D., Prendiville,W. and Chalmers, I. (1988) Choice of oxytocin preparation for routine use in the management of the third stage of labour: an overview of the evidence from controlled trials. *British Journal of Obstetrics and Gynaecology*, **95**, 17–30.

Enkin, M. Keirse, M.J.N.C., Renfrew, M. and Neilson, J.P. (eds) (1993) *Cochrane Database of Systematic Reviews*. Cochrane Updates on Disc, Oxford.

Garcia, J., Garforth, S. and Ayers, J. (1987) The policy and practice of midwifery study: introduction and methods. *Midwifery*, **3**(1), 2–9.

Gytte, G. (1989) Comment on Bristol third stage trial. *New Generation*, **8**(3), 19–20.

Hall, M., Halliwell, R. and Carr-Hill, R. (1985) Concomitant and repeated happenings of complications of the third stage of labour. *British Journal of Obstetrics and*

Gynaecology, **92**, 732–8.

Harding, J. (1988) Problems experienced when running a large randomised controlled trial. *Midwives Information and Resource Service Information Pack*, No.7 (April).

Harding, J., Elbourne, D. and Prendiville, W.J. (1989) Views of mothers and midwives participating in the Bristol randomized, controlled trial of active management of the third stage of labor. *Birth*, **16**(1), 1–6.

Inch, S. (1989) Bristol third stage trial: commentary. *AIMS Quarterly Journal*, **1**(4), 8–10.

Isherwood, K. (1989a) Management of third stage of labour (letter). *Midwives Chronicle and Nursing Notes*, **102**(1215), 310.

Isherwood, K. (1989b) Management of third stage of labour (letter). *Midwives Chronicle and Nursing Notes*, **102**(1217), 205.

Kwast, B.E. (1991a) Maternal mortality: the magnitude and the causes. *Midwifery*, **7**(1), 4–7.

Kwast, B.E. (1991b) Postpartum haemorrhage. *Midwifery*, **7**(2), 64–70.

McDonald, S., Prendiville, W.J. and Blair,E. (1993) Randomised controlled trial of oxytocin alone versus oxytocin and ergometrine in active management of the third stage of labour. *British Medical Journal*, **307**, 1167–71.

Mitchell,G. and Elbourne, D. (1993) the Salford third stage trial: oxytocin plus ergometrine versus oxytocin alone in the active management of the third stage of labour. *Online Journal of Current Clinical Trials*, Doc. No. 83.

Moore, J. and Levy, V. (1983) Further research into the management of the third stage of labour and the incidence of post partum haemorrhage. In Thomson, A. and Robinson, S. (eds). *Proceedings of the 1982 Research and the Midwife Conference.* Department of Nursing, University of Manchester.

Newton, M., Mosey, L.M. Egli, G.E., Gifford, W.B. and Hull, C.T. (1961) Blood loss during and immediately after delivery. *Obstetrics and Gynecology*, **17**, 9–18.

Nikoden, V.C. (1993) Upright vs recumbent position during second stage of labour. In Enkin, M., Keirse, M.J.N.C., Renfrew, M. and Neilson, J.P. (eds), *Cochrane Database of Systematic Reviews.* Review No. 3334. Cochrane Updates on Disc, Oxford.

Nikoden,V.C. (1994) Upright vs recumbent position during second stage of labour. In Enkin, M., Keirse, M.J.N.C., Renfrew, M. and Neilson, J.P. (eds), *Cochrane Database of Systematic Reviews.* Review No. 3335. Cochrane Updates on Disc, Oxford.

Prendiville, W.J., Elbourne, D.R. and Chalmers, I. (1988) The effects of routine oxytocic administration in the management of the third stage of labour. *British Journal of Obstetrics and Gynaecology*, **95**, 3–16.

Prendiville, W.J. and Elbourne, D. (1989) Care during the third stage of labour. In Chalmers, I., Enkin, M. and Keirse, M.J.N.C. (eds), *Effective Care in Pregnancy and Childbirth*. Oxford University Press, Oxford.

Prendiville, W.J., Harding, J. Elbourne, D. and Stirrat, G.M. (1908) The Bristol third stage trial: active versus physiological management of third stage of labour. B*ritish Medical Journal* **297**, 1295–300.

Quinlivan, W.L.G., Brock, J.A. and Sullivan, H. (1970) Blood volume changes, blood associated with labour. 1. Correlation of changes in blood volume measured by I^{131} albumin and Evans blue dye, with measured blood loss. *American Journal of*

Obstetrics and Gynecology, **106**, 843–9.

Simms, C., McHaffie, H., Renfrew, M. and Ashurst, H. (eds) (1994) *The Midwifery Research Database (MIRIAD): A Sourcebook of Information about Research in Midwifery*. Books for Midwives Press, Hale.

Sleep, J. (1989) Physiology and management of the third stage of labour. In Bennett, V.R. and Brown, L.K. (eds), *Myles Textbook for Midwives*. Churchill Livingstone, Edinburgh.

Thiliganathan, B., Cutner, A., Latimer, J. and Beard, R. (1993) Management of the third stage of labour in women at low risk of post partum haemorrhage. *European Journal of Obstetrics, Gynecology and Reproductive Biology*, **48**, 19–22.

CHAPTER TEN

Research into some aspects of postnatal care

Ann M. Thomson

The annual Research and the Midwife conference was first held in the UK in 1978. Its purpose was to present to the profession research that was relevant to the practice of midwifery and the conference has allowed studies of varying sizes to be presented. Some of these studies are not extensive enough to warrant a single chapter each but the studies are of sufficient importance to merit wider dissemination than can be achieved in the conference proceedings. In Volume III of this series some studies of care in labour were presented (Thomson, 1994). In this chapter three studies of care in the postnatal period are described; the development of the FIRST score to assess mother–baby relationships in the early postnatal period (Salariya, 1983), early transfer home from hospital after birth (Whelton, 1992) and an assessment of the value of the six weeks' postnatal examination (Bowers, 1985). Each study is described and the findings are discussed in the light of literature published since the research was undertaken. However, no attempt has been made to undertake a comprehensive review of the literature for each of the study subjects. In the final section lessons which can be learnt and implications for practice and further research are discussed.

MOTHER–CHILD RELATIONSHIP 'FIRST' SCORE

In the late 1970s and early 1980s there was much concern amongst those health professionals involved in the provision of maternity services to identify women who were not relating well with their baby. Poor maternal–baby relationships in the early period after birth were thought to be predictors of babies at risk of non-accidental injury. Observations in the USA about mother–baby interaction made by nurses and doctors working in labour and delivery wards and postnatal care areas were recognized to have value (Kempe, 1976). In the UK Ounsted *et al.* (1982) acknowledged that midwives working in postnatal wards voiced intuitive feelings about mothers and babies who appeared to have a fragile relationship. It was suggested that measures could be instituted to improve the relationship and hopefully prevent non-accidental injury. However, there was no simple, objective tool to quantify the interaction available in the UK. In an attempt to measure objectively mother–baby interaction during the first two weeks after birth Salariya developed a scoring method (FIRST score) similar to the Apgar score that was developed to measure the baby's condition soon after delivery (Salariya, 1983; Salariya and Cater, 1984).

In reviewing the literature at that time Salariya (1983) noted that the first few days after birth were recognized as being a sensitive period when maternal attachment to the baby developed (Kennell, Trause and Klaus, 1975). At birth the baby has what Lorenz (1981) described as the character-istics of 'cuteness'. It is suggested that this 'cuteness' encourages the adult to care for the baby (Lorenz, 1981). The baby born at term has many capabilities. While rudimentary in comparison to those at a few months of age, all sensory abilities are intact and functioning at birth (Packer and Rosenblatt, 1979). Sounds are responded to but those with patterns, for example the human voice, elicit more response than those with a single tone (Hutt *et al.*, 1968). The baby is capable of recognizing its own mother's smell when compared with the smell of another woman (MacFarlane, 1975). Visual capacity is intact at birth although development of capabilities needs to take place (see McGurk, 1979). The newborn baby is also capable of rooting and head turning (MacFarlane, 1975).

Interaction between mother and baby is a two-way process (Lewis and Rosenblum, 1974; Brazelton *et al.*, 1975). That is, the baby often initiates 'conversation' with its mother and this 'conversation' is particularly evident when the mother and baby are *en face* (Brazelton *et al.*, 1975). Salariya utilized this knowledge in designing the FIRST score by basing the score on five factors known to be relevant to mother–baby interaction. The factors were Feeding, Interest, Response, Speech and Touch and the definition of each is shown in Figure 10.1.

Figure 10.1 Definition of factors in FIRST Score

FEEDING	The mother's understanding of her baby's needs, either breast or bottle feeding
INTEREST	The mother's general interest, at all levels, in her baby's needs
RESPONSE	The mother's reaction and the way she responds to her baby's needs
SPEECH	Represents communication, verbal and non-verbal (including eye contact)
TOUCH	Extended touching – more than basic touching carried out during bathing and/or nappy changing

Source: Salariya (1983)

Methods

Development of the tool A scoring sheet was designed with the factors listed and staff were asked to score 0 or 1 for each of the factors depending on the absence or presence of the behaviour (Figure 10.2). Thus the minimum score that a mother–baby pair could achieve was 0, with a maximum of 5. The tool was pilot tested in one of three postnatal wards in the maternity unit. The observers worked in teams of three consisting of two midwives and one student. The initial assessment was made on admission of the mother and baby to the postnatal ward at one to one and a half hours after birth following vaginal delivery, and at three hours after birth following caesarean section. The mother was asked if she would like to hold her baby and she was told that the baby would be put into bed with her. The baby's blanket was removed and the baby was placed on her/his side facing the mother so that eye contact could take place if and when the mother tilted her head. The baby's feet were placed on the mother's thigh. On subsequent days mothers and babies were observed before, during and after feedings.

Figure 10.2 Scoring sheets

Original score		
F	Feeding	0, 1
I	Interest	0, 1
R	Response	0, 1
S	Speech	0, 1
T	Touch	0, 1
Revised score		
F	Feeding	0, 1, 2
I	Interest	0, 1, 2
R	Response	0, 1, 2
S	Speech	0, 1, 2
T	Touch	0, 1, 2

Source: Compiled from Salariya (1983)

Using standardized criteria the observers scored each factor independently on the scoring sheet. It became apparent that there was a need for a range for the score. Therefore the criteria were redefined with three categories for each factor and a potential score of 0, 1 or 2 (Figure 10.2). Thus the minimum possible score was still 0 but the potential maximum was 10.

The revised score was tested with 90 observations of mother–baby interaction on the first, third and fifth days post delivery. The kappa statistic was used to test agreement among observers on the five factors. There was strong agreement ($\kappa = 0.7$–0.8) for the factors Feeding, Interest and Response, but only moderate agreement for the factors Speech and Touch ($\kappa = 0.4$). Discussion with the observers elicited that Speech was being considered literally as the spoken word and non-verbal communication and eye contact were not being scored within this factor. Consequently 'eye contact' was added in brackets to the Speech factor. 'Mother holds baby ventrally, allowing her cheek to touch baby's face' was added to the Touch factor.

A further 60 observations were then made by groups of two midwives on the first, third and fifth days and the following kappa scores were achieved: Feeding $\kappa = 0.92$, Interest $\kappa = 0.86$, Response $\kappa = 0.73$, Speech $\kappa = 0.55$, Touch $\kappa = 0.52$. The kappa scores were considered to suggest a satisfactory level of agreement for the FIRST score (see Figure 10.3 for final version of criteria).

Figure 10.3 Criteria for FIRST score

FEEDING

Score 0 = Mother will give a positive answer when asked how she intends feeding her baby, i.e. breast or bottle.
If *breast feeding*, the mother makes no effort to offer the breast to the baby.
If *bottle feeding,* no choice of formula feed has been made or no interest is shown as to when the baby will be fed.
Mother over-feeds/under-feeds baby.
Has no idea of baby's feeding requirements.
Makes no attempt to sterilize bottles.

Score 1 = If *breast feeding,* mother will make attempt to offer breast to baby, but may require much help and support to do so.
If *bottle feeding*, mother may enquire about feeding regime and at what time baby will be fed; she may require much help and support in this.
Mother's hygiene not good – does not wash her hands.
Careless about the sterilizing of bottles.
Copes with feeding and understands baby's feeding requirements.

Score 2 = Mother will recognize and be able to satisfy baby's feeding needs with minimal or no supervision.
Hygiene (in relation to baby and feeding) good.

INTEREST

Score 0 = Mother is uninterested and does not recognize baby verbally, visually or tactually.
Mother leaves baby to be cared for by others (e.g. husband, mother-in-law, neighbours).
Mother spends much time in day-room, not returning to check that baby is all right.
Makes no comment about baby.

Score 1 = Mother will comment about baby's appearance: colour of hair, closed eyes, dry skin, size or behaviour, e.g. crying, fist-sucking or rooting.
Mother is only concerned about satisfactory or unsatisfactory feeding patterns.

Score 2 = Generally interested in baby's welfare and development, e.g. weight gain, baby's measurements, stools, urinary output, sleeping pattern.

May enquire about attending clinics in the future or about when district mid-wife or health visitor will visit again.

May be interested in vaccinations etc. for baby.

RESPONSE

Score 0 =　Mother does not react to baby's crying. She persistently turns away from baby. Does not look at baby in cot.

Spends much time away from cot later.

Mother will only attend to baby if she/he cries.

Will lead baby unattended for long periods if she/he does not cry.

Score 1 =　Mother responds to baby's crying by soothing utterances.

She may suggest that the baby is hungry.

Mother may spend some time away from cot, but does return periodically to check that all is well.

Mother interprets all crying as hunger.

Score 2 =　Mother is confident in her approach to baby's welfare.

Is realistic and logical in her approach to baby's needs.

Recognizes various cries, e.g. hunger or pain, but allows reasonable time for baby to settle after feeding, changing or 'winding'.

SPEECH (eye contact)

Score 0 =　No eye-to-eye contact attempted.

Baby held in position which makes visual contact with mother meaningless/impossible.

Does not speak to baby.

Score 1 =　Baby held in position making eye contact possible.

Mother may smile to baby.

She may be inhibited about speaking to baby.

Mother may speak 'at baby' not 'to baby'

Score 2 =　Mother holds baby *en face* and speaks to her/him.

She generally treats baby as if capable of understanding conversations and interpreting facial expressions.

Mother sends time speaking to and/or looking at baby after or between feeds.

TOUCH

Score 0 =　No attempt made to touch baby's face, hands, body or feet when given baby to hold.

Minimal touching of baby (by mother) when changing napkins or bathing baby or when feeding baby.

Score 1 =　Mother touches baby's face, hands, body or feet.

Mother encourages baby to 'finger hold'.

Finger-tipping is practised when baby is in cot.

Finger-holding practised at feeding times.

Score 2 =　Mother makes extended contact by touching, stroking, kissing or cuddling baby after or between feeds.

Mother holds baby ventrally allowing cheek to touch baby's face.

Source: Salariya (1983).

Main study　During 17 months 1008 sets of scores were made. Some scores for mother–baby pairs were recorded daily whereas some were only recorded on the first, third and fifth days post delivery. Naturally those mother–baby pairs who had an 'early discharge' only had one or two observations. A sample of 100 was selected from the 1008 by taking every 10th set of scores recorded on the three days, first, third and fifth days post delivery.

Findings

Information was obtained on the distribution of the scores over the three days and the interaction of the mother's age, social class, parity, mode of delivery, sex of baby and baby feeding method with the scores was assessed.

The distribution of scores across the three-day period is shown in Figure 10.4. There was a trend for higher scores to be achieved on days 3 and 5 when compared with day 1. The highest scores achieved were 5 on day 1, 7 on day 3 and 8 on day 5.

Figure 10.4 Scores for days 1, 3 and 5. Day 1□; day 3 ▨; day 5 ■

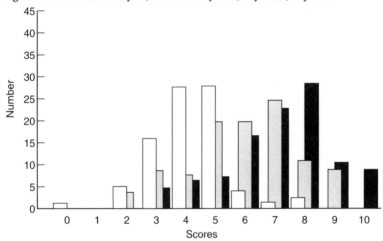

Source: Compiled by Salariya (1983).

When the scores for the three days were cross-tabulated there was a trend for younger mothers (those 19 years and under) to have lower scores than those who were 20 years and older (Table 10.1). Social class was assessed using the Registrar General's Classification of Occupations, with class 6 for those in the armed forces, class 7 unspecified and class 8 for those who had been in class 5 when in employment. There was no difference between the classes for the scores on day 1 but there appeared to be a trend for those in the higher socio-economic groups to have higher scores on days 3 and 5 (Table 10.2). For parity, mode of delivery, sex of baby and baby-feeding method only the scores achieved on day 3 were reported. There was no difference in the scores between primiparae and multiparae, the different methods of delivery and sex of the baby (Table 10.3). However, those women who breast fed achieved higher scores on day 3 when compared with those who bottle fed (Table 10.3).

Table 10.1 FIRST scores on days 1, 3 and 5 by maternal age

	Age	0–2	3–5	6+	No.
Day 1					
	<19	3	12	0	15
	20–24	3	32	3	38
	25–34	2	37	3	42
	≥35	0	5	0	5
Day 3					
	<19	2	7	6	15
	20–24	1	13	24	38
	25–34	0	11	31	42
	≥35	0	2	3	5
Day 5					
	<19	0	7	8	15
	20–24	0	7	31	31
	25–34	0	2	40	42
	≥35	0	1	4	5

Source: Salariya (1983)

Table 10.2 FIRST scores on days 1, 3 and 5 by social class

Social class	No.	Day 1			Day 3			Day 5		
		0–2	3–5	6+	0–2	3–5	6+	0–2	3–5	6+
1	6	0	6	0	0	0	6	0	0	6
2	13	1	10	2	0	3	10	0	0	13
3N	13	1	11	1	0	3	10	0	1	12
3M	27	1	24	2	1	8	18	0	4	23
4	18	2	16	0	0	9	9	0	4	14
5	6	1	5	0	0	4	2	0	2	4
6	6	0	6	0	0	1	5	0	1	5
7	1	0	1	0	0	0	1	0	0	1
8	10	2	7	1	2	5	3	0	5	5

Source: Compiled from Salariya (1983)

Table 10.3 FIRST score on day 3 by parity, mode of delivery, sex of baby and baby feeding method

	Scores No.	0–2	3–5	6+
Parity				
0	60	2	18	40
1+	40	1	16	23
Mode of delivery				
Normal	64	2	24	38
Forceps	21	0	5	16
Caesarean section	15	1	5	9
Sex of baby				
Female	53	3	16	34
Male	47	0	18	29
Feeding method				
Breast	52	0	8	44
Artificial	48	3	26	19

Source: Compiled from Salariya (1983).

Discussion

The potential problem of non-accidental injury to babies and children led a midwife to attempt to develop an objective method of measuring mother–baby relationships in the early postnatal period as it had been suggested that poor relationships at this time were predictive of later non-accidental injury. In order to develop the tool Salariya (1983) first reviewed the literature to ascertain what factors were relevant to mother–baby relationships at this time. Having ascertained the relevant factors she then designed an objective simple tool that could be used in clinical practice. In order to do this she needed the help of the clinical staff. First, in order to test any potential tool and secondly because the tool was intended for clinical use it was important that the tool had clinical credibility. It would be no good developing a tool if it was not feasible to use in clinical practice.

The tool that was designed utilized factors which had been identified in the literature as being relevant to mother–baby interaction (Figure 10.1). Groups of practitioners were asked to score the same mother–baby interaction in order to assess the validity of the tool and the practitioners were asked to make repeated observations of the same mother–baby pair over a period of days, thus testing the reliability of the instrument. While repeated testing and refinements led to what Salariya considered to be satisfactory kappa scores, it has to be questioned whether the way the factors were operationalized were actually relevant to the times when the observations were made and scored. For example, this author would not necessarily expect a first-time mother to know how to breast or bottle feed her baby, to know how much her baby should take or to be interested in sterilizing the equipment within an hour and a half of birth. However, on the FIRST score the mother would be awarded a score of 0 on the Feeding factor at the initial observation in the described situation. Likewise the scoring criteria for the Interest and Response factors are inappropriate to what a mother is expected to be doing so soon after birth. Therefore it is hardly surprising that the scores were lower on day 1 than on days 3 and 5.

Information is given on the mother's age, social class, parity, type of delivery, method of baby feeding and baby's gender and the relationship of these variables to the FIRST score. While there was no difference in scores for parity, mode of delivery or baby's gender there was a difference in scores for the age of the mother, social class and method of baby feeding. Women who were up to 19 years of age had significantly lower scores on days 3 and 5 in comparison to women over 20 years of age. Those women who when they had been in employment were in social class 5 had significantly lower scores on days 3 and 5 when compared with women in the other groups. Women who bottle fed had significantly lower scores on day 3 when compared with women who breast fed. No information is given on the analgesia that the mother might have had during labour and its possible affect on mother–baby interaction. Mothers have described feeling drowsy after birth if given pethidine at the end of the first stage of labour. It is known that pethidine given to a woman in labour interferes with the baby's neurobehaviour. Adverse effects have been shown on a baby's state of alertness and response to stimuli (Hodgkinson and Marx, 1981), visual attentiveness (Stechler, 1964), habituation rate to an auditory stimulus (Brackbill *et al.*, 1974), ability to suck a teat (Richards and Bernal, 1972) and on the ability to breast-feed effectively in the first three days of life (Matthews, 1989). Salariya does not appear to have considered whether analgesia given to the mother in labour has affected maternal–baby interaction in the first few days of life, which would there- fore affect the scores on the FIRST score. Lorenz (1981) described char- acteristics of newborn babies which are thought to elicit caring in parents. In this study there does not appear to have been a consideration of the baby's contribution to the interaction. No information is given on whether any of the babies were, or were not, exhibiting signs of 'cuteness'. If any were not 'cute' then it would be understandable that they were not stimu- lating the mother's caring capabilities and the FIRST score would, under- standably, be low.

In the two papers published on this score (Salariya, 1983; Salariya and Cater, 1984) there is no apparent consideration of whether it matters that the mother–baby pair achieves a low score in the first few days of life. Unfortunately there appears to have been no attempt to follow up the mothers and babies over a period of time to assess whether there is a rela- tionship between a poor score in the early days after birth and difficulties with longer-term mother–baby relationships.

EARLY POSTNATAL TRANSFER HOME

Patterns of care for mother and baby during the postnatal period have, as with patterns of care in other parts of the childbirth continuum, changed dramatically in this author's experience. Whilst multiparous women were allowed to have a 48-hour discharge in the late 1960s, proportionately few took up the option and most women were required to stay in hospital for seven days after birth. In the late 1970s/early 1980s the length of stay gradually shortened to five days for a woman having her first baby, and more multiparous women had a 48-hour discharge. Whelton (1992) had been working in the area of fetal medicine for some years before she returned to general midwifery in the late 1980s. By this time relatively few women at the hospital where she was working were staying in hospital for five days, with 40% transferring home within 72 hours.

Whelton (1992) was concerned at this wholesale change in practice because it did not appear to have been based on research. However, neither was there any research which suggested that it was disadvantageous to the woman and her baby. Whelton wanted to ascertain whether early postnatal transfer offered the mother and baby the best start together and for the purposes of her study defined 'early transfer home' as being within 72 hours of birth.

A review of the literature confirmed that very little work on this topic had been undertaken in the UK. Most of the research was American or Canadian and the emphasis in the studies had been on morbidity and re-admission rates. Of the work that had been undertaken in the UK, that of most value to Whelton was Theobald (1959) and Fenton *et al.* (1985). Theobald's work is considered to be a 'classic' in this area because he is recognized to have been the first person to consider early postnatal transfer home after birth. However, he did not start this practice for the benefit of postnatal women but because he wanted to increase the number of available beds for women needing hospitalization in pregnancy (Theobald, 1959). Fenton *et al.* (1985), a group of student midwives, undertook their study of the views of women who had had their first baby. They were of the opinion that everyone, except postnatal women, was being given the chance to air their views about how long women should stay in hospital after delivery, and these student midwives felt it was important to 'listen to the women'. These first-time mothers were of the opinion that the optimal hospital postnatal stay was four days.

Figure 10.5 Advantages and disadvantages of early transfer home following birth

Advantages	Disadvantages
It offers an earlier return to family life and therefore has	Lack of rest and sleep
– emotional and psychological benefits	Lack of professional help
– a more relaxed atmosphere at home	Risks if medical emergency occurs
– less disruption to family life	Lack of job satisfaction for hospital-based midwives
Parents learn to care for baby in own home	Risk if mother is not suitable for early transfer
Easier to teach parenting skills and health education	Woman may feel lonely or isolated
Continuity of care by community midwife	Abnormalities in the baby may not be detected
Midwife's expertise used	
Treatment of the woman and baby as if well rather than ill	
Better use of resources	
Less self-discharge against medical advice	
Possible longer stay for those who need it	

Source: Compiled from Whelton (1992).

The only study which had systematically evaluated early postnatal transfer home was undertaken in Sweden (Waldenström, 1987a, 1987b, 1987c, 1987d, 1988). As a result of the literature review Whelton (1992) concluded that there were advantages and disadvantages to early postnatal transfer home and these are summarized in Figure 10.5.

Methods

In attempting to answer the question of whether early transfer home, defined as before 72 hours post delivery, offered mother and baby the best start together Whelton (1992) wanted to investigate aspects of both ante- and postnatal care which might have contributed to this style of care. In order to reduce the effect of memory loss Whelton decided that to achieve her aim she needed to collect data in late pregnancy, postnatally while the women were still in hospital and at six weeks post delivery. She decided that the best method to utilize was a questionnaire and three questionnaires were developed for the three data collection time periods.

The women were recruited to the study when they attended the hospital antenatal clinic at 36 weeks gestation. As it is recognized that only mothers and babies who are normal should be going home soon after delivery only women at low obstetric and potential paediatric risk were invited to participate. The inclusion criteria were as follows:

1. No medical complications
2. Parity not greater than 6
3. A singleton pregnancy
4. An uneventful pregnancy to date
5. No previous pre-term labour
6. No previous ante- or postpartum haemorrhage
7. No previous baby with major congenital anomaly
8. No previous baby with intra-uterine growth retardation
9. No previous baby loss (other than 1st trimester spontaneous abortion)
10. Not 'booked' for DOMINO delivery

The population served by the hospital had a diverse ethnic mix. As the study was carried out without additional funding women who could not speak English had to be excluded from the study.

One hundred and fifty women were invited to participate, seven declined the invitation and because of language difficulties a further six were identified as being ineligible. Of the remaining 137 all completed an antenatal questionnaire, while they were waiting to be seen in the clinic. Eleven women had a caesearean section and four others experienced complications which precluded them from having an early transfer home. Of the remaining 122 women, 26 were not given a questionnaire in the hospital because they were admitted and discharged either on the weekend or when Whelton was on annual leave. Thus the final potential sample was 96 women. Ninety (94%) returned the questionnaire before they left hospital and 80 (83%) returned a questionnaire at six weeks post delivery.

Findings

Fifty-three per cent (73/137) of the women who agreed to participate were primiparous and the parity of the other 64 ranged between 1 and 6 (Table 10.4). The length of post-delivery stay was between one and eight days and is shown in Table 10.5. As can be seen, 26% (32) of the women stayed more than 72 hours in hospital following delivery. A greater proportion of multiparae went home within 72 hours of delivery than did primiparae (Table 10.6).

Table 10.4 Parity of women who agreed to participate

Parity	No.
0	73
1	35
2	19
3	6
4	2
5 and 6	2
Total	137

Source: Compiled from Whelton (1992)

Table 10.5 Day of postnatal transfer home

Day	No.
1 (i.e. within 24 hours of delivery)	26
2	37
3	27
Total within 72 hours	90
4	24*=4
5	3*=1
7	3*=3
8	2*=2
Total	122

*Indicates where postnatal stay was determined by medical complications affecting the baby, e.g. raised serum bilirubin requiring phototherapy, excessive weight loss.
Source: Whelton (1992).

Table 10.6 Length of postnatal stay according to parity

Day	Primiparae		Multiparae	
	No.	%	No.	%
1	7	11	19	33
2	17	26	21	37
3	18	28	8	14
Total within 72 hours	42		48	
4	17	26	7	12
5	3	5	0	
7	3	5	0	
8	0		2	4
Total	65		57	

Source: Compiled from Whelton (1992).

Responses to the antenatal questionnaire showed that more than three-quarters of the 137 women who agreed to participate in the study had at some time considered an early transfer home post delivery. However, less than 30% could recall the opportunity to discuss this with either a midwife or doctor. Only 19% (26) of the women had asked for an early transfer home. Their reasons for the request were a desire to be with their family and to return to their 'normal environment'.

Not surprisingly women expecting their first baby were more uncertain, than those who already had at least one baby, about how long they wanted to stay in hospital and how they would feel after delivery. As with women in Ball's (1987) study they felt unable to make a decision about early transfer in case they were not allowed to change their mind after the baby was born.

In response to a question asking for the advantages, as they saw them, of an early transfer home the women gave 'being with family', 'the comfort and privacy of my own home' and 'partner being able to be more involved' as being 'very important'. However, the fact that it might have been easier for visitors to visit at home or that there was the opportunity for continuity of care from a community midwife were not seen to be important. Whelton (1992) gained the impression that many primiparae were unaware that the community midwife would support them at home. Several reported that they had not met the community midwife despite the fact that all were receiving 'shared care' and all were at 36 weeks gestation when recruited into the study. The failure to recognize a midwife as providing antenatal care is not a new phenomenon. In the study of factors affecting successful breast feeding Thomson (1978) found that despite the fact that the women had frequently had a private talk from a midwife about baby feeding immediately prior to being interviewed by Thomson, the women denied having had any health education on baby feeding from a midwife.

When asked to give the potential advantages of a longer hospital stay many women saw 'having help readily available' as the most important aspect. 'Help with feeding' was rated highly and many women saw the hospital as 'potentially restful'. Nine per cent (13) of the women stated that they would not have any help at home following delivery and of those who expected to have help the greater majority would only have it for one week.

When asked if they had had the opportunity to discuss worries during pregnancy with a midwife only just over half reported that they had. The rest suggested that midwives in clinics were too busy or they felt that there was no one person responsible for their care. Just under a third (31%; 42) had attended parentcraft classes at the hospital and 8% (11) had attended classes elsewhere, while a further 8% (11) had decided to keep all their options open and had attended both types of preparation. When asked in the hospital postnatally how they rated the help and support that they had received ante-natally in preparation for transferring home 49% saw it as being of little or no help. Several multiparae commented that 'because it was my second child it was assumed that I would know what to expect' (Whelton, 1992).

It is pleasing to note that a greater proportion of women were satisfied with the help and support they received while in the postnatal ward. Eighty-three per cent (101) of the women felt that the support was of value, but that still leaves 17% of postnatal women dissatisfied with their care. Factors which contributed to the perceived lack of support were 'conflicting advice', a need for more information on 'basic baby care' and on 'what to expect'. It is a sad reflection on the midwifery profession that one mother commented 'No one asked me about my home condition.' It is possible that some staff in the postnatal ward might have presumed that 'basic baby care' had been covered in parentcraft classes. However, of the 15 women commenting on this aspect of their care four had been to classes at the hospital, ten had been to classes elsewhere and only the remaining woman had not been to any parentcraft classes. Even if this topic had been covered during pregnancy it is important to remember that the woman's memory may have been affected by labour, and knowledge base should be ascertained after birth.

Of the 80 returned six-weeks postnatal questionnaires 56% (45) were from primiparae and 44% (35) from multiparae. The distribution between short and long stay is shown in Table 10.7.

The comments on the timing of transfer home of the women who had an early transfer home are shown in Table 10.8. Half of the primiparae (56%; 14) and multiparae (50%; 15) felt that the time of their transfer home was about right. While the proportions of those who felt they would have liked to have gone home sooner (primiparae 24% (6), multiparae 30% (9)) were similar, the proportions of primiparae and multiparae who felt they had gone home too soon were also similar. The reasons the women felt they had gone home too early varied, with primiparous women not feeling confident but multiparous women feeling that they needed longer time to rest. Unfortunately Whelton (1992) does not give any comments on the timing of transfer home of women who remained in hospital for more than 72 hours post delivery.

Table 10.7 Length of postnatal stay by parity

	Primiparae No.	%	Multiparae No.	%	Total No.	%
Short stay						
Possible sample	42		48		90	
Questionnaires returned	25	60	30	63	55	61
Long stay						
Possible sample	23		9		32	
Questionnaires returned	20	87	5	55	25	78

Source: Compiled from Whelton (1992).

Table 10.8. Comments on time of transfer home from those transferring within 72 hours post delivery

	Primiparae No.	%	Multiparae No.	%	Total.
Home sooner	6	24	9	30	15
Timing right	14	56	15	50	29
Home too soon	5	20	6	20	11

Source: Compiled from Whelton (1992).

When commenting about the support offered by community midwives only 15% (12) gave negative comments about the help they had or had not received. The positive comments included:

> She took a real interest in me.
> She saw my family as a whole.
> She made sure I was all right.
> She explained a hell of a lot to me.
> She was fantastic.

When asked what more they would have liked women stated that they would have liked both 'more' and 'less' visits and for the visits to continue on a support basis beyond 10 days post delivery. Women also wanted both longer and shorter stays in hospital and continuity of care between home and hospital from the same midwife.

Discussion

This is a small study which was undertaken in part fulfilment of a course of study. It was undertaken in one hospital in the south of England and had a relatively small sample of women who could speak and write English; therefore the findings are not generalizable. However, that does not mean that there are not some lessons which can be learnt. As with other research, events outside the research overtook the investigator. Since Whelton undertook her study the length of postnatal stay has reduced even further so that a greater proportion of women are now going home within 48 hours of birth and some are going home within 24 hours. This is right if this is what the women want. The comments that the women wanted both shorter and longer stays in hospital and that they wanted more and fewer visits from the midwife postnatally stresses the importance of providing a service that is designed to meet the needs of the individual. In a study of involuntary early discharge home in Sweden Waldenström (1989) found that women who were discharged earlier than they wanted experienced much greater fatigue than did women discharged home at a time of their choice. Not only should the service be designed to meet individual needs but there should be a mechanism to ascertain individual needs. Since Whelton's study was carried out the report of the House of Commons Health Committee (1992) on the maternity services has been published and the government has replied in the *Changing Childbirth* Report (Department of Health, 1993). Both reports have stressed the need to provide services which meet individual needs and continuity of care is seen as being one way to meet those needs.

There is a significant difference between cultural groups within the UK as to the amount of support a woman is given postnatally from her own community. When this author was undertaking her community midwifery experience in the late 1960s in one area in the UK, childbearing women were provided with a home help for the first week after birth if they did not have help, usually from their own mother, in the home. The availability of home helps for childbearing women in the UK in the latter quarter of the twentieth century is virtually non-existent. In the 1990s many women do not live near their own family and even if they do the family may not be able to help because of their own work commitments. However, in some of the ethnic minority communities in the UK women are not expected to undertake housework for the first six weeks postnatally. In their study of morbidity post delivery Glazener, Abdullah and Russell (1994) found that 61% of women did not get what they considered to be enough sleep and rest in the first eight weeks post delivery. Therefore we should bear in mind the comment of one woman in Whelton's study:

You can overdo it with early transfer. It would be nice to go back into hospital after six weeks for a rest.

Looking after a newborn baby is tiring and, while it is understandable that the woman wants to be home with the rest of the family, society has a responsibility to ensure that the woman has adequate support. The support may not have to be expensive. Just giving advice about what is feasible may be all that is needed. For example, another woman stated that her midwife had told her to forget about the housework for the time being; she said she did and it was wonderful! Another woman wrote a sobering comment: 'The midwife should check with each individual woman the amount of help that she will personally have at home beforehand ... there is no other way of knowing.' It is a pity that a woman had to tell the midwives what they should be doing but hopefully with the continuity of care which should result from the *Changing Childbirth* Report (Department of Health, 1993) the midwife will know what support a woman has.

THE SIX WEEKS POSTNATAL EXAMINATION

As with previous studies (e.g. Levy, 1994) the impetus for Bowers's study of the postnatal examination was her own personal experience as a mother of four. These experiences led her to discuss with other women, fellow midwives and doctors what format the six weeks' postnatal examination took. She found that there was a great variation from a general enquiry such as 'How are you?' to a full physical examination including a discussion on the woman's health. At the time that Bowers began to investigate this topic general practitioners (GPs) were paid £6.25p per woman per examination, no matter how much or how little they did. At the time data collection took place there were readily available statistics on the uptake of postnatal examinations undertaken in hospital but no comparable available statistics for the examination performed by GPs (NWRHA, 1983; DHSS, personal communication). The overall aim of the study was to investigate the value of the six weeks' postnatal examination and was undertaken in part fulfilment of an undergraduate degree (Bowers, 1984, 1985).

The postnatal examination at six weeks postpartum is not a recent phenomenon. In her presidential address to the 'Women and Children and the Public Health' section of the Royal Institute of Public Health and Hygiene the Countess of Limerick quoted from the annual reports on the Health of the Nation for 1931, 1932 and 1936 (Countess of Limerick, 1939). In the reports it was recommended that facilities be provided to examine all women following childbirth. The purpose of this examination was seen to be the detection and treatment of physical injury following childbirth (Ministry of Health, 1931, 1932, 1936) and the correction of anaemia and other disorders (Ministry of Health, 1936). The Countess of Limerick (1939) quotes findings from studies which suggested that about 30% of women attending gynaecological clinics had been referred because of physical injury sustained during, or infection acquired as a result of, childbirth. However, the Countess of Limerick (1939) did not just recommend to her audience that the medical profession, for it is they who were to provide the service, should think of the woman as she was at the time of the examination but that they should be thinking to the future. The doctor undertaking the examination should be assessing whether the woman was fit to conceive again or whether it would be better for her, the woman, to have a gap before embarking on another pregnancy. She was telling her audience that they should be providing contraceptive facilities at these clinics. She was obviously a woman of vision because she also stated that at the clinics information on maternal morbidity should be collected to enable measures to be developed for curative action in the future (Countess of Limerick, 1939). More recently authorities have suggested that the purpose of the postnatal examination is to detect and correct any abnormalities (Myles, 1964; Llewellyn-Jones, 1969; Towler and Butler-Manuel, 1973; Garrey *et al.*, 1974), to give advice on baby care, in particular baby feeding (Llewellyn-Jones, 1969; Garrey *et al.*, 1974) and to offer contraceptive advice (Llewellyn-Jones, 1969; Towler and Butler-Manuel, 1973; Garrey *et al.*, 1974). While Myles (1964) raises the topic of contraception and describes the then available methods she does not suggest when this advice should be given.

The incidence of take-up of postnatal examination has increased over the years. In 1937 only 10% of women attended for the examination (Lewis, 1980); Douglas and Rowntree (1949) report an attendance rate of 49% and 15 years ago Cartwright (1979) reports a take-up rate of 83%. However, Bowers (1983) reports rates round the country varying between 45% and 90%. Denison (1979) suggests that in his group practice they have a high attendance rate (93 out of 97 women delivered in the previous year) because they undertake the six weeks' examination of the baby at the same clinic at which the woman is examined and given contraceptive advice, thus saving the woman at least one, if not two trips to the surgery.

The purpose of Bowers's study was to clarify whether women saw the examination as being valuable and whether women's views accorded with those of GPs (Bowers, 1985).

Methods

In an attempt to gain a broader view of the value of the six weeks' postnatal examination the views of both women and GPs were sought. A random sample of 210 women who had delivered in a hospital in the north of England between August and October 1983 were approached and asked if they were willing to be interviewed at home. One hundred and ninety agreed to participate – a response rate of 90%. All the GPs on the obstetric register in the area where data collection took place were sent a questionnaire and 55 (54%) responded.

Findings

Demographic characteristics of women who participated Thirty-six per cent (69) of the women had had their first baby and 64% (121) their second or subsequent baby. Social class was assessed using the Registrar General's Classification on the husband/partner's occupation. The greater proportion (42%, 79) of them were in the manual classes (Table 10.9), but a surprising 30% (58) could not be classified because either the woman did not have a partner or the partner was unemployed. Eighty-two per cent (155) of the women were European and the remaining 18% (35) of Asian origin (from India, Pakistan, Bangladesh or East Africa). Seventy-eight per cent (148) had had a normal vaginal delivery, the other 42 (22%) women experiencing forceps, breech, ventouse or caesarean delivery.

Table 10.9 Social class of participants

Class	No.	%
I	2	1
II	28	15
IIIN	23	12
IIIM	38	20
IV	17	9
V	24	13
Unclassified	58	30
Total	190	100

Source: Compiled from Bowers (1985).

Attendance at postnatal clinic Of the 190 women, 88% (167) had attended for a postnatal examination. Advice from the woman's own doctor or midwife were the two most important factors which had influenced the women in attending for examination (Table 10.10). Of the 23 who had not attended 16 had had a normal and 7 an abnormal delivery. While the proportion of women who had had a normal delivery and had not attended for the postnatal examination (11%) was relatively small, the proportion of women who had had an abnormal delivery and had not attended was a worrying 40%. It could be hypothesized that it is more important for a woman who has experienced an abnormal delivery to attend for a check-up than it is for a woman who has experienced a normal delivery.

Table 10.10 Factors influencing a woman's attendance for postnatal examination

Factor	No.*	%
Own doctor's advice	43	26
Midwife's advice	35	21
Hospital appointment	24	14
Hospital doctor's advice	22	13
Letter from GP	18	11
Previous experience	17	10
Own decision	14	8
Friends had been	9	5
Health visitor's advice	5	3
Other[†]	9	5

*Some women reported more than one influencing factor.

[†]Includes: thought she had to go; doctor's receptionist's advice; advice at relaxation class; sister told her; husband made her go; stitches infected; went with a cough but GP did postnatal!

Source: compiled from Bowers (1985)

The reasons for non-attendance, according to the type of delivery, are shown in Table 10.11. At the time the study was undertaken the uptake of postnatal examination in Oldham by women of Asian origin was low (Bowers, 1985). However, of the 35 Asian women who were interviewed 94% (33) had attended for their postnatal examination compared with 86% (134) of the European women.

Table 10.11 Reasons why women did not attend the six weeks' postnatal examination

	Type of delivery	
Reason for non-attendance	Normal N=16*	Abnormal N=7*
	No.	No.
Going later	6	1
Did not wish to go	6	1
Felt well	2	3
No one to mind children	3	1
No time to go	2	–
Other[†]	4	4

*Some women gave more than one reason.

[†]Includes: still bleeding; may go later; working; appointment mix-up; would go if any problems and baby's assessment carried out at the same time; six weeks too early; doctor did not do much last time and 'went and waited one hour'; baby needed breast feeding, receptionist told her to go home and feed baby and return.

Source: Compiled from Bowers (1985).

Preferred gender of doctor It has been recognized for some time that women of Asian origin are reluctant to see male doctors (Henley, 1979) but there is also evidence from a practice where women of all nationalities have the choice of a male or female doctor that women choose to consult, for any problem, a female doctor more frequently than they choose to consult a male doctor (Challacombe, 1983). Bowers asked the women in her study whether they would prefer to see a male or female doctor for their postnatal examination. While the greater proportion of women of Asian origin preferred to see a female doctor for this intimate examination (Table 10.12), Bowers also found that 35% (54) of the European women would prefer to see a female doctor.

Table 10.12 Preference for male or female doctor at postnatal examination

| Nationality | Preference | | | | | | | |
| | Female doctor | | Male doctor | | Don't mind | | Total | |
	No.	%	No.	%	No.	%	No.	%
European	54	35	8	5	93	60	155	82
Asian	23	65	1	3	11	32	35	18
All women	78	41	10	5	102	54	190	100

Source: Bowers (1985)

Postnatal morbidity At the time of the interview 46% (87) of the women were experiencing at least one problem with their own health, the most common being haemorrhoids (Table 10.13). Haemorrhoids were also causing most concern to the women at this stage (Table 10.13). Despite the fact that almost half of the sample reported problems with their own health only 20% (27) of this group, but 31% of those experiencing health problems, had been asked to return to their GP to check on the situation. Twenty-eight women also reported a range of other worries since their baby's birth. Most of these problems were related to the health of the baby and baby feeding. However, they also included financial and housing problems and fear of another pregnancy.

Table 10.13 Problems still experienced/causing concern to women at time of interview

| Problem | Being experienced (N=190) | | Causing most concern (N=87) | |
	No.	%	No.	%
Haemorrhoids	31	16	15	17
Backache	25	13	11	13
Vaginal discharge	24	13	8	9
Depression	21	11	8	9
Weepiness for no reason	18	9	2	2
Problems with intercourse	10	5	2	2
Bladder trouble	8	4	4	5
Episiotomy	4	2	–	–
Tears	3	2	–	–
Other	25	13	16	18

Source: Bowers (1985)

The GPs were asked to list the most frequently occurring problems that women presented at the postnatal visit. The GPs were also asked to indicate, on a scale of 1–8, with 1 being the most frequent and 8 the least frequent, the problems that women reported. The GPs were not reporting the symptoms that the women who were interviewed for this study experienced but the problems that women in their practice experienced. There is a relatively similar distribution of problems to the women's reports (Table 10.14). However, the women did not appear to be as concerned with an episiotomy scar as the GPs reported that they were, and depression was more of a concern for the women than for the GPs.

Table 10.14 Frequency rating of problems found by GPs at postnatal examination

| Problem | *Frequency rating* | | | | | | | |
	1	*2*	*3*	*4*	*5*	*6*	*7*	*8*
Depression	6	5	5	8	1	7	9	2
Episiotomy problems	9	5	9	6	6	4	3	1
Intercourse problems	2	0	5	8	7	6	4	2
Haemorrhoids	6	13	6	7	6	1	2	1
Hypertension	1	0	3	3	3	5	3	10
Urinary problems	1	2	9	4	10	6	1	6
Backache	11	7	6	6	5	3	3	0
Vaginal discharge	15	9	7	6	4	2	0	0

Source: Bowers (1985).

Format of examination   Both the women and the GPs were asked what was carried out and what was discussed during the postnatal examination and the responses to these questions are shown in Table 10.15. As can be seen, the women's reports of procedures carried out and subjects discussed are consistently lower than the GPs' reports. It is possible that the women had forgotten some of the events which occurred during the consultations. Just over half (58%, N = 33) of the GPs reported that they discuss resumption of sexual relations during a postnatal examination, but none of the women reported that this topic was discussed. Even if only half of the GPs for the women in this study had discussed resumption of sexual relations it is difficult to believe that all of these women would have forgotten the discussion of the topic, unless the manner of the discussion was such that the women did not recognize it as a discussion of resumption of sexual relations.

In an attempt to assess the value of the postnatal examination the women were asked to identify those things which were carried out/discussed which were most important to them and the GPs were asked to identify the major benefits of a postnatal examination. The women were asked to state the most important factor and therefore were only allowed one response. The GPs were asked for the major benefits and most gave more than one. Their responses are shown in Tables 10.16 and 10.17. It is interesting to note that contraception/family planning came top of both lists, but proportionately was not as important to the women as to the GPs. It is possible that the women had received contraceptive advice/prescriptions before they left hospital following delivery and therefore did not feel the need to rely on the postnatal examination for this facility.

Table 10.15 Reports by women and GPs of procedures carried out and subjects discussed during postnatal examination

	Women (N=167)		GPs (N=57)	
	No.	*%*	*No.*	*%*
Carried out				
Blood pressure	135	81	53	93
Urinalysis	38	23	29	51
Weight	77	46	37	65
Vaginal examination	133	80	56	98
Cervical smear	27	16	20	35
Blood test (Hb)	5	3	2	4
Discussed				
Renewal of sexual relations	–		33	58
Contraception	135	81	55	96
Baby feeding	90	54	56	84
How woman feels	130	78	52	91
Menstruation	113	68	47	82
Other	22	13	11	20

Source: Bowers (1985).

Table 10.16 Things carried/out discussed which were most important to the women

	(N=190)	
	No.	*%*
Family planning	42	25
How woman felt	28	17
Baby feeding	22	13
Vaginal examination	15	9
Resumption of menstruation discussed	5	3
Blood pressure	2	1
Everything	3	2
Others	5	3
Nothing special	10	6
No response	35	21

Source: Compiled from Bowers (1985).

Table 10.17 Major benefits of postnatal examination indicated by general practitioners

Benefit	(N=57) No.	%
Contraception	25	51
Discussion about baby	18	37
To ensure return to pre-gravid state	18	37
Prevention/detection of morbidity	13	27
Reassurance	11	22
Detection of worries/depression	7	14

Source: Bowers (1985).

At the end of the interview the women were asked if there was anything else they would like to comment on about the postnatal examination. Several responses were received suggesting ways of improving the examination. Nineteen (10%) of the women stated that the baby assessment should be undertaken at the same time and in the same place as the postnatal examination (Table 10.18), supporting the findings of Denison (1979).

Table 10.18 Comments from women on how postnatal examination could be improved

	(N=190) No.	%
Baby assessment should be done at the same time and in the same place as postnatal examination	19	10
Doctors should give more time and be more considerate	10	5
Completely satisfied	8	4
Nothing achieved by postnatal examination	5	3
Would have liked more information beforehand	4	2
Midwife should do this examination	4	2
Ensures everything 'OK'	3	1
Midwife should be present	2	1
Examination should be done correctly	2	1
Would only go to doctor if she had a problem	2	1
Would like more information about family planning	2	1
Other	4	2

Source: Bowers (1985).

Discussion

The research reported here was undertaken in part-fulfilment for an undergraduate degree. Therefore, Bowers had time and funding constraints as well as the needs of the degree which affected the nature of this study. It was undertaken in one area in the north of England and used a sample of convenience of postnatal women and GPs in the area. Bowers was unable to ensure that the GPs of the women who participated responded to the questionnaire; therefore it is not possible to make strict comparisons between the findings from the two groups. However, there are some lessons which can be learnt from this study. Limerick (1939) stated that one of the objectives of the postnatal examination should be the collection of information on morbidity following childbirth. Almost half of the women (46%) interviewed by Bowers were experiencing a range of problems associated with childbirth. Bowers comments that despite better statistics on mortality associated with childbirth (see Editorial, 1981) statistics on morbidity following childbirth were almost non-existent. The situation is little better 10 years later as the House of Commons Health Committee (1992) was concerned that the medical and midwifery professions had failed to audit the quality of care in terms of maternal morbidity. It is hardly surprising then that a large study of the health of women between 2 and 11 years since their last delivery found that a considerable proportion were experiencing health problems that they attributed to childbirth (MacArthur, Lewis and Knox, 1991). It is of concern that despite the fact that 88% of the women in Bowers's sample had attended for postnatal examination, their health problems did not appear to have been addressed satisfactorily.

It is recognized within the UK health service that women from ethnic minorities prefer to have a female health care worker, be they midwife, nurse or doctor. However, the preferences of all women as to the gender of their health provider are rarely addressed. Bowers asked her respondents if they had a preference and while 65% of women of Asian origin would prefer a woman doctor to carry out the postnatal examination, 35% of those of European origin would prefer to be seen by a woman doctor (Table 10.13). Challacombe (1983) found that 82% of adult patients seen by a female GP in a group practice were female, compared with 62% and 52% seen by the two male partners. This suggests that a greater proportion of women were seeking care from the female GP. The report of the Expert Maternity Group (Department of Health, 1993) states that women should be able to choose who provides them with care during the childbirth continuum. This surely means a health care worker of an acceptable gender.

It is interesting that Bowers (1985) found dissonance between what the women say was discussed/undertaken at the postnatal examination and what GPs state that they do. The most interesting difference is in the proportion of GPs who report that they discuss resumption of sexual relations and the proportion of women who did not report to Bowers that this took place. It is possible that this is due to the fact that the GPs of the women interviewed did not necessarily take part in the study. However, it is also possible that there is a communication problem in that the women did not recognize the discussion on sexual relations.

DISCUSSION

In his evidence to the House of Commons Health Committee on the maternity services Iain Chalmers stated that midwives ask different questions from those asked by obstetricians (House of Commons, 1992). The three studies reported in this chapter illustrate that point. Salariya (1983) wanted to design an objective tool to measure interaction between mother and baby in the first few days after birth. There was a need for a tool in order to be able to identify those mothers and babies at risk of not developing good relationships. The report of this study suggests that further developmental work needs to be carried out on this tool before it can be put to general use but midwives should find the description of the development and testing of the tool of value.

Whelton's desire to investigate whether early postnatal transfer home meets the needs of both mother and baby has been overtaken by factors outside the control of the research. Since her work was undertaken the practice of discharging women home early after childbirth has accelerated. Not only are more women going home early but they are going home sooner after birth. However, that does not mean that midwives should not still be asking whether this practice is meeting needs. The greater proportion of women in Whelton's study anticipated that the most they would have help at home following birth would be for one week. If this is the situation nationally it is hardly surprising that almost two-thirds of postnatal women report inadequate rest and sleep in the first 8–10 weeks after birth (Glazener, Abdullah and Russell, 1994). In the House of Commons Health Committee (1992) report on the maternity services it is stated that 'Linked to women's needs in relation to the length of postnatal stay is the level of social support which women receive when they return home'. While other aspects of maternity care provision have been addressed in the report of the Expert Maternity Group (Department of Health, 1993) the issue of social support provision following transfer home has not been considered.

The six weeks' postnatal examination has never been subjected to systematic evaluation. There is no consideration of this topic in Chalmers, Enkin and Keirse (1989) or in the Cochrane database (Enkin *et al.*, 1994). Recent studies (MacArthur, Lewis and Knox, 1991; Glazener, Abdullah and Russell, 1994) suggest that women do experience morbidity after childbirth but Bowers (1985) and MacArthur, Lewis and Knox (1991) would suggest that attendance at a postnatal examination is doing little to relieve the symptoms. This is supported by a recent survey (Bick and

MacArthur, 1995). A postal questionnaire was sent, six to seven months after delivery, to 1606 women who had delivered in 1992. Of the 1278 who responded 91% had attended a postnatal examination, suggesting that women find attendance for such an examination acceptable. However, Bick and MacArthur (1995) could find no rationale for the examinations performed during the consultation and conclude that whilst a considerable amount of postnatal morbidity is known to exist it is not routinely assessed at the postnatal examination. If this is so it is hardly surprising that in a postal survey conducted by the National Childbirth Trust one woman commented:

> There is still tenderness and occasional discomfort after sexual intercourse. It was six months before sex was anything other than painful and yet at my postnatal (examination) I was pronounced healed.
>
> (Greenshields, Hulme and Oliver, 1993)

Further research is needed into the timing of the examination, its format and who should perform the examination. Bowers (1985) seems to imply that the midwife would make a good second choice in a busy GP surgery. However, it is possible that the two respondents are correct in suggesting that the midwife should be the person to perform the examination. This suggestion is worthy of investigation as midwives in Ghana, Sweden and Uganda are already providing this service for the women they have cared for and it would allow British midwives to complete the 'childbirth care cycle' for women.

REFERENCES

Ball, J. (1987) *Reactions to Motherhood: The Role of Postnatal Care.* Cambridge University Press, Cambridge.

Bick, D. and MacArthur, C. (1995) Attendance, content and relevance of the six week postnatal examination. *Midwifery,* 11(2) 69–74.

Bowers, J.P. (1983) Post natal examination (letter). *Practitioner,* 227(1378), 519.

Bowers, J.P. (1984) Uptake of six weeks postnatal examination by puerperal women in Oldham. Unpublished undergraduate dissertation. Manchester Polytechnic.

Bowers, J.P. (1985) The six week postnatal examination. In Robinson, S. and Thomson, A.M. (eds), *Proceedings of the 1984 Research and the Midwife Conference.* Nursing Research Unit, King's College, University of London.

Brackbill, Y., Kane, J., Manello, R. *et al.* (1974) Obstetric meperidine usage and assessment of neonatal status. *Anaesthesiology,* 40, 116–20.

Brazelton, T.B., Tronick, E., Adamson, L., Als, H. and Wise, S. (1975) Early mother–infant reciprocity. In *Parent–Infant Interaction.* Ciba Foundation Symposium No 33. Elsevier, Amsterdam.

Cartwright, A. (1979) *The Dignity of Labour?* Tavistock, London.

Challacombe, C.B. (1983) Do women patients need women doctors? *Practitioner,* 227, 848–50.

Chalmers, I., Enkin, M. and Keirse, M.J.N.C. (1989) *Effective Care in Pregnancy and Childbirth*. Oxford University Press, Oxford.

Dennison, R.S. (1979) After delivery care (letter) *Journal of the Royal College of General Practitioners* **29**, 499.

Department of Health (1993) *Changing Childbirth: The Report of the Expert Committee*. HMSO, Oxford.

Douglas, J.W.B. and Rowntree, G. (1949) Supplementary maternal and child health services. *Population Studies*, **3**(2), 205–26.

Editorial (1981) Official statistics and women's health. *Journal of the Royal College of General Practitioners*, August, 451–2.

Enkin, M., Keirse, M., Renfrew, M. and Neilson, J. (1994) *The Cochrane Collaboration, Pregnancy and Childbirth Database*. Update Software, Oxford.

Fenton, J., Hartwell, C., Jambaccus, A. *et al.* (1985) Length of stay in hospital after delivery of a first baby. *Midwives' Chronicle*, **98**(1169), 156–9.

Garrey, M.M., Goven, A.D.T., Hodge, C. and Callander, R. (1974) *Obstetrics Illustrated*. Churchill Livingstone, Edinburgh.

Glazener, C.M.A., Abdullah, M. and Russell, I.T. (1994) Postnatal care: a survey of women's and staff experiences. In Thomson, A.M., Robinson, S. and Tickner, V. (eds), *Proceedings of the 1993 Research and the Midwife Conference. School of Nursing Studies*, University of Manchester.

Greenshields, W., Hulme, H. and Oliver, S. (1993) *The Perineum in Childbirth*. National Childbirth Trust, London.

Henley, A. (1979) *Asian Patients*. King Edward's Hospital Fund for London, London.

Hodgkinson, R. and Marx, G.F. (1981) Effects of analgesia–anaesthesia on the fetus and neonate. In Cosmi, E.V. (ed.), *Obstetric Anesthesia and Perinatology*. Appleton-Century-Crofts, New York.

House of Commons Health Committee (1992) *Second Report, Maternity Services* (Chairperson N. Winterton). HMSO, London.

Hutt, S.J., Hutt, C., Lenard, H.G., Bernuth, H.V. and Muntjewerff, W.J. (1968) Auditory responsivity in the human neonate. *Nature*, **218**, 888–90.

Kempe, C.H. (1976) Approaches to preventing child abuse: the health visitor concept. *American Journal of Diseases of Children*, **130**, 941.

Kennell, J.H., Trause, M.A. and Klaus, M.H. (1975) Evidence for a sensitive period in the human mother. In *Parent–Infant Interaction*. Ciba Foundation Symposium Report No 33, Elsevier, Amsterdam.

Lewis, J. (1980) *The Politics of Motherhood*. Croom Helm, London.

Lewis, M. and Rosenblum, L.A. (eds) (1974) *The Effect of the Infant on its Care-Giver*. Wiley, New York.

Levy, V. (1994) The maternity blues in postpartum women and postoperative patients. In Robinson, S. and Thomson, A.M. (eds), *Midwives, Research and Childbirth*, Vol. III. Chapman & Hall, London.

Limerick, Countess of (1939) Postnatal care. Presidential address to the 'Women and Children and the Public Health' section of the Royal Institute of Public Health and Hygiene. *Journal of the Royal Institute of Public Health*, **12**, 358–67.

Llewellyn-Jones, D. (1969) *Fundamentals of Obstetrics and Gynaecology*, Vol 1. Faber & Faber, London, p. 24.

Lorenz, K. (1981) *The Foundations of Ethology*. Springer-Verlag, New York.

MacArthur, C., Lewis, M. and Knox, E.G. (1991) *Health after Childbirth*. HMSO, London.

MacFarlane, A. (1975) Olfaction in the development of social preferences in the human neonate. In *Parent–Infant Interaction*. Ciba Foundation Symposium Report No 33. Elsevier, Amsterdam.

Matthews, M.K. (1989) The relationship between maternal labour analgesia and delay in the initiation of breast feeding in healthy neonates in the early neonatal period. *Midwifery*, **5**, 3–10.

McGurk, H. (1979) Visual perception in young infants. In Oates, J. (ed.), *Early Cognitive Development*. Croom Helm, London.

Ministry of Health (1931) *Annual Report on the Health of the Nation*. HMSO, London.

Ministry of Health (1932) *Annual Report on the Health of the Nation*. HMSO, London.

Ministry of Health (1936) *Annual Report on the Health of the Nation*. HMSO, London.

Myles, M. (1964) *Text Book for Midwives* (5th edn). E. & S. Livingstone, Edinburgh.

North West Regional Health Authority (1983) *Document No. SH3*. NWRHA, Mersey.

Ounsted, C., Roberts, J.C., Gordon, M. and Milligan, B. (1982) Fourth goal of perinatal medicine. *British Medical Journal*, 284, 879–82.

Packer, M. and Rosenblatt, D. (1979) Issues in the study of social behaviour in the first week of life. In Shaffer, D. and Dunn, J. (eds), *The First Year of Life*. Wiley, Chichester.

Richards, M.P.M. and Bernal, J. (1972) An observational study of mother–infant interaction. In Blurton-Jones, N. (ed.), *Ethological Studies in Child Behaviour*. Cambridge University Press, Cambridge.

Salariya, E. (1983) Mother–child relationships: FIRST score. In Thomson, A.M. and Robinson, S. (eds), *Research and the Midwife Conference Proceedings for 1982*. Department of Nursing Studies, University of Manchester.

Sarariya, E. and Cater, J. (1984) Mother–child relationships: FIRST score. *Journal of Advanced Nursing*, **9**, 589–595.

Stetchler, G. (1964) Newborn attention as affected by medication during labor. *Science*, **144**, 315–17.

Theobald, G.W. (1959) Home on the second day: the Bradford experience, the combined maternity scheme. *British Medical Journal* ii, 1364–7.

Thomson, A.M. (1978) *Why don't women breast feed?* Unpublished report to the Scottish Home and Health Department, Edinburgh.

Thomson, A.M. (1994) Research into some aspects of care in labour. In Robinson, S. and Thomson, A.M. (eds), *Midwives, Research and Childbirth*, Vol. III. Chapman & Hall, London.

Towler, J. and Butler-Manuel, K. (1973) *Modern Obstetrics for Student Midwives*. Lloyd-Luke, London.

Waldenström, U. (1987a) Early and late discharge after hospital birth: health of mother and baby in the post-partum period. *Uppsala Journal of Medical Science*, **92**, 301–14.

Waldenström, U. (1987b) Early and late discharge after hospital birth: a comparative study of parental backgrounds. *Scandinavian Journal of Social Medicine*, **15**, 159–67.

Waldenström, U. (1987c) Early and late discharge after hospital birth: breastfeeding. *Acta Paediatrica Scandinavica*, **76**, 727–32.

Waldenström, U. (1987d) Early and late discharge after hospital birth: father's involvement in infant care. *Early Human Development*, **17**, 19–28.

Waldenström, U. (1988) Early and late discharge after hospital birth: fatigue and emotional reactions in the post-partum period. *Journal of Psychosomatic Obstetrics and Gynaecology,* **8,** 127–35.

Waldenström, U. (1989) Early discharge as voluntary or involuntary alternatives to a longer post-partum stay in hospital: effects on mother's experience and breast feeding. *Midwifery,* **5**(4), 189–96.

Whelton, J.M. (1992) Early postnatal transfer: does it offer the mother and her baby the best start together? In Thomson, A.M., Robinson,S. and Tickner, V. (eds), *Proceedings of the 1991 Research and the Midwife Conference.* School of Nursing Studies, University of Manchester.

CHAPTER ELEVEN

Supporting families with a very low birthweight baby*

Hazel E. McHaffie

That having a baby in hospital undergoing neonatal intensive care is a stressful event is beyond dispute. Ample evidence of its traumatic effect is to be found in parents' own accounts (e.g. Stinson and Stinson, 1983; Hill, 1989), from observers' records (e.g. Gustaitis and Young, 1986; Knepfer and Johns, 1989) and from scientific investigation (e.g. Jeffcoate, Humphrey and Lloyd, 1979; McHaffie, 1988). Increasing numbers of smaller and sicker babies are being admitted to neonatal units and babies are being discharged home earlier. These changes have obvious implications for both professional staff and families, since resources are finite, but parents of these children need help to adjust and cope. In this prospective study formal and informal sources of support for families of very low birthweight (VLBW) babies were investigated and current visiting policies in neonatal units were evaluated.

BACKGROUND

In Scotland, approximately seven in every 1000 live births are VLBW babies weighing 1500 g or less (Scottish Health Service Common Services Agency, 1990a). More and more of these babies are surviving although risks increase dramatically with decreasing weight (Scottish Health Service Common Services Agency, 1990b). However, the increasingly sophisticated technology which has improved the prognosis of this group has produced its own effects. Many survivors have long-term iatrogenic medical problems although exact figures are difficult to obtain. In addition, a growing number of premature babies remain in hospital for long periods of time and seriously tax limited resources. In spite of impressive developments in physiological management of this group of babies, there is a paucity of systematic investigation of the psychological impact on families. In one in-depth study of 21 mothers of VLBW babies it was found that mothers of these babies felt very vulnerable and inadequate (McHaffie, 1988). An initial surge of support at the times of maximum excitement and anxiety – the birth and the discharge home – diminished rapidly and there was an inadequate amount of help available during the long periods of time after these crises when the mothers were tired, anxious and lacking in confidence.

Clearly the stress of having a small sick baby affects many members of the family, not just the parents. Another study, in Seattle, USA, included grandparents in an exploratory study (Blackburn and Lowen, 1986). The sample consisted of 50 parents and 83 grandparents of premature babies who had spent up to 12 weeks in a neonatal intensive care unit. A very low response rate (only 32% from parents) and the retrospective design, limit the value of the data but the authors did reveal a deficiency in the amount of emotional support the family members received. The stress the grandparents felt detracted from the effectiveness of the support they could themselves offer to the parents.

In spite of limited understanding of the impact on families, visiting policies have changed to allow more family members into neonatal units. Most units in Scotland now permit grandparents and siblings to enter but there are various restrictions on what each may do once there. These restrictions appear to have no foundation in research and to be at least partially determined by constraints of time and space, but it often falls to the midwifery and nursing staff to enforce such policies (Pottle, 1990).

Building on the earlier work (McHaffie, 1988) which had identified inadequacies in the existing support systems, the present author undertook a study as part of a core programme of research under the broad theme of 'Coping' in the Nursing Research Unit at Edinburgh University. This Unit was funded by the Scottish Office Home and Health Department, so my salary and the costs of the full project were subsumed in the rolling grant to the Unit.

METHODS

This was a prospective study employing both quantitative and qualitative approaches. Midwives, nurses, doctors, parents and grandparents were all surveyed in order to obtain a comprehensive view of available support, the role of grandparents and the appropriateness of current visiting policies.

Aims

The purpose of this study was to provide information on sources of support for families of VLBW babies in order to improve or enhance the contribution of midwives and nurses in this area. The aims of the study were to answer the following questions:

1. What support do grandparents offer to the parents of VLBW babies?
2. How do parents perceive this support?
3. How do midwives/neonatal nurses and doctors rate enjoyment of aspects of their work and what do they perceive the role of grandparents to be?
4. How appropriate to relatives' needs are the visiting policies of neonatal units?
5. How appropriate to the needs of the family do the medical, midwifery and nursing staff find these policies to be?
6. How do parents and grandparents perceive professional support offered and how can midwives, neonatal nurses and medical staff improve the support offered to the families of VLBW babies?

Plan of investigation

The setting For reasons of expediency the sample for the main study was drawn from the seven largest neonatal units in Scotland, situated in Aberdeen, Dundee, Bellshill, Glasgow (two units), Irvine and Edinburgh. These units were comparable in terms of the population of babies they admitted and the level of care they could provide. They were also the units admitting the largest number of VLBW babies. To accommodate a parallel study, recruitment to this project was limited to six months in the four units common to both. In the remaining three, recruitment spanned the originally targeted 12 months, May 1988 to April 1989.

The sample Data collection was in two phases, the first focusing on staff and the second on families. At the commencement of the study 265 qualified midwives and nurses, and 63 doctors were employed in the seven neonatal units and all were invited to participate as respondents. In the second phase the sample comprised the mothers of all consecutive admissions of VLBW babies who met the following inclusion criteria:

1. English speaking
2. No previous VLBW baby
3. The baby must
   – weigh 1500 g or less
   – be a singleton
   – have no congenital abnormality

The mothers themselves nominated the fathers and any grandparents if they wished them to be involved.

Access and ethical considerations Access was negotiated through both medical and midwifery/nursing hierarchies. Research Ethics Committee approval was obtained separately from each of the Ethics Committees for the seven units involved. No approach was made to the women until seven days after delivery in order to exclude those babies who died in the first few days and to be sensitive to the impact of the event on parents. Where family members or babies died after recruitment to the study a personal letter of condolence was sent to the bereaved relatives. Confidentiality of all information and anonymity were assured.

Tools Questionnaires were designed specifically for this study. As well as both open and closed questions, these included Likert scales for measurement of attitudes and simple linear scales for the measurement of support. The staff questionnaires explored:

1. The background and experience of the participants
2. Their enjoyment of various aspects of the work in neonatal units
3. Their perception of policies and practices relating to family visiting
4. Their perception of the needs of each family member
5. Their perception of the role of grandparents

The parents and grandparents questionnaires investigated:

1. Ease of visiting
2. Involvement in care of the baby
3. Sources, nature and effectiveness of both formal and informal support
4. Perceptions of the role and needs of grandparents.

Table 11.1 Structure of the study

Time	Activity
April 1988	Postal questionnaires to staff
Throughout study period (May 1988–April 1989)	Liaison staff identify eligible families Liaison staff give fortnightly update
One month after birth	Postal questionnaire to parents and grandparents
One month after discharge	Second postal questionnaire sent to parents and grandparents

Source: Compiled by the author.

Procedure The structure of the study is shown in Table 11.1 In the first phase, postal questionnaires were sent to the health professionals during the month of April 1988 with one reminder as necessary after two weeks. Family members were recruited in the second phase. One week after the birth of a VLBW baby, one of the liaison people in each unit gave the mother an envelope containing a letter explaining the research and the form for nomination of relatives. This form was returned directly to me.

One month after delivery, the first questionnaire was sent to all named family members with a covering letter, and a reminder sent where necessary after two weeks. Liaison staff supplied fortnightly updates on progress, until the baby's discharge from hospital, to enable me to keep abreast of discharges, transfers, deterioration and deaths. One month after the baby's discharge home, the second questionnaire was sent, again with a covering letter. These two points in time were selected to relate to the two periods shown in other studies to be of maximum anxiety (Bidder, Crowe and Gray, 1974; McHaffie, 1988).

Pilot study The tools and procedures for the first phase of the study were pilot tested with staff in three smaller neonatal units, and 17 midwives and nurses and six doctors responded. Pilot testing of the family questionnaires took place in the same seven units which were to take part in the main study, and involved all families of babies born in the month of April who met the inclusion criteria. A total of 19 parents and 23 grandparents from 10 families took part at this stage of the process. Only very minor amendments were necessary before the main study could commence.

Response rates Response rates achieved are shown in Table 11.2. Of the 265 midwives and nurses eligible to participate 198 (75%) responded. Thirty-three of the 63 (52%) eligible doctors responded. The response rates of the members of the families and the responses at the various stages of the study were as follows. One hundred and twenty-two families were eligible to take part in the study; 97 (80%) mothers agreed to take part initially. Usable information was supplied by at least one member in all except four of the families, giving an actual response rate of 76% (93/122). In the first round, 147 out of 181 parents (81%) returned their questionnaires: 81 mothers and 66 fathers. Fewer questionnaires were sent out in the second round because of the death of five of the babies. Failure to respond to the first questionnaire did not preclude involvement at the second point of enquiry. In the second round, 65% (112/172) returned their forms: 60 mothers and 52 fathers.

One hundred and three maternal grandparents and 79 paternal grandparents (105 grandmothers and 77 grandfathers) responded to the first questionnaire (75% response rate). Fewer questionnaires were sent out in the second round, because as well as those babies who died, a number of grandparents themselves died or became seriously ill or incapacitated. Those grandparents who did not respond to the first round for other reasons were not excluded from participation at the second point of enquiry. Thus 231 questionnaires were sent out one month after the baby's discharge from hospital; 149 (64%) usable questionnaires were returned: 80 from grandmothers and 69 from grandfathers.

Table 11.2 Response rates during the study

Staff questionnaires

Participants	No. sent	No. returned	Response rate
Midwives and Nurses	265	198	75%
Doctors	63	33	52%

Family questionnaires

	No. eligible	No. participated	Response rate
Families	122	93	76%

Individuals

	No. sent	No. returned	Response rate
One month after birth			
Parents	181	147 [81 mothers] [66 fathers]	81%
Grandparents	242	182 [105 grandmothers] [77 grandfathers]	75%
One month after discharge			
Parents	172	112 [60 mothers] [52 fathers]	65%
Grandparents	231	152 (3 too incomplete for use) [80 grandmothers] [69 grandfathers]	66%

Source: Compiled by the author.

Coding and analysis Coding frames were designed for each of the questionnaires to enable storage on a mainframe computer and analysis using SPSSX (Statistical Package for the Social Sciences, Version X). Recognized checks for rigour were included at each stage and included:

1. Staff being blind to those families which were participating and those which were not
2. 10% of questionnaires coded independently, as a check on accuracy of researcher's coding
3. Rigorous testing of Likert scale items
4. Data sets grouped in different ways to verify the strength of statistical differences

Most of the data were categorical in nature; therefore the non-parametric chi square test was applied. The data from the Likert scales were approximately normal in distribution; therefore Student's *t*-test was used to examine differences between mean scores for the various groups of respondents. A two-tailed test was used to establish levels of significance for the *t* values. The null hypothesis of no difference or no association was rejected if the significance level of the observed result was 5% or less.

FINDINGS

A wealth of data was generated by this study and a full report of the findings has been published (McHaffie, 1991). Those findings relating to the role of grandparents, the effectiveness of professional and family support, and opinions on current visiting policies are presented in this chapter.

The midwives' and the nurses' perspective

Whilst all grades of midwifery and nursing staff were represented in the sample of health professionals, the greater proportion were midwives (Table 11.3). Therefore, the term 'midwife' will be used to refer to all midwives and nurses in this study.

Table 11.3 Grades of midwifery and nursing staff participating

Staff grade	*No.*	*%*
Nursing officer	5	2
Senior sister	10	5
Sister	51	26
Staff midwives	112	57
Staff nurses	20	10
Total	198	100

Source: Compiled by the author.

Since enjoyment of the various aspects of the work of neonatal staff might reasonably affect their attitudes and opinions, participants were asked to rate, on a scale of 1–7, how much they enjoyed different aspects of their work. On the scale, 7 indicated 'really enjoy' and 1 indicated 'intensely dislike'. A score of 4 was taken to be neutral.

Whilst the overwhelming majority of midwives (97%, 192) enjoyed the hands-on care of the babies, working with grandparents was the least liked aspect of the job, with less than half (41%, 81) rating it between 5 and 7 (Table 11.4). Finding time to speak with them was one very real problem.

Most midwives considered that parents should be given information about the baby first wherever possible and many considered that parents should determine how much grandparents were told. Sometimes, however,

Table 11.4 Rating of neonatal staff's enjoyment of various aspects of work (7 = really enjoy, 1 = intensely dislike)

	7 %	6 %	5 %	4 %	3 %	2 %	1 %	No answer %
Midwives (N=198)								
Working with								
baby	76	15	6	1	1	1	–	–
parents	30	36	25	7	2	–	–	–
grandparents	17	24	32	18	6	–	–	3
siblings	23	26	26	15	4	2	–	4
'high tech'	29	27	22	11	6	3	1	1
Doctors (N=33)								
Working with								
baby	55	21	21	3	–	–	–	–
parents	24	34	15	24	3	–	–	–
grandparents	9	21	9	24	28	9	–	–
'high tech'	21	31	24	24	–	–	–	–
Hours job entails	–	6	15	24	6	31	18	–

Source: Compiled by the author.

circumstances made this difficult or impossible. Concern was also expressed about the accuracy and adequacy of information passed on to the grand-parents via the parents. Many midwives made reference to the need for grandparents to understand the situation if they were to offer adequate help and support to the parents:

> I have noted that there is a great number of grandparents unable to appreciate the condition of the baby. I am aware of several situations where parents have been encouraged and reassured by staff; grand-parents have raised doubts and have caused parents distress.

Midwives' and nurses' views on visiting policies When data on visiting policies in the seven different units were analysed some internal inconsistencies were found in that staff from the same unit sometimes held different views as to what the policy entailed – a fact which may well have important ramifications for parents. All seven units had open access for parents, with only one limiting the timing of visits in some instances. There were more restrictions on grandparents. The midwives were alive to the problems in their units and made many suggestions for improvements. They also instanced many and various situations in which the normal rules were waived.

Overall 74% (147) of the midwives considered that their current policies met parental need. Of the 22% (44) who felt their policies did not meet needs, the main specific reasons cited related to pressure of work and environmental deficiencies.

Only 58% (116) considered that the grandparents' visiting policies met the needs of the grandparents and 20% (40) felt that they were unsuitable from the parents' viewpoint too. The restrictions placed on the grandparents' access were given as the main cause of deficiencies. In those units where visiting was more restricted, midwives were more likely to consider that visiting policies did not meet needs compared with midwives in those units with more open access to grandparents ($\chi^2 = 10.0$, d.f. $= 1$, $p < 0.001$).

Midwives' perceptions of the role of grandparents In considering the needs of the different family members a more focused enquiry in the form of a list of items was made to determine what midwives perceived the role of grandparents to be in these families. Supporting parents emotionally was seen to be the key role identified, with practical help enabling them to be with the baby part of this function. It should be noted that many midwives spontaneously commented on the necessity for grandparents to be informed and involved if they were adequately to fulfil a supportive role.

The doctors' perspective

Among the 33 doctors participating each rank was represented, with 11 being consultants, 16 registrars and six senior house officers. A number of respondents acknowledged the fact that they had never addressed the topics under investigation before and so had difficulty in responding.

When doctors were asked to rate their enjoyment of the different aspects of their work on the same 1–7 scale as the midwives, they too almost all enjoyed the hands-on care of the baby (Table 11.4). However, while about three-quarters of the doctors enjoyed working with the parents to some degree, only about a third enjoyed contact with the grandparents.

It will be readily appreciated that the numbers of respondents in each unit were small. Their reporting of quite divergent ideas on what the current visiting policies were, therefore, made analysis problematic. Perhaps the main conclusion which could be drawn was that there was much uncertainty amongst the medical staff about how involved parents and grandparents could be. This uncertainty raises questions about communication within units. It is against this background that views of the effectiveness of current policies are set.

Doctors' views on visiting policies Most of the doctors considered that the policies for parents' visiting met the needs of both the parents and the baby. Some however, linked 'communication' with visiting policies and considered that this was deficient. The parents were not considered to be sufficiently involved in the practical care, and facilities were thought to be inadequate.

There was less satisfaction expressed with the policies for grandparents, with only 54% (18) feeling that they met the needs of the grandparents themselves and 64% (21) that they were satisfactory from the parents' point of view. The main reason cited for this unease was the restrictions on the grandparents' access to the unit. Although a number of the respondents alluded to the limitations of space and time which made such restrictions necessary, many suggestions were made for improving the situation and the doctors gave examples of exceptions to the rules being made in every unit to accommodate a variety of circumstances. It was this very variety that made fixed policies so difficult to determine. A number qualified their responses by pointing out the prior rights of the parents:

> We must balance allowing grandparents to see the children against undermining the parents' role.

Doctors' perceptions of the role of grandparents All of the doctors considered supporting the parents to be the main role of grandparents. Facilitating their being with the baby by practical means was part of this support:

> Support without intrusion should be the motto.

The parents' perspective

Characteristics of the parents

Of the 81 mothers who responded, 9% (7) were teenagers, 67% (54) were in their twenties and 25% (20) in their thirties (Table 11.5). The fathers (*N*=66) were slightly older, with more than half (34) in their twenties and 38% (25) in their thirties.

Table 11.5 Ages of parents

	Teens		Twenties		Thirties		Forties		Total
	No.	%	No.	%	No.	%	No.	%	No.
Mothers (*N*=81)	7	9	54	67	20	25	–		81
Fathers (*N*=66)	3	5	34	51	25	38	4	6	66

Source: Compiled by the author.

Sixty-four per cent (52) of the mothers were primiparous. The other 36% (29) had from one to four other children (mean 2), ranging in ages from 1 to 12 years (mean 5 years).

Social class was assigned using the Registrar General's Classification of Occupation (1981) with each parent assessed independently. Less than half the mothers (44%, 36) were in the manual classes when assigned by their own occupations but two-thirds of the fathers were in manual employment.

Eighty-three families supplied information on the distance they lived from the unit where their baby was being nursed; two fathers supplied information when the mother did not. The mean distance was 18 miles; some, however, lived up to 200 miles away.

The babies The babies weighed between 535 g and 1500 g, with a mean of 1130 g. Their length of stay in hospital ranged from 26 days to 421 days, with a mean duration of 74 days (Figure 11.1). Two of the 'veteran prems' were in hospital for more than a year but one of these died at 14 months of age. In all, five babies died after recruitment to the study; three while in the neonatal intensive care unit and two after discharge home. In spite of the outcome, information at some point was supplied by all except one of these families.

Figure 11.1 Duration of hospital stay for babies (*N*=93)

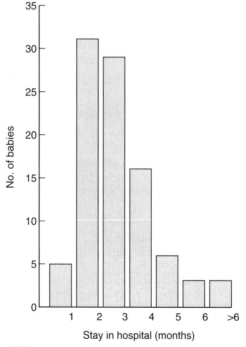

Source: McHaffie, 1991

Parents' perceptions of the visiting policies Parents' perceptions of what visiting policies in the units entailed in general matched those of the midwives, although since few parents instanced all the restrictions exact comparison was not possible. The vast majority expressed satisfaction with the open policies for the parents themselves, but more unease about the restrictions which applied to others. The overall sense conveyed by many of the comments made was that families accepted that certain limitations were necessary in the interest of the babies, but that rules too strictly applied failed to take account of the very different circumstances of each set of relatives.

Professional support At both points of enquiry parents were asked to rate the support they had had from the midwives and from the medical staff in the unit on a scale of 1 to 7, where 1 indicated 'of no value' and 7 'of great value'. A low score, then, indicated a low level of support. The majority of parents rated professional support highly. As many as 85% (125) of the parents felt that midwifery staff could not have been more supportive. However, a slightly smaller proportion regarded the medical staff as supportive (79%, 116).

As well as ascertaining the amount of support parents received, it was also important to establish the nature of the help they wanted in order to gain an understanding of how these families could be helped. The types of support both expected and received from staff were explored by asking parents to tick the appropriate activities on a provided list (details in McHaffie, 1991). The expected help varied over time: initially they would have liked better explanations with less conflicting information from the midwives; later they looked for more emotional support, with staff having time to listen attentively to them. As far as the help they actually received was concerned, a difference was seen in the support provided by the two groups of professional staff. Parents found that midwives gave information concerning the baby (97%) instruction on the care of the baby (93%) and emotional support (88%). Doctors, however, were seen to concentrate their effort on giving information (92%) rather than on giving emotional support (69%) or instructing parents on how to care for the baby (63%). There were only minor differences in the perceptions of mothers and fathers on this issue. Ineffective communication was the main criticism levelled at the doctors.

Following a baby's discharge, professional help is provided principally by health visitors and general practitioners. There were no reports of parents receiving specialist services from the neonatal units although schemes are in existence for such a service. Seventy seven per cent (51) of the 66 families who had taken part in the second round of the study, and who had seen a health visitor, had found her as supportive as she could have been. The principal components of her support were seen to be giving advice on the care of the baby (78%) and listening to the mothers (76%). Less than half (46%) felt that the health visitor gave emotional support but since listening can reasonably be seen as a part of emotional support this finding needs to be interpreted with caution.

A quarter of the families felt the health visitor could have been more supportive and their comments reflected a perceived lack of interest indicated partly by too few visits (28 of 36 comments):

> The liaison between the hospital and her should have been immediate as she should have visited the first few days when things were very difficult and nerve-wracking. I didn't see her for a few weeks, by then I'd sorted myself out. I'm not the sort of person to ask for help ... I feel there should be someone come to you at home ... all in all I suppose home support from outsiders has been *nil!*

General Practitioners (GPs) do not have a statutory obligation to visit VLBW babies following their discharge from hospital but the GPs of half of the families participating in this study had done so. In addition, three-quarters of the parents had taken their baby to see the GP at some point for a variety of reasons.

Overall, 85% (55) of the 65 families who had taken part in the second part of the study and who had seen their GP, had been satisfied with his/her support. The main ways cited in which they, the GPs, had helped were by listening to them and giving them advice on the care of the baby. The GP taking a more active and knowledgeable interest in the baby would, in the parents' opinion, have helped for the 15 parents who instanced ways in which medical support could have been improved.

Both age and social class were found to be associated with perceptions of professional support. Younger fathers (less than 30 years of age) were more likely to see the midwives as supportive than were the older fathers ($\chi^2 = 9.65$, d.f. = 1, $p < 0.005$). Fathers employed in manual occupations were also more likely to have felt supported by professional staff than were fathers belonging to the professional/managerial occupations ($\chi^2 = 10.42$, d.f. = 2, $p < 0.01$). Mothers from social classes 3, 4 and 5 were significantly more likely than those in classes 1 and 2 to perceive the health visitor as supportive emotionally ($\chi^2 = 5.05$, d.f. = 1, $p < 0.05$). It is generally recognized that professional people are more critical of professional services and less accepting of advice, and the differences outlined may well be explained by this reality (McIntosh, 1989).

Informal support The number of members of a family participating in this study varied between one and six. Therefore in this section information is reported as coming from a 'family' even if only one member of the family responded.

The partners All except four of the parents lived with their partners. Only 10% (8) of the 81 women considered that their partner could have been more supportive, and only one father expressed dissatisfaction with the help his partner had given him. Following the baby's discharge home, very few respondents detailed any problem area with their partner's help, and those which were cited were attributed to differences in expectation. They were seen to tackle most tasks and to offer emotional support as well.

The grandparents More paternal than maternal relatives were unavailable to the parents because of either death or not being in touch. The overwhelming majority of the parents' (91% (74) of mothers and 85% (56) of fathers) looked to the grandparents to provide emotional support and there was general agreement from both genders about the type of help they wanted from the older generation: principally emotional support and help with visiting the baby.

Singled out for special mention was the value that parents placed on grandparents showing that the new baby was a high priority in their lives. One set of maternal relatives suffered a major fire which destroyed most of their farm buildings, injured stock and extensively damaged their home. But they still managed to visit the baby at least once every two days and clearly enormously impressed the parents by the strength of their commitment.

At one month after delivery, parents were asked to rate the support they had received from any or all of the four grandparents individually. The same scale ranging from 1 to 7 was given. Here important differences were seen between the parents, with mothers rating their own parents more highly than their partner's parents but fathers rating both grandmothers more highly than the grandfathers. A similar picture emerged when the parents were asked to reflect back over the whole time their baby was in hospital, and again in the period following the baby's discharge home.

Parents were well aware of the complexities of the grandparents' position and some suspected that the paternal relatives were more interested than they appeared to be but because they held themselves distant they were not perceived as supportive. In some instances direct conflict was reported. The paternal grandmother in one family phoned every day in the initial weeks for a progress report on her first grandchild in spite of being expressly asked not to. This baby subsequently died and for the mother a major stressor was 'that phone call'.

Since fathers, too, were rating their own parents quite low on the support scale, this appeared to be tapping something more than merely an 'in-law' phenomenon. A number of possible explanations may be posited. Since the mother is inevitably more involved initially, paternal relatives may hold back to allow her own family to be given priority. They may assume a closeness between the mother and her own mother. It is also possible that the fathers were less communicative with their parents than the mothers were with theirs.

The nature of the help that parents wanted from grandparents was also explored and top of the list again was being available to listen and support the parents emotionally. In this regard both mothers and fathers found their own mothers most supportive. It is noteworthy that advice was one area of help that was definitely in the professional domain as far as parents were concerned; they did not want ill-informed opinions thrust upon them in his very specialized situation:

> Grandparents should ... try not to keep giving their opinion of what is happening. They should try to remember that what held true when they had children is not true now. Medicine has advanced ... [their advice] is 30 to 40 years out of date and neither actually knew better than the doctors and nurses.

During the time the baby was in hospital there was a general tendency for both parents to find both sets of grandparents more supportive if the parents had no other children. In particular a significant association was found between parity and the support of the maternal grandmother (χ^2 = 10.4, d.f. = 1, p < 0.005). Presumably this was a measure of the focus of attention being on this only child and not spread over several children. In addition it is well known that a first child often brings a new understanding and bond between a mother and her own mother.

This picture, however, changed following the baby's discharge home. The maternal grandmother was still a key figure but, in this period, she was more likely to be perceived as supportive if there were other children (χ^2 = 10.4, d.f. = 1, p < 0.005). It would seem likely that the increased responsibility and work associated with more children meant that there was more for grandmothers to do to help. As might be expected younger mothers (< 30 years of age) were more likely than older women to feel supported by the grandmothers (χ^2 = 6.68, d.f. = 1, p < 0.05). Possible explanations for this are that older mothers were presumably more keen to maintain their independence. Their mothers were in all probability older people and in many cases less able bodied. In addition their own expectations of themselves and of others were likely to be quite different.

A consistent picture of perceived lack of interest from the paternal relatives continued into this period. Although detailed analysis by family in the cases of lack of support revealed individual views as to why this assessment was made, it was not possible to draw conclusions since the two generations often reported quite different things. For instance, a father conveyed his annoyance at his mother-in-law's interference with his plans to decorate a room and to name the baby; understandably the grandmother mentioned neither incident. Expectations, responsibilities and perspectives varied between the two generations and between the genders.

Other sources of support   Just over half of the parents reported having also received help from other people. Friends and relatives were cited equally frequently. It was clear that the main ways in which these others supported was by offering practical assistance with an element of emotional support underlying their actions. The cushioning effect of a variety of sources of help and different expressions of support was much appreciated.

The grandparents' perspective

Characteristics of the grandparents

The respondents' ages ranged from the thirties to the sixties, with the grandfathers ($N=77$) slightly older than the grandmothers ($N=105$). They had from one to 11 children (mean 3.4) and up to 13 grandchildren (mean 3.4). The ages of the grandchildren ranged from the baby in the study up to 24 years (mean 5.5).

Using the Registrar General's Classification of Occupations (1981) social class was determined for each individual. Rather more were grouped in the manual classes than the non-manual (58% as against 30%). As will be noted, the social class of parents was higher than that of grandparents.

Information provided by the grandparents indicated that some lived up to 600 miles away from the parents, with maternal relatives on average living nearer than the paternal ones (mean: 31 and 68 miles). Similar differences were seen in the data on distance from the unit where the baby was being nursed.

Almost all of the grandparents in this study had visited the baby in the first month of his/her life in the neonatal unit (92%, 168). Ill-health and distance were the main reasons cited for not having done so. A few observed that they felt the rules in the unit discouraged them from being involved and a number specifically commented that they would have liked to give the parents a break from visiting, but the hospital did not allow them to be substitutes.

One grandfather in his forties demonstrated the urgency of his need to see his grandson by travelling 15 miles each way flat on his back on a mattress in the back of a van. He had had spinal fusion and was in a full body plaster. Although his son had given him a lot of information, he felt a great need to actually see the baby. Himself the youngest of nine this grandfather had weighed only 2 lb 2 oz at birth and had been cared for in a size 12 shoe box by the side of the fire. His story encapsulates something of the dilemma for grandparents dependent on the baby's parents for information second hand.

Grandparents' perceptions of the visiting policies Asked for their views on the visiting policies in the units, the grandparents' overwhelming response was positive. Only 33 made negative comments. Restrictions in their access and involvement were their main criticism and fluctuating rules made them feel very insecure.

Although most of the suggestions for improvement called for a lifting of restrictions, many commented that they were satisfied that the policies were made for good reasons and were necessary:

> I was originally very vexed that I could not touch the baby when she was in the incubator but, of course, understood why, but that was the thing that really upset me ... I know from 'germs', etc., it would be inadvisable for grandparents to touch baby but ...

Professional support   The majority of grandparents found the midwifery staff supportive and only 2% rated support as of no value. Over time their support diminished to an extent, as would be expected when the baby's condition improved and the family's needs for expert help declined. Doctors were perceived as slightly less supportive but since they were seen less frequently this is not a surprising finding. A number did make reference to their feeling of being excluded not just by existing rules but by staff attitudes and behaviours:

> Nursing and medical staff always talk directly to the parents when giving information about the baby. As a grandparent I very much feel the need to be included even if only with eye contact.

Tapping sources of professional support for the grandparents following the baby's discharge proved more complicated than with the parents since grandparents did not fall into any specific system of professional care. How much professional support the grandparents received varied greatly and depended on how involved the grandparents were with the baby and the parents after the baby's discharge from hospital. The grandparents only met the health visitor or GP if they happened to be in the home when either called. Some of the comments from grandparents on the professional support provided for the family may have been reports of the parents' comments.

Informal support   *The partners*   Grandparents were asked to rate the support of their own partners on the scale of 1 to 7 in order to give a fairly complete picture of their sources of support. Just over three-quarters were supported from this source and the remaining quarter included those whose partner was dead or not in touch.

The baby's parents   Almost all the grandparents felt supported by the baby's mother while the baby was in hospital. Remarkable consistency was found across each of the four groups of grandparents and the mother was clearly supportive of her partner's parents as well as of her own. Following the baby's discharge home no paternal relatives or maternal grandfathers rated the mother as anything other than supportive but two maternal grandmothers were critical of their own daughters and reported that they were unsupportive.

Although all except 20 of the grandparents found the father supportive to some degree over the period of the baby's hospitalization, he was seen to be more supportive of his own rather than the mother's parents. It is note-worthy that six of the maternal relatives specifically gave a low score for the father at this time. The picture changed somewhat after the baby had gone home, however, when the maternal relatives found him much more helpful. Presumably by this time the fathers were more secure in themselves, less shocked by events and more at ease with their own role. They were not try-ing to juggle trips to the hospital, domestic commitments and many enquiries, nor were they separated from their partner. Being less stressed they could be more available for people other than the new mother and baby.

Some of the comments grandparents made demonstrated an awareness that they depended on the parents to give them information and in a sense 'allow' them to be involved. Where this failed they were left hurt, isolated or resentful. Geographical proximity was not essential in this matter; rather, a close confiding relationship was a prerequisite.

Other sources of support Having established levels of support from the clos-est relatives, questions were then posed which explored other sources of sup-port. For 58% (105) of the 182 grandparents there had been additional help. In this, other relatives featured most frequently (88%, 92) and friends were cited by 35% (37). These additional people helped the grandparents to cope by supplying both emotional and physical support. Inherent in these offers was a sense of being interested and concerned for the family. The very fact that needs were recognized was supportive.

One month after the baby's discharge from hospital, 36% (53) of the 149 grandparents who returned a questionnaire at this stage were supported by people other than the named individuals. The majority of others cited were relatives (56) and friends (19). Their support was again expressed by an iden-tification of practical ways in which to help. A few grandparents mentioned the need to confide in others outside the immediate family circle in order not to further burden the parents with their own worries.

The grandparents' own needs

When grandparents were asked an open question about their own needs, supporting the parents was clearly identified as the most commonly per-ceived need (65/136 citations). Expressions of practical help (41) were sepa-rately itemized but clearly contained elements of such support.

Some grandparents were juggling with many and competing demands on their time and resources, and some acknowledged that they were simply not able to devote the amount of attention they wished to the new family.

> The only support I have given is listening ... I would have liked to have given more ... but my wife has had a stroke arising when the baby was still in hospital. So we were all trying to rally round for my daughter, baby and wife.

Other respondents made reference to the problems inherent in balancing their own needs, parents' needs, competing rights and their own perception of their role.

Logically it seemed important to ascertain how effectively grandparents had felt they could provide the support they considered so important. The 136 grandparents who offered comment on this point between them instanced 305 ways in which they had, in their judgement, been supportive. Almost a third of these referred to offering emotional support. However, many of the practical demonstrations of help held an underlying sense that they were a manifestation of care and understanding. Thus, where a grandmother knitted specially small clothes for the baby, she is classified as providing practical help but in reality her action is an expression of her concern. Overall more grandmothers than grandfathers on both sides were seen to be offering help and some of the men themselves commented on the more active role of their partners.

Interestingly, giving advice or information was less often cited as a help in the first month (10) than over the whole period (24). A number did add a proviso that the advice should be asked for and not thrust upon parents. But it would seem that as the situation became more 'normal' and within grandparents' experience their advice was more acceptable. It could also have been tolerated more easily when parents were less stressed.

Throughout the period following the baby's discharge home, 27 grandparents felt they had been unable to help the parents compared with only 16 while the baby was still in hospital. In addition the reasons had now changed. The main reason cited after discharge was that the parents did not want the help, or the grandparents considered it wise not to intervene.

For the 122 who felt that they had been able to help there was often an underlying sense expressed that they tried hard to be sensitive to the parents' needs:

> The role of a grandparent should be unobtrusive and subtle. A new mother needs to feel that she is not alone with her new baby until her confidence grows. A forceful, dominating attitude, however, will alienate both new parents and will prove counterproductive to the baby's welfare.

By this time practical help had taken precedence over emotional support and tasks like baby-sitting and taking care of the baby topped the list. Once again maternal grandmothers were the principal source of help. A few grandparents recounted incidents where parents had wanted to be independent and thwarted their efforts to help but most expressed pride and pleasure in seeing the family confidently coping and caring after their difficult experience. It was clearly this sense of understanding the prior rights of the parents in this event that helped the grandparents to accept their role of waiting in the wings most of the time, accepting that they were not always needed but ready to move into play if they were called upon.

LIMITATIONS OF THE STUDY

There is no such thing as the perfect study in the natural world and this study had its limitations. Not all eligible relatives were nominated by the women, so the views of all the family members were not represented. Limiting the period of recruitment to six months in four units meant that the total number of families approached was less than it might have been had these limitations not been necessary. A poor response rate (52%) from doctors was not unexpected since questionnaires are known to yield a lower response rate than interviews (Hedges and Ritchie, 1987) and doctors tend to respond less frequently than others. Had there been opportunity to approach them individually and discuss the importance of the study the response rate in that group might have improved, but as with most projects this one was limited by financial and temporal constraints. A postal strike in September 1988 probably reduced the family response rate to a degree. This was not anticipated and was clearly outside the present author's control. However, it should be noted that the populations studied were not different from those which might reasonably be expected to be found in any large regional neonatal unit. The fact that they were drawn from seven different units further strengthens the applicability of these findings.

DISCUSSION

The discussion of the findings is organized round three main topics: the support grandparents can provide, an assessment of current visiting policies, and ways in which support might be improved for families of VLBW babies.

The support of grandparents

Every individual, no matter how well developed her/his own personal resources, depends to some extent on the co-operative effort of people in their network to transcend stressful encounters (Mechanic, 1974). The nature and source of such help may well vary. Having a VLBW baby is a particularly stressful experience where support is vitally important.

Both parents and grandparents of VLBW babies felt that the principal role of grandparents was to support the parents. Simply being available to listen and respond appropriately was an invaluable function and the older generation, by virtue of their own investment in this baby, were uniquely placed to devote themselves to this effort. Giving priority to the parents' needs conveyed a sense of the esteem in which they were held.

Visiting is one very specific way in which interest and concern may be demonstrated but restrictive policies can thwart grandparents' intentions in this matter. Grandparents in this study were already very aware that they depended on the parents to allow them to be informed and involved. Both a lack of information and rejection of proffered help can limit their ability to support. To have outside agencies further restricting their potential must be particularly difficult.

There are, of course, many other constraints which limit grandparents' potential to help, and parents do appear to be aware of these problems. Other competing demands, age and infirmity, work, distance, resources, values and relationships all feature. A real understanding, saying and doing the right thing at the right time and conveying a sincere care and concern can, however, be enormously supportive and can be available irrespective of mobility, distance, health or other commitments. Paternal relatives, though, do seem to be particularly disadvantaged.

Bearing in mind all the problems family members have overcome, it is important to look carefully at the messages they receive when they arrive at the neonatal unit. The remarkable tolerance seen in the grandparents, and well recognized in the older generation (Qureshi and Walker, 1989), should not be allowed to blind the staff to their true feelings of hurt or vexation.

Another limitation that is more subtly conveyed is the amount of support the grandparents themselves have. Their personal major investment in this baby was clear. If their own support system is inadequate they will have less resources to help others and indeed may well become an additional burden on the already stressed parents. Staff have a responsibility not to undermine their confidence or diminish their role. In this respect, the low numbers in this study who felt accepted and supported by the doctors are noteworthy and their comments about being excluded even in eye contact are to be taken seriously.

The fact that the baby's mother was seen to be so universally supportive raises questions about the strain imposed on this key figure. Here, once again, the women appeared to bear the heaviest load since the fathers were not perceived to be as supportive in general in the period while the baby was in hospital. It is perhaps in recognition of this fact that many of the grandparents shared their own burdens with others outside the immediate family circle.

Being included and informed is an essential element in grandparents' equipment for their supportive role. Grandmothers in particular are key figures in terms of support, but because of the complex emotional tensions of this situation family members sometimes need help to translate their concern into appropriate action.

At times the grandparents' emotions placed an added burden on the parents but most seemed able to cope with this. Perhaps this was a feature of the reciprocity of their relationships. If the grandparents were supporting with their love and concern, parents were willing to take on board some of their anxiety. Too big a burden can be caused, however, where grandparents try to advise. The grandparents were not perceived by parents as having the appropriate experience or knowledge to pass comment in these very specialized circumstances. Clearly, expectation varied across grandparents, with much less expected of the men. This is consistent with the findings of other studies of social support which have concluded that women have better resources and are superior at giving and receiving support (Vaux 1985; Qureshi and Walker, 1989).

In summary, it was shown in this study that there was a general need amongst the parents for the grandparents to be unobtrusively available, ready to help if called upon to do so but content to stay on the periphery if the parents were coping adequately on their own.

Visiting policies in neonatal units

There was general satisfaction among parents with the open policies for their visiting in the units. The wisdom of having some restrictions to safeguard the interests of the babies was accepted and applauded. There was, however, considerable frustration with the restrictive policies for other visitors being too rigidly applied, and they were perceived as denying the special circumstances of individual families.

Similarly, parents were unhappy with blanket policies which limit their own choices. The overriding message was that parents themselves wish to decide who may visit and support, and what is right and appropriate for different people to do when there. Being conscious themselves of strengths and weaknesses in their relationships, they were understandably less than satisfied when others dictated the involvement of these people.

Families appreciated the need for certain restrictions, but grandparents, if they are to be supportive, need to be included and informed. Flexibility which takes account of preference and circumstances in individual families is called for by the family members.

Doctors and midwives were aware of the potential conflicts and tensions which arise in families with a sick neonate and the problems in accommodating competing demands and rights. They expressed widespread unease about the restrictions imposed in units, and freely acknowledged the inadequacies of existing facilities, pressure of work and low staffing quotas which all limit care-giving. Although many of these constraints are outside the scope of individual practitioners to remedy, communication is one area which is in their power to change to some extent. Doctors especially need to improve their skills in this respect. For the midwives the inability to make time for lengthy in-depth listening is a further cause of stress and frustration in an already highly charged environment.

The staff recommended constant vigilance to guard against possible infringement of rights and takeover bids but pointed out that making exceptions has the potential for resentment and hostility. Providing, however, that priority is given to the safety of the babies, individual tailoring of access and involvement is the only way to respond to the changing needs and inherent strengths and weaknesses within each individual network.

Improving the support offered to families of VLBW babies

Visiting policies Certain practical changes could readily be implemented in line with the recommendations from the respondents in this study. To begin with, notices dictating who may and may not enter neonatal units might be revised in order to create an atmosphere of understanding about different types of family structures and to be more welcoming. To a great extent midwives determine the milieu in the neonatal unit; this is one way in which they could effect change. The main way visiting itself could be improved is clearly by staff having time and opportunity to really listen to parents, and being careful in word, deed and attitude not to add to the stress these relatives are under.

The grandparents' delicate position has already been clearly outlined. It would seem likely that if some of the restrictions on them were eased midwives would have less ground to defend and more space to work sensitively with them. Midwives' own clear appraisal of the potential hazards of a flexible approach should be a safeguard. In addition, if they are listening carefully to all sides, the wishes of the parents should help them to prioritize needs and steer a sensitive course in difficult circumstances. Such an emphasis necessitates much collaboration and team effort and there is no place for individuals retaining the monopoly on decisions.

Attitudes Once visitors are in the unit there are other opportunities for improvement. It is all too easy, in the rarified atmosphere of intensive care, to limit the family's world to the confines of the incubator. In reality, of course, family members are often grappling simultaneously with many stressors and many competing demands. Parents value concern being shown for their total circumstances; they are hurt when criticism is given or implied which fails to acknowledge their other roles and special circumstances. Care must be taken in dealing with these very vulnerable families.

If the focus of midwives becomes truly family-centred, they will be uniquely placed to identify those individuals who are supportive and those who introduce conflict. By listening sensitively they will be better able to present alternatives, mobilize resources or facilitate resolution of difficulties. In this way the potential of each family's support system may be realized or enhanced. Those closely involved, stressed or defensive may well be unable to consider such options alone. A perceived lack of interest from health visitors has been identified. The immediate weeks after a baby's discharge home are anxious ones in most cases until the mother feels confident about accepting responsibility for this vulnerable baby. Community staff, however, have problems both in finding time to support the family and in keeping abreast of a rapidly advancing speciality – neonatology. Closer liaison between hospital and community and integrating formal and informal networks could provide a better support structure for the parents, at the same time relieving the pressure on professional staff and helping to loosen the apron strings tying parents to specialist help.

IMPLICATIONS FOR PRACTICE

It has been clearly established that adequate support of families with VLBW babies is not always achieved. By adopting a flexible, integrated approach, helping families to realize their own full potential, midwives could assist parents and grandparents to become self-sufficient, confident and competent, mutually supporting of each other and capitalizing on their individual strengths and acknowledged roles. The essential theories of social support and the role of families in integrated care need to be included in education and practice.

Inadequately preparing families to cope with the heavy responsibility of caring for these vulnerable babies is rather like failing to train staff in the use of essential equipment.There will be casualties. Both hospital and community staff have a responsibility in this preparation. It is equally unacceptable to deny the very special rights, needs and roles of parents, grandparents and other relatives at a time of major stress and at a time when they feel very insecure and powerless. They are already dependent on the professionals for the very life of their baby; to deprive them further of a say in the management of their own care and support is to infringe their individual and collective rights.

It may be concluded that all those who are involved in neonatal intensive care and its sequelae should look again at policies for and attitudes towards families in receipt of their services. There is no place for rigid rules or fixed attitudes. Each case has to be assessed on its own merits. Where gaps in care are identified, extra resources must be mobilized. Midwives, because of their unique and privileged position in the system of care-giving, are ideally placed to be key workers in the support of these families. To really listen to the needs of the consumers takes time and resources; both managers and practitioners are involved in determining priorities in this respect and must weigh in the balance the costs and benefits of support for these special families.

FUTURE RESEARCH

With the groundwork established in the area of support for these families a next step would be to explore the effectiveness of specific practices aimed at giving help to these families. At the time of completion of this research a number of initiatives are in operation such as neonatal sisters going out into the community to help the mother to adjust to her new responsibility; care being given by community midwives with expertise in looking after babies who have been in the neonatal intensive care unit; liaison health visitors forming an administrative link between hospital and community; and specialist health visitors providing follow-up care in the home. Investigation of all these schemes is long overdue. Their value to families as well as their cost-effectiveness need to be evaluated.

Huge sums of money are spent on increasingly sophisticated neonatal care. For many years these technical and managerial advances outstripped understanding of the psychological and social impact of this event. The gap must not be allowed to widen again. No one is better equipped to ensure this does not happen than neonatal midwives and nurses. They must determine that the research is undertaken and that the findings are disseminated. It is part of their professional responsibility to the babies and families in their care.

ACKNOWLEDGEMENTS

This study was conducted while the author was a Research Fellow in the Nursing Research Unit, University of Edinburgh. The unit was funded by the Scottish Office Home and Health Department. The opinions expressed are those of the author and do not necessarily reflect those of the department. The generous contribution of both medical and midwifery and nursing staff in the neonatal units and of the families who participated is gratefully acknowledged.

REFERENCES

Bidder, R.T., Crowe, E.A. and Gray, O.P. (1974) Mothers' attitudes to preterm infants. *Archives of Disease in Childhood,* **49**, 766–770.

Blackburn, S. and Lowen, L. (1986) Impact of an infant's premature birth on the grandparents and parents. *Journal of Obstetric Gynecological and Neonatal Nursing,* **15**(2) 173–178.

Gustaitis, R. and Young, E.W.D. (1986) *A Time to be Born, a Time to Die.* Addison Wesley, Massachusetts.

Hedges, B. and Ritchie, J. (1987) *Research Policy: The Choice of Appropriate Research Methods.* Social and Community Planning Research, London.

Hill, S. (1989) Family. Michael Joseph, London.

Jeffcoate, J.A., Humphrey, M.E. and Lloyd, J.K. (1979) Role perception and response to stress in fathers and mothers following pre-term delivery. *Social Science and Medicine*, **13A**, 139–145.

Knepfer, G. and Johns, C. (1989) *Nursing for Life*. Pan Books, Australia.

McHaffie, H.E. (1988) A prospective study to identify critical factors which indicate mothers' readiness to care for their very low birthweight baby at home. Unpublished PhD thesis, University of Edinburgh.

McHaffie, H.E. (1991) *A Study of Support for Families with a Very Low Birthweight Baby*. Nursing Research Unit Report, University of Edinburgh.

McIntosh, J. (1989) Models of childbirth and social class: a study of 80 working class primigravidae. In Robinson,S. and Thomson, A. (eds), *Midwives, Research and Childbirth*, Vol. I. Chapman & Hall, London.

Mechanic, D. (1974) Social structure and personal adaptation: some neglected dimensions. In Coehlo, G.V., Hamburg, D.A. and Adams J.E. (eds) Basic Books, New York.

Pottle, A. (1990) To visit or not to visit. *Nursing Practice*, **3**(2), 7–11.

Qureshi, H. and Walker, A.(1989) *The Caring Relationship: Elderly People and their Families*. Macmillan, Basingstoke.

Scottish Health Service Common Services Agency (1990a) *Scottish Health Statistics, 1990*. CSA, Edinburgh.

Scottish Health Service Common Services Agency (1990b) *Scottish Stillbirth and Neonatal Death Report, 1989*. CSA. Edinburgh.

Stinson, R. and Stinson, P. (1983) *The Long Dying of Baby Andrew*. Little, Brown & Co., USA.

Vaux, A. (1985) Variations in social support associated with gender, ethnicity and age. *Journal of Social Issues*, **41**(1), 89–110.

Index